# Find instructive videos and additional figures on MediaCenter.thieme.com!

| | WINDOWS | MAC | TABLET | |
|---|---|---|---|---|
| **Recommended Browser(s)*** | Microsoft Internet Explorer 8.0 or later, Firefox 3.x | Firefox 3.x, Safari 4.x | HTML5 mobile browser. iPad — Safari. Opera Mobile — Tablet PCs referred. | |
| | *all browsers should have JavaScript enabled* | | | |
| **Flash Player Plug-in** | Flash Player 9 or Higher** \*\* *Mac users: ATI Rage 128 GPU does not support full-screen mode with hardware scaling* | | Tablet PCs with Android OS support Flash 10.1 | |
| **Minimum Hardware Configurations** | Intel® Pentium® II 450 MHz, AMD Athlon™ 600 MHz or faster processor (or equivalent) 512 MB of RAM | PowerPC® G3 500 MHz or faster processor Intel Core™ Duo 1.33 GHz or faster processor 512MB of RAM | Minimum CPU powered at 800MHz 256MB DDR2 of RAM | |
| **Recommended for optimal usage experience** | Monitor resolutions: • Normal (4:3) 1024×768 or Higher • Widescreen (16:9) 1280×720 or Higher • Widescreen (16:10) 1440×900 or Higher DSL/Cable internet connection at a minimum speed of 384.0 Kbps or faster WiFi 802.11 b/g preferred. | | 7-inch and 10-inch tablets on maximum resolution. WiFi connection is required. | |

T0329759

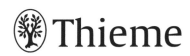

# Atlas of Peripheral Regional Anesthesia

**Anatomy and Techniques**

3rd Edition

**Gisela Meier, MD**
Former Head of the Department of Anesthesia and Interventional Pain Therapy
Oberammergau Center for Rheumatology
Oberammergau, Germany

**Johannes Buettner, MD**
Former Head of the Department of Anesthesia
Trauma Center
Murnau, Germany

780 illustrations

Thieme
Stuttgart • New York • Delhi • Rio de Janeiro

**Library of Congress Cataloging-in-Publication Data**

Meier, Gisela, 1954- , author.
  [Atlas der peripheren Regionalan?sthesie. English]
  Atlas of peripheral regional anesthesia : anatomy and techniques / Gisela Meier, Johannes Buettner. – 3rd edition.
      p. ; cm.
  "This book is an authorized translation of the 3rd German edition published and copyrighted 2013 by Georg Thieme Verlag, Stuttgart."
  Includes bibliographical references and index.
  ISBN 978-3-13-139793-5 (alk. paper) – ISBN 978-3-13-164973-7 (eISBN)
  I. Buettner, Johannes, 1950- , author. II. Title.
  [DNLM: 1. Anesthesia, Conduction–Atlases. 2. Nerve Block–methods–Atlases. 3. Pain Management–methods–Atlases. WO 517]
  RD84
  617.9'640222–dc23

                                                    2015016781

This book is an authorized translation of the 3rd German edition published and copyrighted 2013 by Georg Thieme Verlag, Stuttgart. Title of the German edition: Atlas der peripheren Regionalanästhesie. Anatomie-Sonografie-Anästhesie-Schmerztherapie

Translator: Melanie Nassar, Beit Sahour, Palestine
Illustrator: Nikolaus Lechenbauer and Gerhard Schlich (for Astra Zeneca); Peter Haller, Stuttgart, Germany; Gay & Rothenburger, Sternenfels, Germany

**Important note:** Medicine is an ever-changing science undergoing continual development. Research and clinical experience are continually expanding our knowledge, in particular our knowledge of proper treatment and drug therapy. Insofar as this book mentions any dosage or application, readers may rest assured that the authors, editors, and publishers have made every effort to ensure that such references are in accordance with **the state of knowledge at the time of production of the book.**

Nevertheless, this does not involve, imply, or express any guarantee or responsibility on the part of the publishers in respect to any dosage instructions and forms of applications stated in the book. **Every user is requested to examine carefully** the manufacturers' leaflets accompanying each drug and to check, if necessary in consultation with a physician or specialist, whether the dosage schedules mentioned therein or the contraindications stated by the manufacturers differ from the statements made in the present book. Such examination is particularly important with drugs that are either rarely used or have been newly released on the market. Every dosage schedule or every form of application used is entirely at the user's own risk and responsibility. The authors and publishers request every user to report to the publishers any discrepancies or inaccuracies noticed. If errors in this work are found after publication, errata will be posted at www.thieme.com on the product description page.

Some of the product names, patents, and registered designs referred to in this book are in fact registered trademarks or proprietary names even though specific reference to this fact is not always made in the text. Therefore, the appearance of a name without designation as proprietary is not to be construed as a representation by the publisher that it is in the public domain.

© 2016 Georg Thieme Verlag KG

Thieme Publishers Stuttgart
Rüdigerstrasse 14, 70469 Stuttgart, Germany
+49 [0]711 8931 421, customerservice@thieme.de

Thieme Publishers New York
333 Seventh Avenue, New York, NY 10001, USA
+1-800-782-3488, customerservice@thieme.com

Thieme Publishers Delhi
A-12, Second Floor, Sector-2, Noida-201301
Uttar Pradesh, India
+91 120 45 566 00, customerservice@thieme.in

Thieme Publishers Rio, Thieme Publicações Ltda.
Edifício Rodolpho de Paoli, 25° andar
Av. Nilo Peçanha, 50 – Sala 2508,
Rio de Janeiro 20020-906 Brasil
Tel: +55 21 3172-2297 / +55 21 3172-1896

Cover design: Thieme Publishing Group
Typesetting by Thomson Digital, India

Printed in China by Everbest Printing Ltd, Hong Kong          5 4 3 2 1

ISBN 9783131397935

Also available as an e-book:
eISBN 9783131649737

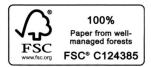

FSC
www.fsc.org

100%
Paper from well-managed forests

FSC® C124385

# Contents

**Part I General Aspects of Ultrasound-Guided Peripheral Regional Anesthesia**

**Part II Upper Limb**

# Contents

# Contents

## Part IV Peripheral Regional Anesthesia in Pediatrics

# Contents

# Foreword

Compared to general anesthesia, regional anesthesia can provide anatomically selective anesthesia with less interference with the patient's vital functions and a reduced need for opiates. Using a continuous catheter technique, the regional block can be transformed into a likewise selective analgesia with similar advantages for postoperative and other pain management.

Regional anesthesia is sometimes considered an art; this art can, however, be learnt by any interested anesthesiologist who has access to professional instructions and a good training program. The most exclusive form of regional anesthesia is peripheral nerve blockade, and for colleagues interested in practicing peripheral nerve and plexus blocks, this Atlas is an excellent source of clear and instructive descriptions of most clinically relevant extremity blocks. The art of peripheral nerve blockade is based on good anatomical understanding, careful handling of needles, catheters and patients, and good knowledge of pharmacology of local anesthetics. All these components are well presented in this Atlas.

Today's technology offers advanced assistance in localizing the target nerve; however, the use of electrostimulation or ultrasonography, for example, does not reduce the importance of anatomical knowledge. In my opinion, a competent anesthetist should also be able to find most peripheral nerves without this special equipment. And those readers who have carefully studied this Atlas will certainly be able to do that!

*Dag E. Selander[†]*
*Nösund, Orust, Sweden*

[†]This foreword to the 2nd English Edition was written in 2007 by Dag Selander, who sadly passed away 4 July 2013. In memory of this truly marvelous clinician, scientist, teacher, and above all human being, we decided to take over this foreword for the 3rd Edition, especially since it has lost none of its relevance.

# Acknowledgements

The authors of this book consider themselves lucky to have had the continued support for many years of trusted colleagues and numerous friends. In the last decade we have been actively involved, both as speakers and tutors, in courses on anatomy for regional anesthesia and pain management at Innsbruck University and at the Medical University of Graz, Austria. Thanks to Drs. Christoph Huber, Gottfried Mitterschiffthaler, and Asst. Prof. Herbert Maurer and their courses, the field of anatomy has been opened up for special clinical and anesthesiological questions. Later on Professor Feigl started to arrange similar courses at the Institute for Anatomy, Medical University of Graz (Head Professor Dr. Anderhuber). During this time we were able to discuss various questions pertaining to peripheral blocking techniques. Together we carried out scientific research at the Department of Anatomy in order to clarify specific problems. Our special thanks go to all our colleagues and friends at Innsbruck University and the Medical University of Graz.

Other colleagues in Germany and Austria, both in Anesthesia and in Anatomy, have kindly cooperated with the authors over years. There has been a long-standing exchange of experience among them Profs. J. Jage and Stofft (Mainz University, Germany), Profs. Kessler and H.-W. Korf (Frankfurt University, Germany), Profs. T. Standl and Z. Halata (HamburgUniversity, Germany), Dr. M. Gründling and Prof. Fanghänel (Greifswald University, Germany), and Prof. B. Freitag and Dr. S. Rudolph (Klinikum Südstadt Rostock, Germany) were very collegial and helpful and their cooperation lead to many new findings. In these institutes the authors also had the chance to regulary clarify anatomical details relevant to peripheral blocking. We received support from numerous colleagues and apologize that we are unable to mention all of them here. We thank all the members of the institutes.

We are especially grateful that the anatomists allowed us to take photographs of their specimens. Many of the anatomical drawings for this book were produced by Mr. N. Lechenbauer. This was only possible with the support of B. Schmalz and R. Ploenes (AstraZeneca Co.). We also received active support in our own hospitals. Surgeons patiently waited for clinical pictures to be taken and members of staff made themselves available as test persons. Special thanks go to our staff. Dr. M. Neuburger (Klinikum Achern, Germany) has been kind enough to let us have research results and took additional photographs and performed extra examinations. Drs. D. Lang, F. Reisig. T. Geiser (Trauma Center, Murnau) and B. Bünten, A. Heuckerodt (Oberammergau Center for Rheumatology, Germany) have supported us in taking clinical pictures. Support from our own and other departments of our hospitals was so great that it is impossible to name everybody. We received a great deal of encouragement and many useful tips. This book is the result of many years of cooperation between anatomy and anesthesia. We would like to express our thanks to all those who have supported us along the way.

The *Atlas of Peripheral Regional Anesthesia* has won a lot of approval and recognition within the first month of publication in the German-speaking world. We thank Thieme Publisher's, notably Angelika Findgott and Joanne Stead, for their excellent cooperation and for making an English edition of this Atlas possible. We are proud to have acquired Dr. Dag Selander for revision of the translation of the 2nd Edition. Dr. Selander was internationally renowned for his many publications in the field of regional anesthesia, including his article *Catheter technique in axillary plexus block* (Acta Anaesth Scand 1977; 21:324-329). He was the first to describe continuous percutaneus axillary brachial plexus anesthesia. We are honored that Dr. Selander agreed, as a specialist in this field, to edit the translation of the 2nd Edition and also supported us amicably with competent suggestions. We are grateful for this special support without which an English edition would have been impossible.

Panta rhei (Everything is in flux)

Heraklit (540-480 BC)

*Gisela Meier, MD*
*Johannes Buettner, MD*

# Contributors

**Editors:**

**Gisela Meier, MD**
Former Head of the Department of Anesthesia
   and Interventional Pain Therapy
Oberammergau Center for Rheumatology
Oberammergau, Germany

**Johannes Buettner, MD**
Former Head of the Department of Anesthesia
Trauma Center
Murnau, Germany

**Contributors:**

**Georg Feigl, MD**
Associate Professor
Institute for Anatomy
Medical University of Graz
Graz, Austria

**Ralf Hillmann, MD**
DESA
Pediatric Center Olga Hospital, Klinikum Stuttgart
Department of Anesthesia and Intensive Care Medicine
Stuttgart, Germany

# List of Videos

**General Aspects of Ultrasound-guided Peripheral Regional Anesthesia**
General Principles of Ultrasound-guided Peripheral Nerve Blocks

**Upper Limb**
General Overview
Interscalene Techniques of Brachial Plexus Block
Supraclavicular and Infraclavicular Techniques of Brachial Plexus Block
Suprascapular Nerve Block
Axillary Block
Selective Blocks of Individual Nerves in the Upper Arm, at the Elbow and Wrist

**Lower Limb**
General Overview
Psoas Block
Inguinal Paravascular Lumbar Plexus Anesthesia (Femoral Nerve Block)
Proximal Sciatic Nerve Blocks
Blocks at the Knee
Peripheral Blocks (Conduction Blocks) of Individual Nerves of the Lower Limb
Peripheral Nerve Blocks at the Ankle

**General Aspects**
General Principles for Performing Peripheral Blocks

# Abbreviations

| | |
|---|---|
| a. | artery |
| ACT | activated clotting time |
| ASS | acetyl salicylic acid |
| BART | blue away, red toward |
| CFM | color flow modus |
| CNB | central neuraxial block |
| COPD | chronic obstructive pulmonary disease |
| CRPS | complex regional pain syndrome |
| CW | continuous wave |
| ECT | ecarin clotting time |
| IP | in plane |
| IV | intravenous |
| LAST | local anesthetic systemic toxicity |
| LAX | long axis |
| LMH | low molcular weight heparin |
| LOR | loss of resistance |
| MRI | magnetic resonance imaging |
| OOP | out of plane |
| PCA | patient-controlled analgesia |
| PNS | peripheral nerve stimulation |
| PONV | postoperative nausea and vomiting |
| PRF | pulse repetition frequency |
| PW | pulsed wave |
| SAX | short axis |
| TAP | transversus abdominis plane |
| TGC | time gain concentration |
| THI | tissue harmonic imaging |
| v. | vein |
| VIB | vertical infraclavicular (plexus) block |

# Part 1

## General Aspects of Ultrasound-Guided Peripheral Regional Anesthesia

1

# 1 General Principles of Ultrasound-Guided Peripheral Nerve Blocks ▶

## 1.1 Technical Requirements

### 1.1.1 Equipment

Portable, high-resolution ultrasound machines with interchangeable transducers now constitute devices that are well suited for use in anesthesiology and intensive medicine.

### Types of Visualization

▶ **B-mode (brightness mode).** Every signal received from the transducer is displayed in a certain gray tone depending on its amplitude (intensity). The B-mode is used only in conjunction with the two-dimensional (2D) real-time mode. A two-dimensional image is made from the numerous ultrasound waves transmitted and received (▶ Fig. 1.1). Depending on the penetration depth and the type of probe used, just a few images or up to 200 images per second can be visualized.

▶ **M-mode (or TM-mode, time–motion).** An impulse is transmitted with a high pulse repetition rate (1,000–5,000/s). The amplitudes of the signals received are displayed on the vertical axis (one dimensional) in various gray tones; the horizontal axis is the time axis on which the signals received over time are displayed at short intervals according to frequency.

| Note |
| --- |
| The M-mode has almost no role in ultrasound-guided regional anesthesia. |

The M-mode can be helpful for diagnosing pneumothorax (see below). When the visceral pleura glide normally along the parietal pleura, a homogeneous granular pattern can be visualized below the pleura in M-mode—in contrast to the horizontal lines that can be seen above the pleura in immobile tissue (▶ Fig. 1.2). If pneumothorax is present, the granular pattern below the pleura is replaced by horizontal lines (▶ Fig. 1.3).

### Transducers

Linear array and curved array transducers are used (▶ Fig. 1.4).

▶ **Linear array transducer.** The *standard transducer* is the high-frequency linear array transducer. A multi-frequency transducer (e.g., 4.0–16 MHz), with the option of varying the frequency depending on the penetration depth required, is generally used. A special form of high-frequency linear probe known as a hockey stick linear array transducer is shaped so that it can be used in small anatomical situations. Modern multi-frequency linear broadband transducers use an electronic phased array technique, allowing the beam to be directed at various angles (sector scanning by electronic pan both in the transmission and the receptor field).

▶ **Curved array transducer.** The curved array transducer (2.0–6.0 MHz) is used for blocks of deeper nerves.

| Practical Note |
| --- |
| The higher the frequency, the better the resolution—but the lower the penetration depth. |

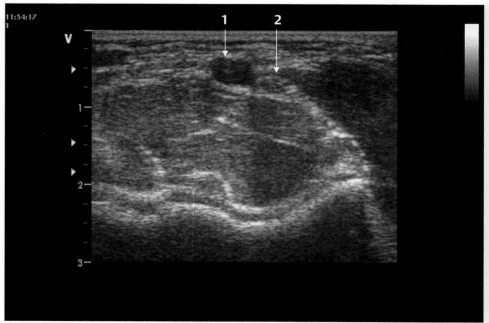

**Fig. 1.1** Visualization of the elbow in B-mode (2D real-time mode).
1 Brachial artery
2 Median nerve

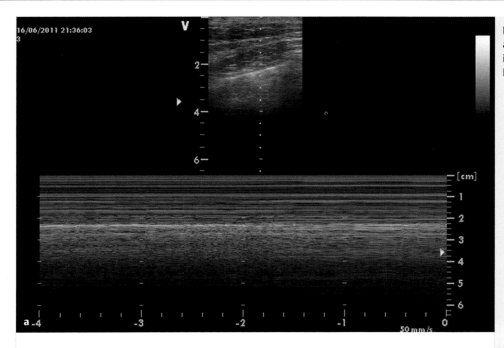

**Fig. 1.2** Intact pleura in M-mode.
**a** Small image at top: Pleura in B-mode indicating the ultrasound beam in which the M-mode was recorded.

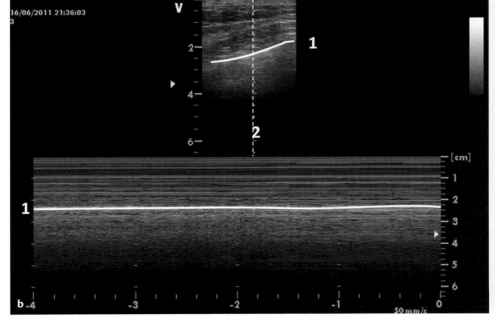

**b** Intact pleura in M-mode labeled.
1 Pleura
2 Ultrasound beam with which the M-mode was recorded

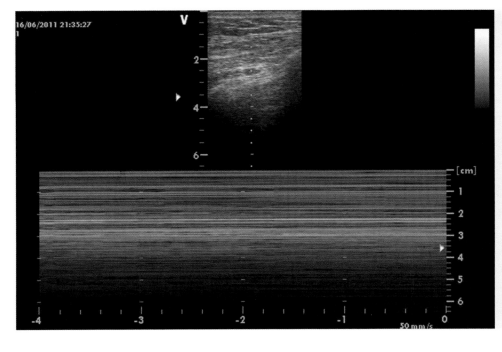

**Fig. 1.3** Pleura in pneumothorax.

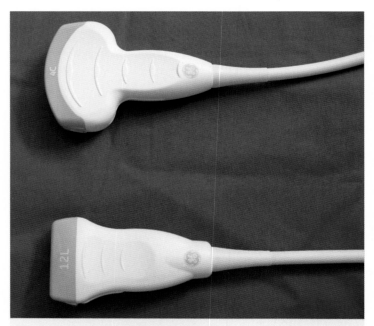

**Fig. 1.4** Linear and curved array transducer.

## 1.1.2 Optimizing the Ultrasound Image

Newer generations of ultrasound machines have numerous options for optimizing the image, some of which are mentioned here; the designations sometimes vary depending on the manufacturer.

### Penetration Depth

The penetration depth should be adjusted depending on the target structures. Increasing penetration depth leads to attenuation of amplitude and thus to poorer image quality. High frequencies are subject to strong attenuation and therefore do not penetrate tissue as well; low frequencies are attenuated to a lesser degree when penetrating tissue and are therefore better suited for visualizing deeper structures.

↑ Frequency = ↑ Signal attenuation
↑ Signal attenuation = ↓ Penetration

> **Practical Note**
>
> The higher the frequency, the higher the resolution!
> The highest possible frequency that still results in a usable image at the required penetration depth should always be selected.
> The target object should be approximately in mid-field when performing peripheral regional nerve blocks.

### Frequency

The penetration depth is also relevant for the frequency.

> **Note**
>
> High frequency = high resolution, limited penetration depth.
> Low frequency = greater penetration depth, poorer resolution.

▶ **High frequency range (e.g., 8–12 MHz).** Optimal for penetration depths of 3 to 4 cm—for example, interscalene, supraclavicular, axillary, femoral, peripheral nerve blocks of the upper limb.

▶ **Medium frequency range (e.g., 6–10 MHz).** Optimal for penetration depths of 4 to 8 cm—for example, axillary, infraclavicular, femoral nerves in obese patients, distal sciatic nerve block.

▶ **Low frequency range (e.g., 2–5 MHz).** Optimal for penetration depths of > 8 cm—for example, proximal sciatic nerve blocks, psoas block.

### Gain (Amplification)

The gain function amplifies the signals returning to the device. The amplification determines how bright (hyperechoic) or dark (hypoechoic) the image appears on the monitor. All signals received can be amplified equally over the entire field (overall gain). Too high overall gain leads to overexposure of the image and should be avoided.

> **Note**
>
> As a guide, the fluid in the vessels should appear black.

Using the "slide controls" available in most ultrasound machines (time gain compensation, TGC), the signals returning from various depths can be amplified to different degrees. This allows increased amplification of the attenuated signals received from deeper levels so a homogeneous image can be produced.

Modern ultrasound machines generally have a feature for *automatic image optimization* that produces the best possible balance between the overall gain and depth compensation settings. In particular, this feature makes it unnecessary to set the slide controls separately (they are all set at the same level when automatic image optimization is activated).

▶ **Focus.** The focus area should be set for the target structures, as the best image quality is achieved in the focus area. The number of foci can be varied.

> **Note**
>
> The more foci, the poorer the image quality.

### Compound Imaging

Depending on the manufacturer, this technique is also known as "Cross Beam," "M(ulti)View," "SonoMB," and "SonoCT." Several two-dimensional images taken simultaneously from different angles (due to different beam angles, linear phased array, see above) are electronically compounded to one image for higher contrast resolution with sharper contours. Scatter echoes, speckle noise, and mirror artifacts are reduced.

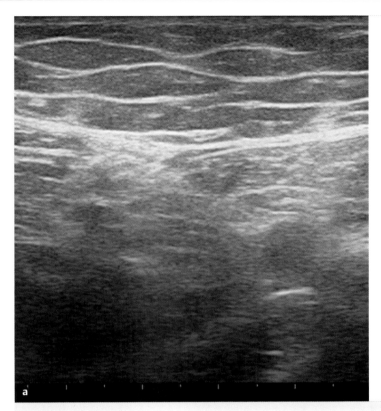
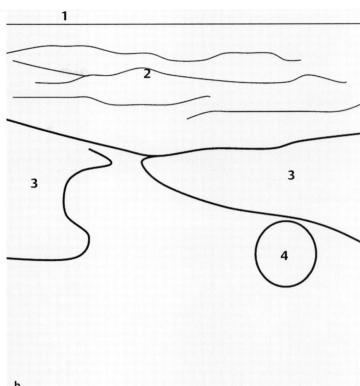

**Fig. 1.5** Subcutaneous fat tissue.
**a** Ultrasound image.
**b** Diagram.
1 Dermis
2 Subcutaneous tissue
3 Muscle tissue
4 Artery

## Tissue Harmonic Imaging (THI)

Also called tissue enhancement imaging (TEI), this method is based on the fact that only those signals that return to the transducer with a frequency twice as great as the signals transmitted by the transducer (harmonic waves) are used for imaging. These high-frequency signals are generated by nonlinear propagation in tissue. This method allows improved contrast and spatial resolution ("lower noise" images). In particular, the artifacts that are caused by superficial fatty tissue are eliminated, as the harmonic waves are generated only with increasing penetration of the tissue (not usually used in peripheral regional nerve blocks).

## Dynamic Range (Compression)

The dynamic range regulates the conversion of echo intensities to gray tones, for which the adjustable contrast range is enlarged. The dynamic range is useful for optimizing the texture of various anatomical tissues. The contours with the highest amplitudes should appear white, while the lowest amplitudes, for example blood, are still just visible.

Both in moving images, as film and video, and in still images, the dynamic range designates the ratios of the largest and smallest discernible brightness levels of noise and grain.

Many other functions are available from various manufacturers today. When the numerous functions are used optimally, an optimal image for peripheral regional anesthesia can usually be visualized.

Most machines have the option of saving the settings for various nerve blocks such as frequency, penetration depth, anticipated focus area, etc. (preset), which speeds up the procedure.

## 1.1.3 Structural Features in Ultrasound

### Skin and Subcutaneous Fat Tissue

The skin (epidermis and dermis) is approximately 1 to 4 mm thick and can be readily differentiated as a narrow strip. Subcutaneous fat is hypoechoic with septa that are mainly parallel to the surface (▶ Fig. 1.5).

A subcutaneous edema has a "riverbed-like" structure (▶ Fig. 1.6).

▶ **Lymph nodes.** Lymph nodes have a hyperechoic center with a hypoechoic border. They can often be visualized in the inguinal region (▶ Fig. 1.7).

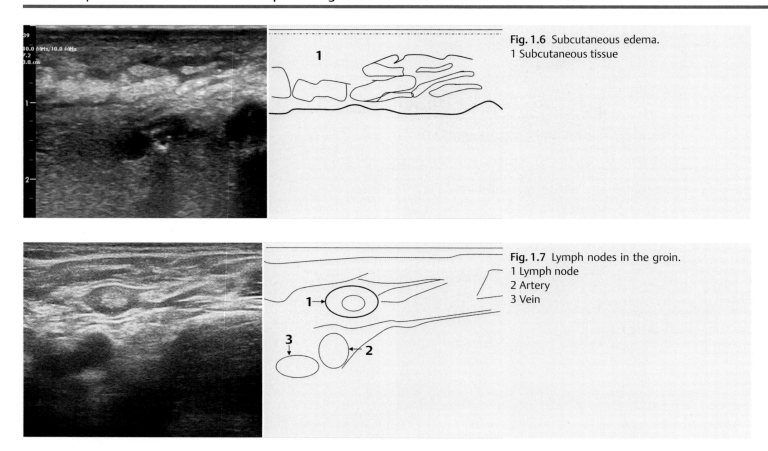

**Fig. 1.6** Subcutaneous edema.
1 Subcutaneous tissue

**Fig. 1.7** Lymph nodes in the groin.
1 Lymph node
2 Artery
3 Vein

**Fig. 1.8** Structure of a nerve (Source: Schünke et al 2011).

Connective and fat tissue

Unmyelinated fibers (vegetative)

Myelinated fiber (somatosensory or sensory)

Endoneurium

Perineurium

Blood vessels     Epineurium

## Peripheral Nerves

Peripheral nerves consist of nerve fibers (axons) that are covered by a myelin sheath and are embedded in delicate layer of connective tissue, the endoneurium. Several nerve fibers are bundled together to form a fascicle surrounded by the perineurium. Several fascicles and connective tissue together form a peripheral nerve and are surrounded by the epineurium (► Fig. 1.8).

Centrally located parts of the nerve fiber on the upper limb (nerve roots, trunks, and fascicle proximal to the clavicles) have a lower percentage of (hyperechoic) connective tissue than the infraclavicular nerve segments and therefore appear "monofascicular" or "oligofascicular" in the ultrasound image, that is, with a uniformly *hypoechoic* cross-section (dark round structures; ► Fig. 1.9, see also Chapter 3.2.3). Distal to the clavicles, the percentage of connective tissue increases in relation to the neurogenic part, leading to the characteristic "honeycomb" pattern in the cross-section of nerves located further peripheral in the upper limbs (Moayeri et al 2008). The fascicles (or rather several

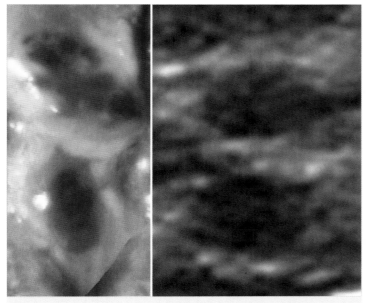

**Fig. 1.9** Roots C6 and C7: hypoechoic structure, centrally located nerve (left: anatomical cross section; right: ultrasound image.

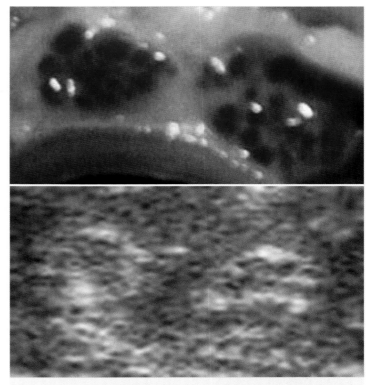

**Fig. 1.10** Nerves in the infraclavicular area (top: anatomical cross-section; bottom: ultrasound image).

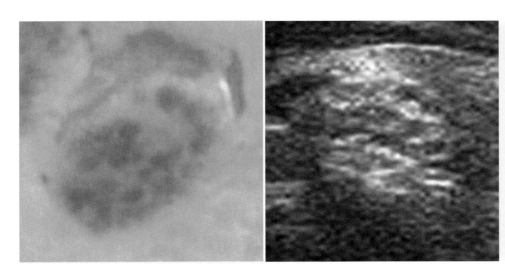

**Fig. 1.11** Distal sciatic nerve: hyperechoic structure of further distal segments of the nerve (left: anatomical cross-section; right: ultrasound image).

bundles of fascicles) appear as hypoechoic (dark), round structures within the hyperechoic connective tissue (▶ Fig. 1.10).

The nerves in the lower limbs that can be visualized by ultrasound appear *hyperechoic* due to the relatively high percentage of connective tissue (▶ Fig. 1.11; Moayeri et al 2010).

For novices, the median nerve in the forearm is the ideal object for visualizing this nerve structure in an ultrasound image (▶ Fig. 1.12).

## Tendons

It is not always easy to differentiate between tendons and nerves. Tendons do not have the typical "honeycomb" structure. Nerves can be best identified by following the course. Tendons have stronger anisotropy (see below) than nerves (▶ Fig. 1.13).

## Vessels

Vessels can be readily visualized in an ultrasound image and are often used as orientation. They are hypoechoic (i.e., dark) in the ultrasound image (▶ Fig. 1.14).

- Veins can be compressed by applying pressure.
- Arteries pulsate (this is especially visible when the artery is compressed.
- Nerves move in response to probe compression and do not pulsate (▶ Fig. 1.14).

## Doppler Methods

If there is any uncertainty in identifying vessels, the Doppler function can be used. One-dimensional methods (pulsed wave

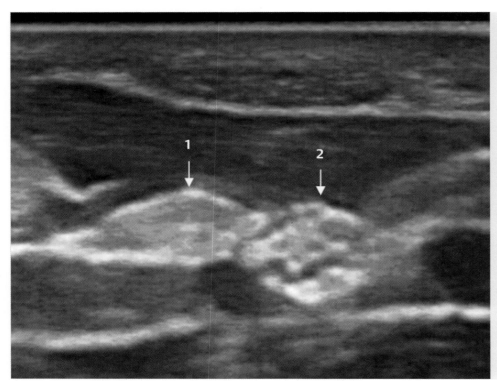

**Fig. 1.12** Typical structure of a peripheral nerve using the example of the median nerve.
1 Tendon
2 Nerve (median nerve near the wrist)

Doppler, continuous wave Doppler) are distinguished from two-dimensional, color-coded methods (color Doppler). The Doppler method is based on the fact that sound waves sent from a stationary transmitter change frequency when they meet a moving reflector. The velocity of the moving object (usually red blood cells) can be calculated from the change in frequency of the reflected wave compared with the transmitted wave, which is also detected by the transducer acting as receiver in order to determine blood flow velocity.

▶ **Pulsed Wave Doppler.** In the pulsed wave Doppler method (*PW Doppler*, "pulsed" Doppler), short intermittent ultrasonic pulses are transmitted and then received. A transducer functions as both transmitter and receiver. This allows the velocity to be measured at a selected location in a conventional ultrasound (B-mode), that is, a point in the conventional ultrasound can be determined where the velocity is to be measured. This is usually visualized as a curve in a velocity–time diagram (▶ Fig. 1.16).

▶ **Continuous Wave Doppler.** In the continuous wave Doppler method (*CW Doppler*), a transmitter and a receiver in the transducer operate simultaneously and continuously, that is, signals are constantly transmitted and received simultaneously. The disadvantage of this method is that the depth of the Doppler echo cannot be determined. However, unlike PW Doppler, relatively high velocities can be registered. As in PW Doppler, visualization is in the form of a time–velocity diagram. This method *is not generally used* for regional anesthesia.

▶ **Color Doppler.** In the color Doppler method, the areas where movement is registered are visualized in a two-dimensional area (a window to be specified in a B-mode image) via Doppler analyses pulsed to thousands of individual points. Conventionally, movements along the beam axis toward the transducer are displayed as red and movements in the opposite direction (away from the transducer) are displayed as blue (BART: "blue away, red toward," ▶ Fig. 1.15).

### Practical Note

The visualization of flow movements is worst when the transducer is held perpendicular (90°) to the flow movement (e.g., to the cross-section of the vessel). The sound waves should thus always be directed at an oblique angle to the flow movement. To optimize the image, color gain must be at an optimal setting. Over-regulation results in the color appearing not only in the vessel, but in the entire color window! The pulse repetition frequency (PRF) must be adjusted to the anticipated flow velocity in the vessel. Arteries can be distinguished from veins based on color behavior and rhythmic behavior (artery) or more even movement (vein) of the signals received.

### Note

The Doppler function is at the expense of the remaining image quality and should therefore be used only temporarily to identify vessels.

Some machines have what is called *power Doppler*. This function allows vessels to be detected that can be visualized using normal color Doppler only with difficulty, if at all. In contrast to color Doppler, power Doppler is almost independent of the beam angle. Due to its greater sensitivity, movement artifacts are more frequently displayed; the flow direction cannot be visualized.

The combination of B-mode and PW Doppler is also known as *duplex sonography*. In the *color duplex method*, the B-mode is combined with color Doppler and PW Doppler (▶ Fig. 1.16).

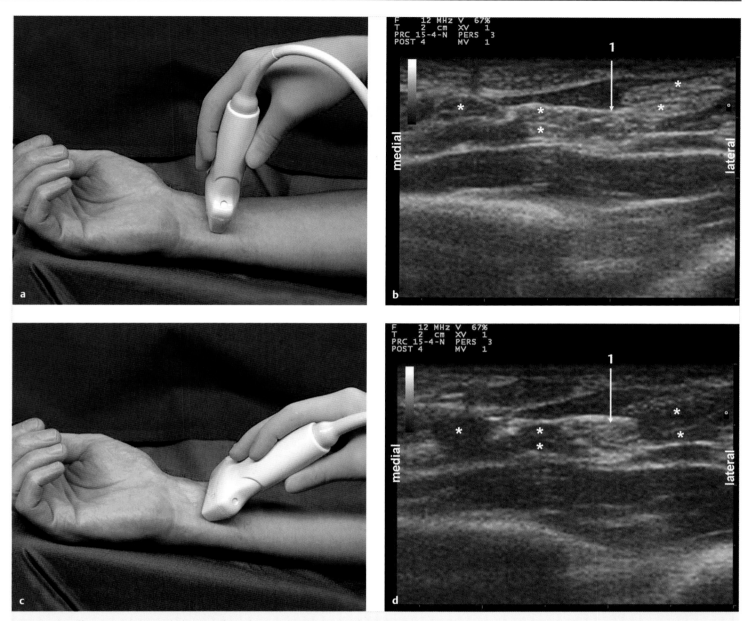

**Fig. 1.13** Different anisotropic behavior of tendons and nerves. Visualization of the median nerve at the fold of the wrist (short axis).
1 Median nerve (short axis), * tendons
**a** Tendon and nerve can hardly be distinguished with a perpendicular beam.
**b** Visualization in ultrasound image.
**c** When the beam is at an angle to the structures (transducer tilted), the reflection disappears through the tendons, while that of the nerves remains longer. This corresponds to the greater anisotropic behavior of nerves compared with tendons (see also anisotropic behavior in this chapter).
**d** Ultrasound image.

## Pleura

The pleura is highly reflective. It thus appears as a light line in the ultrasound scan. Comet tail reverberation artifacts (white streaks spreading downward) that move horizontally with respiration are caused by small vessels in the visceral pleura. The pleural line is interrupted by the osseous structures of the ribs (► Fig. 1.17). ►

Pneumothorax can be diagnosed by the absence of the back and forth movement of these artifacts. The M-mode can be useful for better differentiation (see ► Fig. 1.2 and ► Fig. 1.3).

## Bones

The sound waves are reflected completely at the border to bones. This results in a bright line with an acoustic shadow behind it (see ► Fig. 1.32).

## Air

Air results in strong reflection of sound waves and an acoustic shadow (► Fig. 1.18).

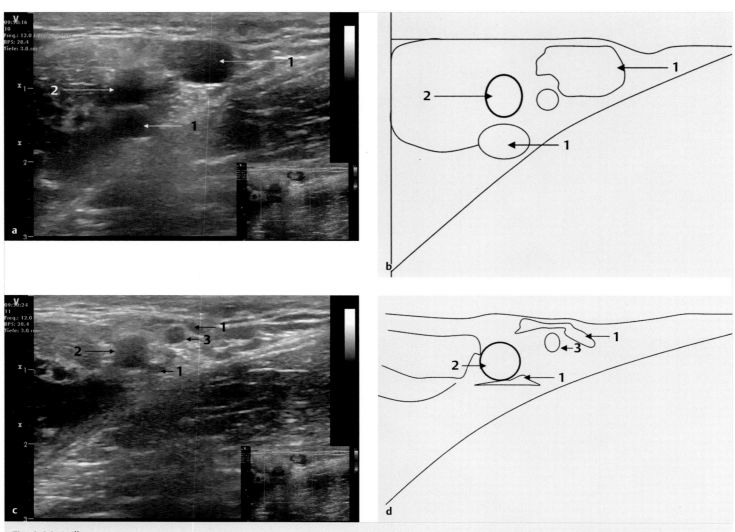

**Fig. 1.14** Axilla.
**a** Axillary scout view imaging.
1 Veins
2 Artery
At the lower right is an identical section with color Doppler.
**b** Diagram.
**c** Axilla with compression in the ultrasound image.

1 Veins (due to compression, visible only as a narrow gap or no longer visible at all)
2 Artery (pulsating in the moving image)
3 Nerve (hypoechoic structure, not compressible, not pulsating)
At the lower right is an identical section with color Doppler without compression.
**d** Diagram.

---

> **Note**
>
> Air is the "enemy" of ultrasound.

When performing nerve blocks, avoid injecting air, as it severely impairs visibility.

# 1.2 Ultrasound-Guided Needle Approach

▶ **Settings.** In contrast to the *conventions for diagnostic imaging* that were adopted for ultrasonography from the interpretation of CT images, it is helpful to set up and position the monitor for needle insertion so the practitioner can view the monitor with the sides corresponding to reality. For example, for an interscalene nerve block, the monitor should be positioned next to the patient so it can be seen easily by the practitioner.

> **Practical Note**
>
> The image should be set so that the patient's left side is also at the left on the monitor. Every transducer has a mark on the side that is displayed on the monitor. "Top/bottom" can also be adjusted to the actual circumstances.

For a distal sciatic nerve block, for example, if the transducer is held against the thigh of a supine patient from posterior direction, the image on the monitor can be set so that the patient's posterior side is displayed at the bottom of the monitor. This makes it easier to position the needle.

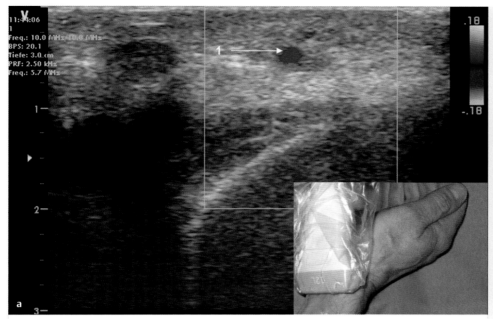

**Fig. 1.15** Color Doppler.
**a** Radial artery (red), transducer tilted against flow direction.
1 Radial artery

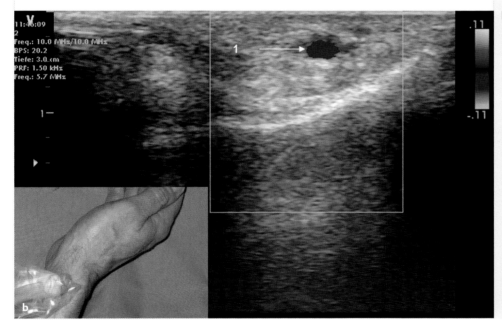

**b** Radial artery (blue), transducer tilted toward flow direction.
1 Radial artery

▶ **Contact of the transducer with skin.** To ensure good contact between transducer and skin, (sterile) ultrasound gel (or alcohol-based disinfectant if the transducer is protected with a sleeve) can be used.

> **Practical Note**
>
> Avoid direct contact of the transducer with alcohol-based disinfectants, as long-term exposure can damage the transducer.

For cleaning the transducer, use only disinfectants and cleaning solutions recommended by the manufacturer. For continuous procedures, there are sterile sheaths for covering the transducer and cable (CIV-Flex Transducer Cover [CIVCO], Flexasoft Ultrasound Cover [Udo Heisig GmbH], ▶ Fig. 1.19.) It is important that there are no air bubbles between the transducer and the sheath. For this reason, there must be gel between the transducer and the sheath. Alternatively, an adhesive film can be applied to the transducer, strictly avoiding air bubbles (Flexasoft Ultrasound Cover, Udo Heisig GmbH).

▶ **Single shot.** For a single-shot block it is possible to cover the transducer with a sterile film (e.g., Tegaderm); in this case, no ultrasound gel is used between the film and the transducer. Alternatively, the transducer can be covered with a (sterile) one-way glove (gel is used between the transducer and glove).

## 1.2.1 Ultrasound Techniques for Needle Insertion

All ultrasound images are combined with a position image that indicates the exact position of the transducer.

### In-plane Technique (Needle Insertion in the Ultrasound Plane)

The needle is inserted in the same plane as the ultrasound beam (▶ Fig. 1.20). Transducer and needle must always be coordinated so that the entire needle can be visualized. The transducer and/or the needle may have to be tilted or rotated slightly for this. The needle must not be at an angle to the long axis of the transducer.

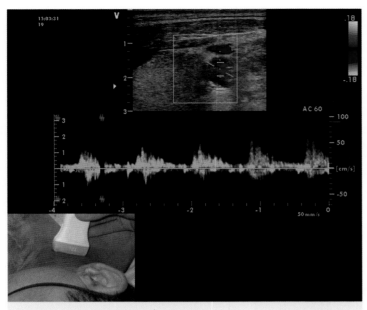

**Fig. 1.16** Color duplex ultrasound (PW Doppler in conjunction with color Doppler in B-mode) using the right carotid artery (red in the color Doppler) as an example.
Blue: internal jugular vein; bottom: visualization of the PW Doppler signal in the time–velocity graph; x-axis: sweep speed (mm/s), y-axis: blood flow velocity (cm [m]/s).

**Note**

The steeper the needle insertion angle with respect to the transducer, the poorer the visualization of the needle (▶ Fig. 1.21).

A special surface design has been developed that makes it possible to visualize needles in an ultrasound image even when the insertion angle is steep (Stimuplex D Plus, B. Braun; SonoPlex Needle, Pajunk GmbH; ▶ Fig. 1.22 and ▶ Fig. 1.23). Using special software, newer ultrasound machines can also make ordinary needles, not fashioned with special processing, visible at steeper angles (e.g., Sonosite).

## Out-of-Plane Technique

The needle is inserted perpendicular to the ultrasound beam. This means that it can be visualized in the ultrasound image only as a dot (▶ Fig. 1.24). It is not possible to determine how far the tip of the needle has already passed the transducer. Small rhythmic movements when advancing the needle (local tissue movement; Marhofer and Chan 2007; "tissue dancing") can provide indirect information on the position of the tip of the needle. Simultaneous use of a nerve stimulator can interfere with this technique.

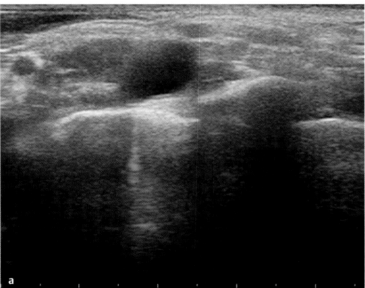

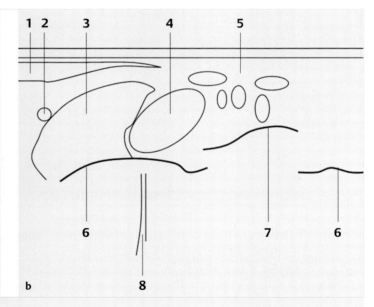

**Fig. 1.17** Pleura.
a Ultrasound image.
b Diagram.

1 Sternocleidomastoid muscle
2 Phrenic nerve
3 Anterior scalene muscle
4 Subclavian artery (with posterior acoustic enhancement)
5 Brachial plexus
6 Pleural cavity
7 Rib (with acoustic shadow)
8 Comet tail phenomenon

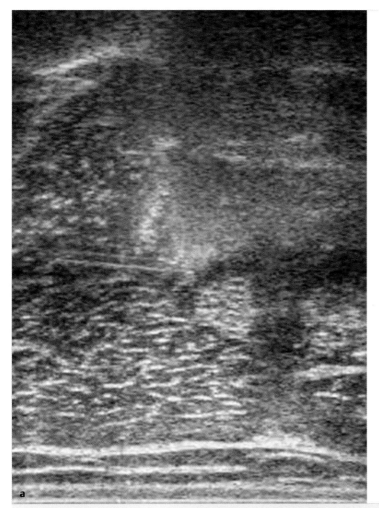

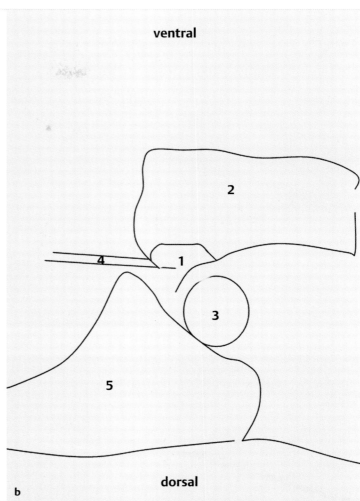

**Fig. 1.18** Air injection: a distal sciatic nerve block as an example.
**a** Supine position, beam from posterior direction.
**b** Diagram.

1 Air bubbles at the tip of the needle
2 Fluid containing air with sound attenuation behind it
3 Sciatic nerve
4 Needle with lumen
5 Long head of the femoral biceps muscle

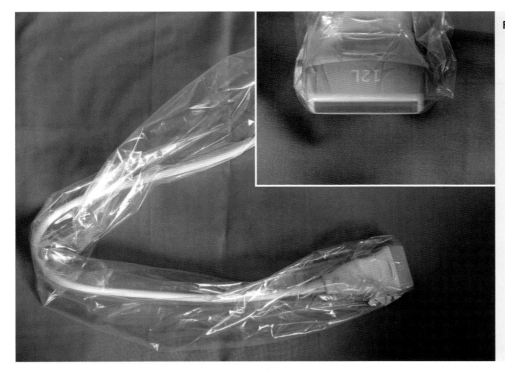

**Fig. 1.19** Sterile sheath for the transducer.

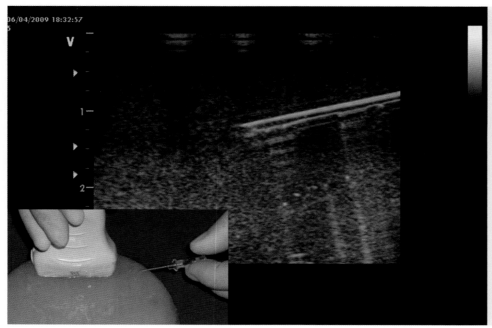

**Fig. 1.20** In-plane needle placement (note the reverberation artifact below the needle).

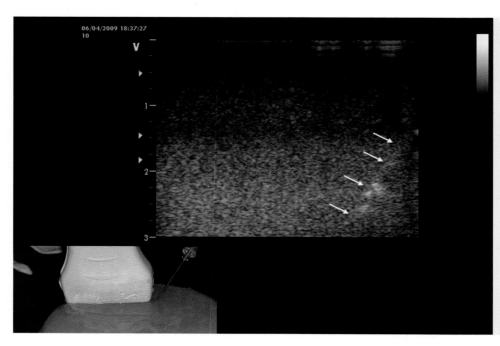

**Fig. 1.21** Ultrasound image. In-plane needle insertion: If the angle is steep, visualization of the needle in the ultrasound is markedly poorer. The arrows indicate the position of the needle.

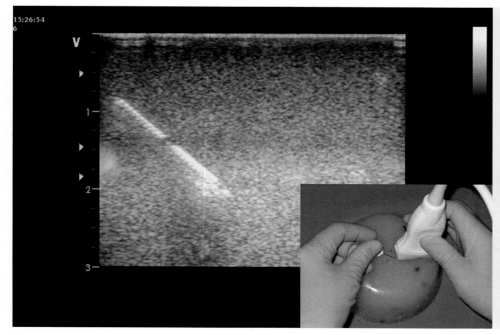

**Fig. 1.22** Special "Sono" needles are readily visible in plane in the last 2 cm even when the insertion angle is steep (SonoPlex Needle; Pajunk GmbH).

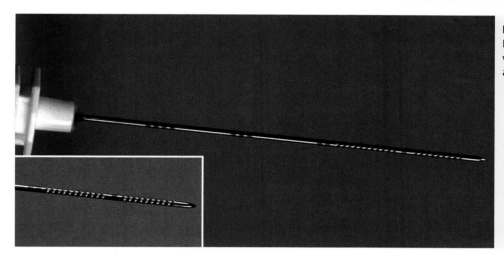

**Fig. 1.23** SonoPlex Needle (Pajunk GmbH). Notches on the surface make the needle easily visible in the ultrasound even when the insertion angle is steep.

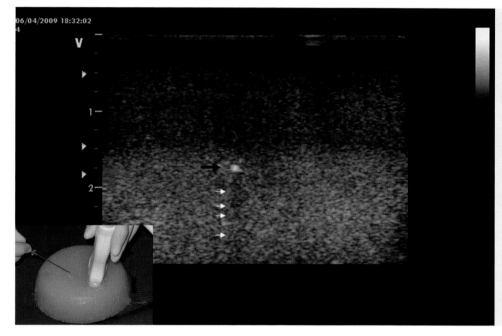

**Fig. 1.24** Out-of-plane needle insertion. The needle can be visualized only as a dot (note the acoustic shadow below the needle). Information on the position of the tip of the needle can be obtained only by shifting the transducer (the white point disappears at the tip of the needle).
The black arrow indicates the needle; the white arrows mark the acoustic shadow.

The repeated administration of small quantities of fluid ("hydrolocation" technique) allows the location of the tip of the needle to be determined. A local anesthetic or normal saline solution can be used for this.

If the nerve stimulator is used simultaneously, glucose 5% should be used, as both local anesthetic and saline solution impair the response to the nerve stimulator (Tsui and Kropelin 2005).

> **Note**
>
> The key to ultrasound interpretation is a moving image.

The tip of the needle should always be followed by tilting and/or sliding the transducer. The transducer is generally positioned perpendicular to the structures to be examined (visualization in the short axis, see below). The target object should be in the middle of the image.

## Visualization of the Target Structures

The desired structures can be visualized in the *short axis* (transducer at a right angle to the object; ▶ Fig. 1.25) or in the *long axis*

(visualization of the target object in the longitudinal axis; ▶ Fig. 1.26).

> **Note**
>
> Visualization in the short axis is usually used for peripheral regional nerve blocks.

The following abbreviations are commonly used:
- SAX: short axis
- LAX: long axis
- OOP: out of plane
- IP: in plane

## Visualization of Neural Structures

Depending on the surrounding tissue, peripheral nerve structures appear hypoechoic (darker than the surroundings, e.g., interscalene nerve, ▶ Fig. 1.27) or hyperechoic (brighter than surroundings, e.g., sciatic nerve, ▶ Fig. 1.28).

> **Note**
>
> A moving image is key to visualizing nerves in an ultrasound scan.

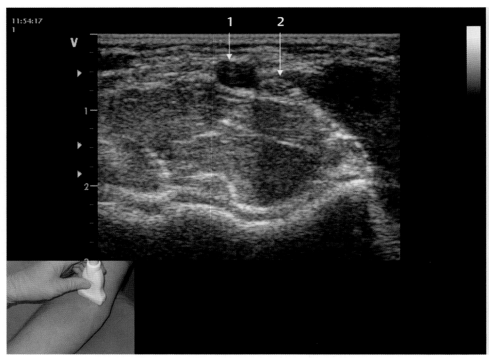

**Fig. 1.25** Visualization of the median nerve in the short axis right cubital fossa (perpendicular to the object).
1 Brachial artery
2 Median nerve
V lateral

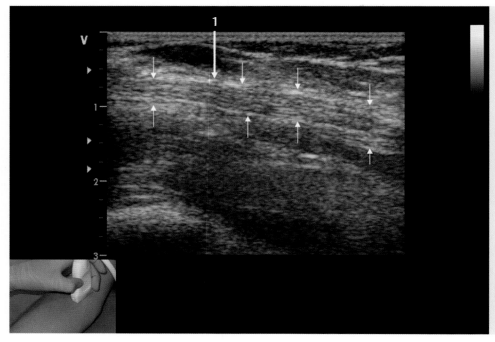

**Fig. 1.26** Visualization of the median nerve in the cubital fossa in the long axis (parallel to the object).
1 Median nerve (arrows)
V proximal

It is important to direct the ultrasound beam at the nerves at the correct angle. Just tilting the transducer slightly can change the visualization entirely (anisotropy of nerves).

The anisotropic behavior of nerves sometimes makes it difficult to visualize nerve and needle optimally at the same time.

**Note**

Isotropic behavior: Visualization of the structure is independent of the angle of insonation.
Anisotropic behavior: Slight changes in the angle of insonation can make the structure disappear entirely (see ▶ Fig. 1.13).

▶ **Distinguishing nerves from tendons** . Tendons have stronger anisotropy than nerves (see ▶ Fig. 1.13). The appearance of tendons changes with even very small changes in the angle (approx. 2°); that of nerves when the angle of insonation is changed by about 10°. This difference can be used to distinguish between nerves and tendons. ▶

When in doubt about whether the target nerve really has been located, the structure must be followed in proximal and distal directions to ensure that it is possible to follow it over a longer distance. It is often useful to locate a neural structure where it can be readily identified and then follow the nerve from there to the desired injection site. For example, the two branches of the sciatic nerve (tibial nerve, common fibular nerve) are often easy to identify in the popliteal fossa. From there, the nerve can be followed proximally. The same applies to many other neural structures (e.g., interscalene block, radial nerve of the upper arm, median nerve of the forearm).

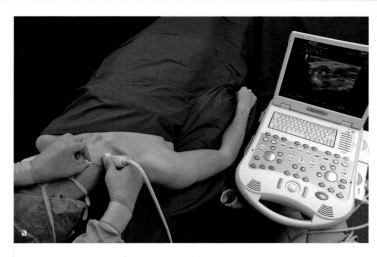

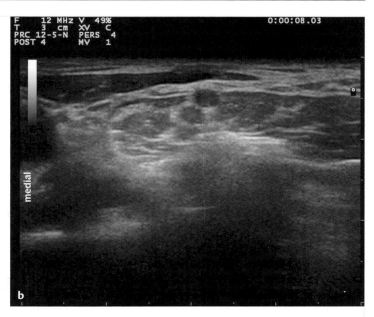

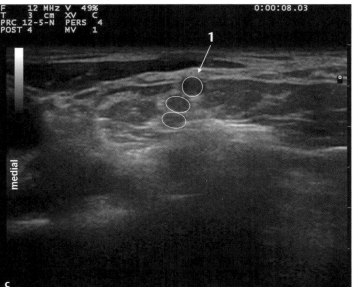

**Fig. 1.27** Hypoechoic visualization ("black" structure) using the example of the interscalene brachial plexus.
1 Brachial plexus (3 "balls" in a row correspond to the trunks).
**a** Clinical setting.
**b** Unlabeled.
**c** Labeled.

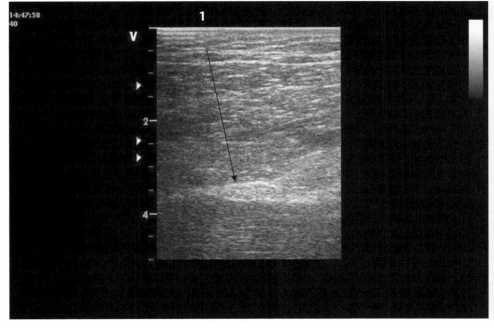

**Fig. 1.28** Hyperechoic visualization ("white" structure) using the example of the sciatic nerve.
1 Sciatic nerve (proximal)

The following manipulations of the transducer may be useful for optimizing the visualization of a peripheral nerve:
- Sliding (visualizing the nerve in the short axis and then following it over a certain distance)
- Tilting
- Rotating
- Compressing

Compressing in particular often leads to improved visualization of the neural structures.

Practical Note

A pragmatic approach to using ultrasound in regions in which the neural structures are located in the immediate vicinity of an artery is to apply local anesthetic around the artery (e.g., infraclavicular nerve block, axillary nerve block), without needing to visualize the nerves in detail. Vessels are generally easy to visualize (see above). When in doubt, Doppler ultrasound can be used.

## Spread of the Local Anesthetic

Ultrasound also provides important information on the spread of the local anesthetic. When using ultrasound, it should therefore always be checked whether the local anesthetic has spread around the neural structures (halo or donut sign, e.g., sciatic nerve, ▶ Fig. 1.29) or into the target compartment (e.g., femoral nerve, axillary plexus; ▶ Fig. 1.30). If this is not the case (e.g., fascia between the needle and tip of the needle), the position of the needle must be corrected.

## Risk Structures

In addition to visualizing the target region, ultrasound can also be used to avoid complications like puncturing a kidney when performing a psoas compartment block, or pleura in blocks near the clavicles (▶ Fig. 1.31).

## Artifacts

*Acoustic shadows* occur when the ultrasound waves at interfaces are completely reflected or absorbed (e.g., bone ▶ Fig. 1.32, needle see ▶ Fig. 1.24). Air can also cause a distal acoustic shadow!

▶ **Posterior amplification.** Posterior amplification (bright structures) occurs following the spread of fluids due to lower attenuation of sound waves in the fluid compared with tissue (▶ Fig. 1.33). In circular objects, the marginal beams can be reflected away; the marginal structures are then missing in the image, causing lateral shadowing.

Note

Amplification behind vessels occasionally leads to misinterpretations when identifying nerve structures.

▶ **Reverberation artifacts (repeating echoes; ▶ Fig. 1.34).**
These occur, for example, when a needle is inserted perpendicular to the ultrasound beam. (In the in-plane technique, the needle is parallel to the linear array transducer. This allows the best visualization of the needle.) The needle is imaged several times in the region lying below it. Reverberation artifacts can also be caused by strongly reflective structures of the body and occasionally result in misinterpretations.

▶ **Bayonet artifacts.** When a needle which is inserted in plane perpendicular to the ultrasound beam penetrates two tissues with slightly different conduction speeds (e.g., muscle and fatty tissue), the part of the needle in the medium with a slower transmission speed (fatty tissue) appears to be further from the transducer. The sound waves reflected through fat arrive later and appear to come from a greater distance, as the distance in the ultrasound is determined in proportion to the time of an assumed fixed conduction velocity in the human body (1540 m/s). This causes the needle to appear bent (▶ Fig. 1.35).

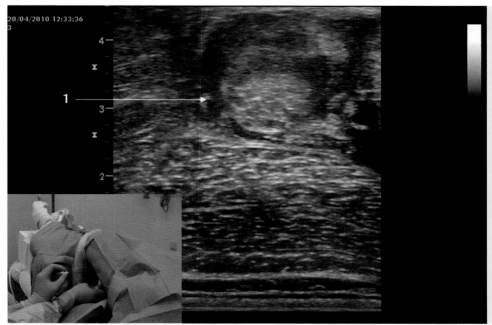

**Fig. 1.29** Distal sciatic nerve surrounded by local anesthetic (halo or donut sign).
1 Sciatic nerve

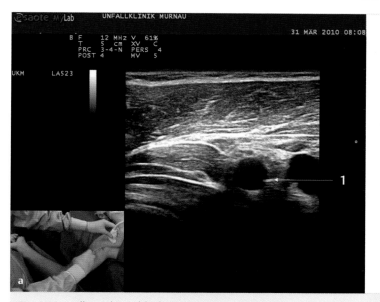

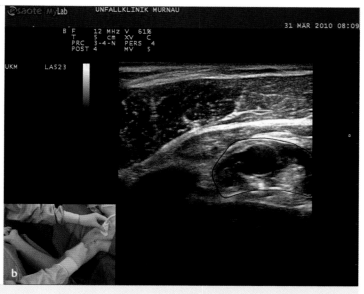

**Fig. 1.30** Axillary plexus block (perivascular technique).
**a** Before injecting the local anesthetic.
1 Tip of the needle
**b** After injecting the local anesthetic.

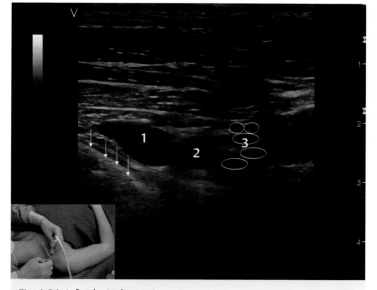

**Fig. 1.31** Infraclavicular region.
1 Subclavian vein
2 Subclavian artery
3 Brachial plexus
Arrows: Pleura
V Caudal

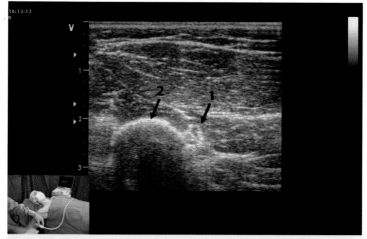

**Fig. 1.32** Visualization of the radial nerve at the middle of the upper arm—note the acoustic shadow (black) behind the bone.
1 Radial nerve
2 Humerus

## Limitations of Ultrasound

Techniques using ultrasound for finding deep nerves are difficult to apply in obese patients. A curved array transducer must be used for this purpose.

Ultrasound is especially suitable for novices for the following nerve blocks:

- Interscalene block
- Femoral nerve block
- Axillary nerve block
- Distal sciatic nerve block
- Blocks of all more peripheral individual nerves (Mariano et al 2009)

## 1.3 Ultrasound for Continuous Block Techniques

The technique for inserting a catheter is not fundamentally different from that for a single-shot block. Theoretical considerations make the out-of-plane technique appear to be more favorable for catheter placement, as the catheter can be advanced along the longitudinal axis of the nerve, making it easier to position. However, several articles also report on successful catheter insertion using the in-plane technique, for example, for the following nerve blocks:

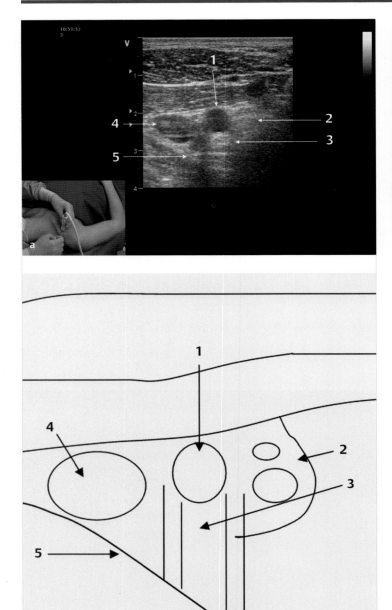

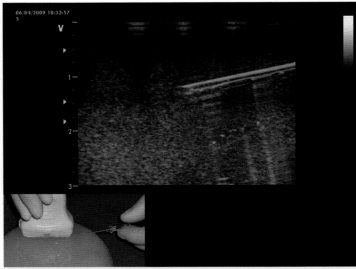

**Fig. 1.34** Reverberation artifacts (occurrence of several echoes at equal distances) due to 1) limited contact between the transducer and the medium (superficial), 2) the needle.

Another method of checking the correct position of the catheter is to apply fluid (local anesthetic, glucose 5%, or normal saline solution). To improve visualization, it is recommended that the fluid be shaken beforehand (Dhir and Ganapathy 2008).

Some authors also use air (1 mL) for better visualization of the position of the tip of the catheter (Heil et al 2010).

A new catheter has been developed with a metal knob and "Cornerstone" reflectors on the tip for better visualization by the ultrasound.

## 1.3.1 Learning Ultrasound-Guided Needle Placement Techniques

Various methods have been recommended for learning ultrasound-guided needle placement (Kessler et al 2007, Sites et al 2007a, 2007b, 2007c, Sites et al 2009).

The following conditions must be met:

- Exact anatomical knowledge of the target region. Courses are offered in various anatomy institutes that enable you to get an overview of the structures on donor bodies.
- Exact knowledge of the functions of the machine.
- Distinguishing the different structures (nerves, muscles, vessels, pleura, intestine, bones, etc.)
- Precise needle positioning under ultrasound guidance. It is important to coordinate the transducer and tip of the needle so that the position of the tip is always visible in the image. In the in-plane technique, the entire length of the needle in the ultrasound beam must be visible.
- These skills can be learned using a model. Training models are available for this (e.g., Blue Phantom); alternatively, a "cornstarch cake" can be made (see text box below for recipe, also ► Fig. 1.37), through which a Redon tube can be pulled for the target structure, for practicing using the transducer and needle. Blocks of tofu or agar (Agar-Agar) can also be used as a phantom for learning ultrasound techniques.
- Exact knowledge of artifacts and problems that can be expected (pitfalls: Sites et al 2007a, 2007b).

**Fig. 1.33** Posterior amplification.
**a** (Relative) amplification behind a vessel (here, infraclavicular region).
**b** Diagram.
1 Subclavian artery
2 Brachial plexus
3 Amplification behind the vessel, acoustic shadow at the edges
4 Subclavian vein
5 Pleura
V Caudal

- Femoral nerve block (Aveline et al 2010, Niazi et al 2009, Wang et al 2010)
- Distal sciatic nerve block (Mariano et al 2010)
- Supraclavicular nerve block (Heil et al 2010)
- Infraclavicular nerve block (Mariano et al 2009)
- Interscalene nerve block (Mariano et al 2010).

The catheter can sometimes be visualized, especially in the in-plane technique (► Fig. 1.36). The catheter can then be positioned under ultrasound guidance.

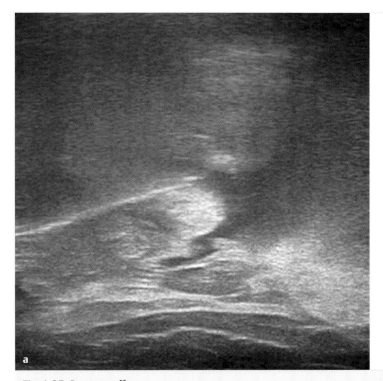

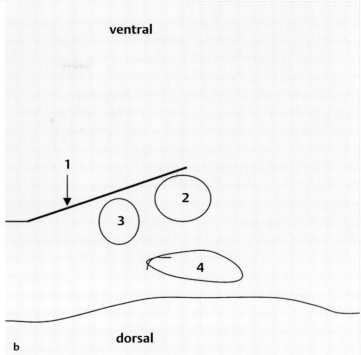

**Fig. 1.35** Bayonet effect.
**a** Bayonet effect in a distal lateral sciatic nerve block.
**b** Diagram.

1 Seemingly bent needle
2 Tibial nerve
3 Common peroneal (fibular) nerve
4 Muscle
Note: The bottom of the ultrasound image is near the transducer. The needle appears to be bent anteriorly in the perineural fat tissue.

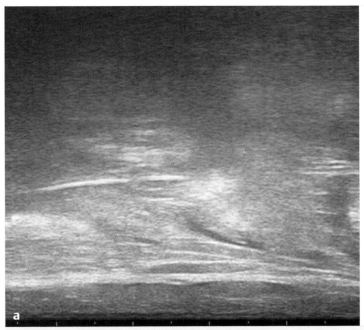

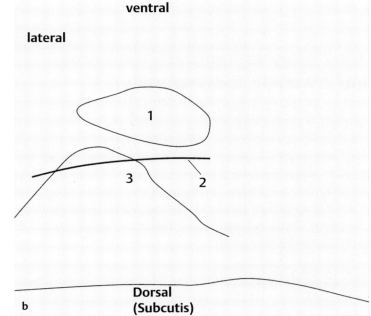

**Fig. 1.36** Visualization of a catheter.
**a** Visualization of a catheter in a lateral distal sciatic nerve block using an in-plane approach.
**b** Diagram.

1 Sciatic nerve
2 Catheter
3 Long head of the biceps femoris muscle

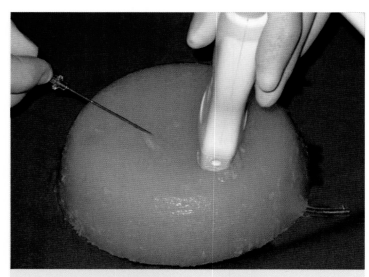

**Fig. 1.37** "Cornstarch cake" for learning ultrasound-guided needle placement.

---

**Tips and Tricks**

"Cornstarch cake" as a model for learning how to position a needle under ultrasound guidance:

1300 mL water

78 g cornstarch

65 g gelatin

Stir cornstarch and gelatin separately in cold water. Then mix first the cornstarch into hot water, then add the gelatin, bring to the boil and stir vigorously!

Pour into a mold—allow to cool—put a Redon tube through it (for the target structure)—finished!

---

## 1.3.2 How to Approach the Nerve? Intraneurally, Extraneurally?

The use of ultrasound has led to the necessity of rethinking some factors that were previously assumed to be true. For example, the assumption that an intraneural injection can be ruled out for nerve blocks performed using nerve stimulation for stimuli that do not go below a certain lower limit (e.g., 0.5 mA, 0.1 ms) is probably not sustainable. There are an increasing number of reports of accidental (Russon and Blanco 2007) or intentional (Bigeleisen 2006) intraneural injections that were detected or performed using ultrasound.

---

**Note**

The goal of every ultrasound-guided nerve block should be not to damage the perineurium, that is, to avoid an intrafascicular injection!

---

▶ **Local anesthetic.** The local anesthetic should be distributed in a circle around the nerve. The tip of the needle should not be pointed directly at the nerve, but be located laterally (out-of-plane technique, short axis) or above and/or below the nerve (in-plane technique, short axis). It is important to ensure that the spread of the local anesthetic around the nerve or in the correct compartment is not obstructed by fascia. If this occurs, the position of the needle must be corrected.

▶ **Nerve stimulator.** A combination with the nerve stimulator is possible, but the practitioner will soon abandon the practice of attempting to reach a certain stimulus level by correcting the needle position and rely mainly on the visualization in the ultrasound. The nerve stimulator can be useful if it is unclear whether the structure found is actually the target nerve.

## 1.3.3 Ultrasound in Any Event—What is the Available Evidence?

According to current knowledge, ultrasound-guided nerve blocks do not ensure greater patient safety in the sense of preventing complications (Neal et al 2010).

Current data suggest a moderate improvement in onset time and quality of ultrasound-guided nerve blocks compared with other techniques (evidence level 1 b, recommendation grade A, Liu et al 2010).

For the upper limb, some studies have found superiority with respect to the onset time and success rate (Liu et al 2010, McCartney et al 2010); for the lower limb, only a few studies found advantages for nerve blocks regarding onset time and a better sensory success rate. Corresponding studies for the lower limb are available only for the femoral nerve and distal sciatic nerve block (popliteal sciatic nerve block; Liu et al 2010, Salinas 2010).

Overall, currently available data do not allow ultrasound-guided nerve blocks to be declared the gold standard. The previously used techniques, in particular blocks performed with a nerve stimulator, are still important in peripheral regional anesthesia.

---

**Tips and Tricks**

With the proper needle position, ultrasound-guided nerve block makes it possible to work with much less local anesthetic. Atraumatic needles should also be used for ultrasound-guided nerve blocks.

---

# References

Aveline C, Le Roux A, Le Hetet H, Vautier P, Cognet F, Bonnet F. Postoperative efficacies of femoral nerve catheters sited using ultrasound combined with neurostimulation compared with neurostimulation alone for total knee arthroplasty. Eur J Anaesthesiol 2010; 27: 978–984

Bigeleisen PE. Nerve puncture and apparent intraneural injection during ultrasound-guided axillary block does not invariably result in neurologic injury. Anesthesiology 2006; 105: 779–783

Dhir S, Ganapathy S. Use of ultrasound guidance and contrast enhancement: a study of continuous infraclavicular brachial plexus approach. Acta Anaesthesiol Scand 2008; 52: 338–342

Heil JW, Ilfeld BM, Loland VJ, Mariano ER. Preliminary experience with a novel ultrasound-guided supraclavicular perineural catheter insertion technique for perioperative analgesia of the upper extremity. J Ultrasound Med 2010; 29: 1481–1485

Kessler J, Marhofer P, Rapp HJ, Hollmann MW. Ultrasound-guided anaesthesia of peripheral nerves. The new challenge for anaesthesiologists. [In English] Anaesthesist 2007; 56: 642–655

Liu SS, Ngeow J, John RS. Evidence basis for ultrasound-guided block characteristics: onset, quality, and duration. Reg Anesth Pain Med 2010; 35(2, Suppl): S26–S35

Marhofer P, Chan VWS. Ultrasound-guided regional anesthesia: current concepts and future trends. Anesth Analg 2007; 104: 1265–1269

Mariano ER, Loland VJ, Bellars RH et al. Ultrasound guidance versus electrical stimulation for infraclavicular brachial plexus perineural catheter insertion. J Ultrasound Med 2009; 28: 1211–1218

Mariano ER, Loland VJ, Sandhu NS et al. A trainee-based randomized comparison of stimulating interscalene perineural catheters with a new technique using ultrasound guidance alone. J Ultrasound Med 2010; 29: 329–336

McCartney CJL, Lin L, Shastri U. Evidence basis for the use of ultrasound for upper-extremity blocks. Reg Anesth Pain Med 2010; 35 Suppl: S10–S15

Moayeri N, Bigeleisen PE, Groen GJ. Quantitative architecture of the brachial plexus and surrounding compartments, and their possible significance for plexus blocks. Anesthesiology 2008; 108: 299–304

Moayeri N, van Geffen GJ, Bruhn J, Chan VW, Groen GJ. Correlation among ultrasound, cross-sectional anatomy, and histology of the sciatic nerve: a review. Reg Anesth Pain Med 2010; 35: 442–449

Neal J M, Brull R, Chan VWS et al. The ASRA evidence-based medicine assessment of ultrasound-guided regional anesthesia and pain medicine: Executive summary. Reg Anesth Pain Med 2010; 35 Suppl: S1–S9

Niazi AU, Prasad A, Ramlogan R, Chan VWS. Methods to ease placement of stimulating catheters during in-plane ultrasound-guided femoral nerve block. Reg Anesth Pain Med 2009; 34: 380–381

Russon K, Blanco R. Accidental intraneural injection into the musculocutaneous nerve visualized with ultrasound. Anesth Analg 2007; 105: 1504–1505

Salinas FV. Ultrasound and review of evidence for lower extremity peripheral nerve blocks. Reg Anesth Pain Med 2010; 35 Suppl: S16–S25

Schünke M, Schulte E, Schumacher U. Prometheus. LernAtlas der Anatomie. Allgemeine Anatomie und Bewegungssystem. Illustrationen von M. Voll und K. Wesker. 3rd ed. Stuttgart: Thieme; 2011: 75

Sites BD, Brull R, Chan VWS et al. Artifacts and pitfall errors associated with ultrasound-guided regional anesthesia. Part I: understanding the basic principles of ultrasound physics and machine operations. Reg Anesth Pain Med 2007a; 32: 412–418

Sites BD, Brull R, Chan VWS et al. Artifacts and pitfall errors associated with ultrasound-guided regional anesthesia. Part II: a pictorial approach to understanding and avoidance. Reg Anesth Pain Med 2007b; 32: 419–433

Sites BD, Spence BC, Gallagher JD, Wiley CW, Bertrand ML, Blike GT. Characterizing novice behavior associated with learning ultrasound-guided peripheral regional anesthesia. Reg Anesth Pain Med 2007c; 32: 107–115

Sites BD, Chan VW, Neal JM et al. American Society of Regional Anesthesia and Pain Medicine. European Society of Regional Anaesthesia and Pain Therapy Joint Committee. The American Society of Regional Anesthesia and Pain Medicine and the European Society Of Regional Anaesthesia and Pain Therapy Joint Committee recommendations for education and training in ultrasound-guided regional anesthesia. Reg Anesth Pain Med 2009; 34: 40–46

Tsui BCH, Kropelin B. The electrophysiological effect of dextrose 5% in water on single-shot peripheral nerve stimulation. Anesth Analg 2005; 100: 1837–1839

Wang AZ, Gu L, Zhou QH, Ni WZ, Jiang W. Ultrasound-guided continuous femoral nerve block for analgesia after total knee arthroplasty: catheter perpendicular to the nerve versus catheter parallel to the nerve. Reg Anesth Pain Med 2010; 35: 127–131

# Part 2

## Upper Limb

# 2 General Overview

## 2.1 Anatomy

The brachial plexus is formed by the anterior rami of the C5–C8 and T1 spinal nerves. The brachial plexus also contains contributions from C4 in over 60% of people and from T2 in over 30% (► Fig. 2.1).

► **Trunks.** The roots of the spinal nerves exit from the spinal canal behind the vertebral artery and cross the transverse process of the corresponding vertebra. They then join to form three trunks and run together toward the first rib.
- The upper trunk arises from the union of the roots of C5/6, where the suprascapular nerve arises immediately as a lateral branch from the upper trunk.
- The middle trunk is formed by the root of C7.
- The lower trunk is formed by the roots of C8/T1.

The trunks, which here lie on top of one another, pass through the interscalene groove (posterior interscalene groove) between the scalenus anterior and scalenus medius muscles; the subclavian artery is positioned in front of the lower trunk in the caudal area of the space and thus also passes through the space.

► **Cords.** Just above the clavicles, each of the trunks splits into an anterior and a posterior division. The three posterior divisions join to form the posterior cord, the anterior divisions of the upper and middle trunks form the lateral cord, and the medial cord is the continuation of the anterior division of the lower trunk.

In the interscalene region, we thus have the trunks and in the immediate supraclavicular and infraclavicular regions initially still the trunks, then their branches, and then the cords.

The cords lie very close together in the infraclavicular region:
- The lateral cord is the most superficial (lateral to and in front of the subclavian artery).

- The posterior cord is a little deeper and in the immediate infraclavicular region slightly lateral to the lateral fascicle!
- The medial cord lies deep (behind the subclavian artery).

The subclavian artery and brachial plexus pass into the axillary cavity medial to the coracoid process (► Fig. 2.2, ► Fig. 2.3, ► Fig. 2.4, ► Fig. 2.5).

Here, the cords rotate by about 90° around the axillary artery, with the medial cord passing under the artery. It is now positioned medial to the artery and then gives off a medial root that unites with the lateral root of the lateral cord to form the median nerve. The median nerve is usually located lateral to the axillary artery. When the chords enter the axillary region, they are actually located medially, laterally, and posteriorly in accordance with their names.

► **Nerves.** The ulnar nerve, the medial cutaneous nerve of the arm and the medial nerve of the forearm, and the medial root of the median nerve arise from the medial cord. After the musculocutaneous nerve has arisen from the lateral cord, it combines with parts of the medial cord to form the median nerve (► Fig. 2.6, ► Fig. 2.7, ► Fig. 2.8). The posterior cord divides into the axillary nerve and radial nerve (see ► Fig. 2.1 and ► Fig. 2.5).

► **Prevertebral fascia.** From its passage through the (posterior) interscalene groove as far as the axillary region, the entire brachial plexus is surrounded by a firm sheath of connective tissue (► Fig. 2.9). This sheath, which encloses the anterior neck muscles, is called the prevertebral fascia. It continues in lateral and caudal direction and covers the trunks like a cloth. The space below it continues in caudal direction to the infraclavicular region, but in medial and cranial direction to the intervertebral foramen and in the broader sense to the epidural space.

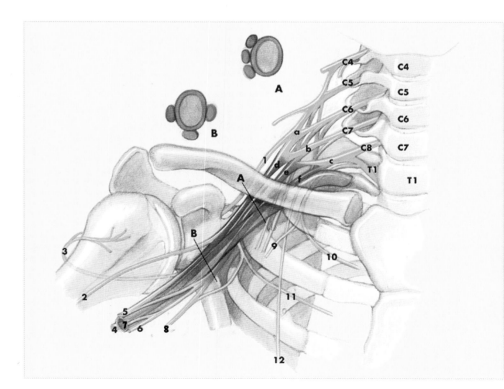

**Fig. 2.1** Anatomy of the brachial plexus.
a Upper trunk (anterior rami of C5 and C6).
b Middle trunk (anterior ramus of C7).
c Lower trunk (anterior rami of C8 and T1).
d Lateral cord.
e Posterior cord.
f Medial cord.
1 Suprascapular nerve
2 Musculocutaneous nerve
3 Axillary nerve
4 Radial nerve
5 Median nerve
6 Ulnar nerve
7 Medial cutaneous nerve of forearm
8 Medial cutaneous nerve of arm
9 Intercostobrachial nerve I
10 Intercostal nerve I
11 Intercostal nerve II
12 Long thoracic nerve
A and B: Sections in the infraclavicular and axillary region (note position of cords)

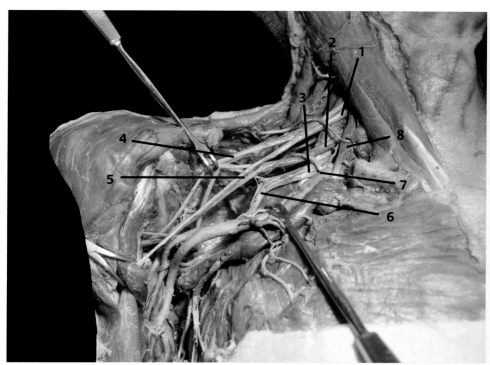

**Fig. 2.2** Anatomy of the brachial plexus.
1 Upper trunk
2 Middle trunk
3 Lower trunk
4 Posterior cord
5 Lateral cord
6 Medial cord
7 Subclavian artery
8 Scalenus anterior

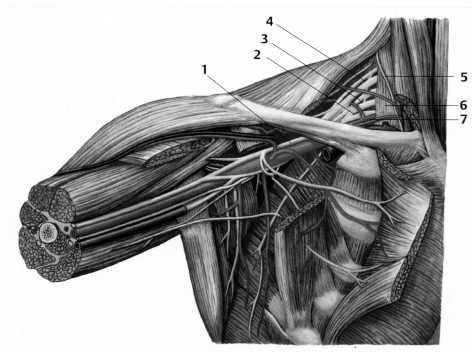

**Fig. 2.3** Anatomy of the brachial plexus.
1 Lateral cord
2 Lower trunk
3 Middle trunk
4 Upper trunk
5 Phrenic nerve
6 Scalenus anterior
7 Subclavian artery

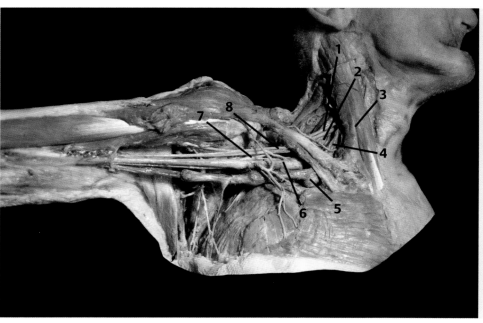

**Fig. 2.4** Anatomy of the brachial plexus.
1 Upper trunk
2 Middle trunk
3 Sternocleidomastoid
4 Scalenus anterior
5 Subclavian vein
6 Subclavian artery
7 Posterior cord
8 Lateral cord

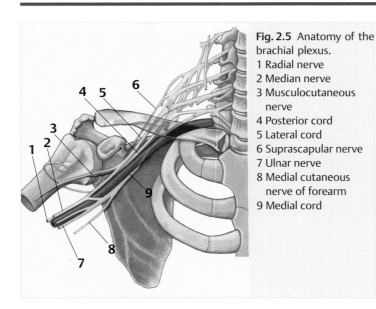

**Fig. 2.5** Anatomy of the brachial plexus.
1 Radial nerve
2 Median nerve
3 Musculocutaneous nerve
4 Posterior cord
5 Lateral cord
6 Suprascapular nerve
7 Ulnar nerve
8 Medial cutaneous nerve of forearm
9 Medial cord

As well as the nerves, this sheath also contains the blood vessels (axillary artery and vein). The subclavian artery passes with the brachial plexus through the (posterior) interscalene groove, while the subclavian vein does not join them until after they pass through the anterior interscalene groove (between the sterno-cleidomastoid located in front and the scalenus anterior positioned adjacent and to the rear). Variations in the branches of the subclavian artery in the supraclavicular fossa may increase the incidence of vascular puncture or intravascular injection of local anesthetic while performing the block (Kohli et al 2014).

**Note**

There are connective-tissue septa inside this neurovascular sheath. However, in the majority of people, these do not appear to impede the steady spread of local anesthetic, so that a complete block of the brachial plexus is possible with a single injection, particularly in the supraclavicular, infraclavicular, and also axillary regions.

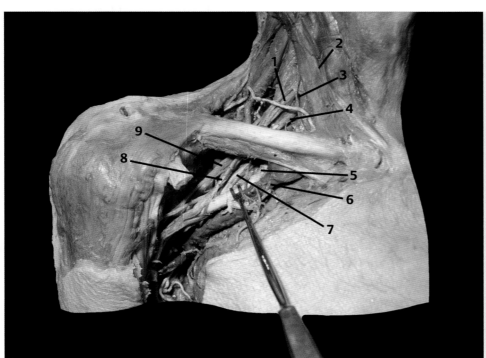

**Fig. 2.6** Anatomy of the infraclavicular region.
1 Upper trunk
2 Sternocleidomastoid
3 Phrenic nerve
4 Middle trunk
5 Subclavian artery
6 Subclavian vein
7 Medial cord
8 Lateral cord
9 Posterior cord

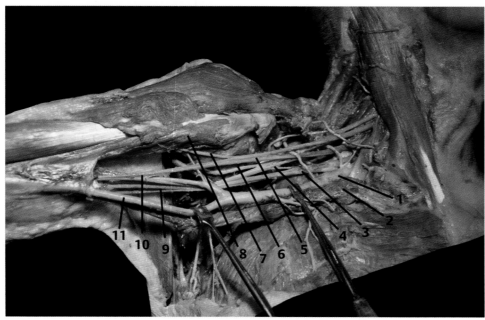

**Fig. 2.7** Brachial plexus in the axillary region: anatomical overview. Note: two roots of the median nerve behind the brachial artery.
1 Subclavian artery
2 Subclavian vein
3 Medial cord
4 Posterior cord
5 Lateral cord
6 Axillary nerve
7 Musculocutaneous nerve
8 Coracobrachialis
9 Ulnar nerve
10 Median nerve with its two roots
11 Brachial artery

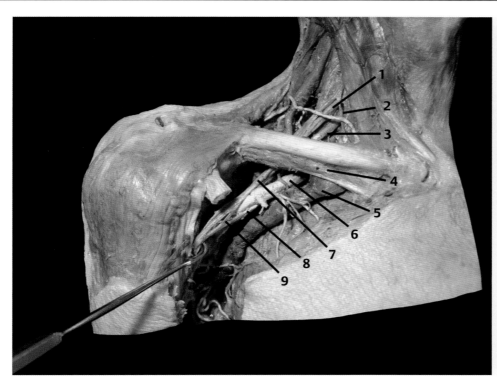

**Fig. 2.8** Brachial plexus in the axillary region: anatomical overview.
1 Upper trunk
2 Phrenic nerve
3 Middle trunk
4 Subclavius
5 Subclavian vein
6 Subclavian artery
7 Lateral cord
8 Medial cord
9 Median nerve with its two roots

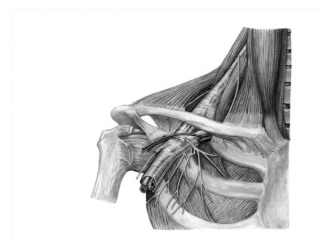

**Fig. 2.9** Neurovascular connective-tissue sheath of the brachial plexus.

## 2.2 Important Topographical Anatomical Relations in the Region of the Brachial Plexus

▶ **Phrenic nerve.** The phrenic nerve runs on the belly of scalenus anterior enclosed in the prevertebral fascia described above (see ▶ Fig. 2.2, ▶ Fig. 2.3, and ▶ Fig. 2.10). If a response to stimulation of the phrenic nerve is produced during interscalene block (contraction of the diaphragm), the position of the needle tip must be corrected laterally and posteriorly. Phrenic nerve paresis can be produced by the local anesthetic effect.

▶ **Recurrent laryngeal nerve.** Recurrent laryngeal nerve block with hoarseness occurs occasionally (▶ Fig. 2.10), which is a sign of the block spreading medial to the scalenus anterior.

▶ **Cervical and thoracocervical sympathetic ganglia.** These ganglia are in the immediate vicinity of the brachial plexus

(▶ Fig. 2.10 and ▶ Fig. 2.11), but always medial to the interscalene groove and in the same region as the recurrent laryngeal nerve. *Horner syndrome* (miosis, ptosis, enophthalmos) can be triggered by the local anesthetic effect. It is argued that *bronchospasm* can be triggered in asthmatic patients by the sympatholytic effect, but this is not undisputed.

▶ **Dome of the pleura.** The dome of the pleura extends clearly above the body of the first rib, but never above the neck of the first rib and is in the immediate vicinity of the structures described here (▶ Fig. 2.11). The risk of pneumothorax must therefore be borne in mind with the corresponding techniques in the supraclavicular and infraclavicular space.

▶ **Vertebral artery.** The vertebral artery lies anterior to the exit of the spinal nerves through the intervertebral foramina (▶ Fig. 2.11). After arising from the subclavian artery medial to the scalenus anterior, it runs in cranial direction and disappears in the transverse foramen of the transverse process of the sixth cervical vertebra and continues with the transverse part ($V_2$ segment) in cranial direction.

> **Caution**
>
> If the needle is inserted in the wrong direction during interscalene block using the Winnie approach or in deep cervical plexus block, intravascular injection of the local anesthetic can occur. Only a few milliliters are sufficient to cause a seizure as the local anesthetic reaches the brain directly through the artery.

▶ **Cervical epidural and subarachnoid space.** The vertebral artery can be accidentally reached or punctured through the intervertebral foramina. Cervical epidural or high spinal anesthesia can occur. Permanent cervical spinal cord injuries with tetraplegia have also been described after interscalene plexus block, but only when this technique was used under general anesthesia.

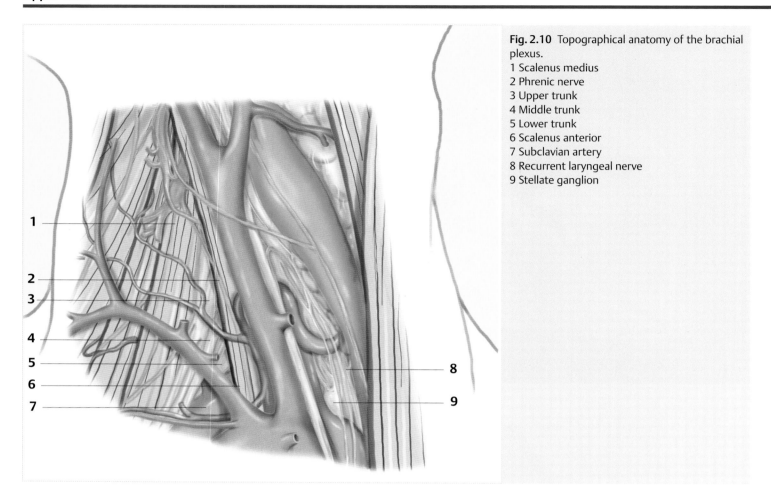

**Fig. 2.10** Topographical anatomy of the brachial plexus.
1 Scalenus medius
2 Phrenic nerve
3 Upper trunk
4 Middle trunk
5 Lower trunk
6 Scalenus anterior
7 Subclavian artery
8 Recurrent laryngeal nerve
9 Stellate ganglion

## 2.3 Motor and Sensory Supply of the Upper Limb ▶

▶ Fig. 2.12 shows the different areas of sensory innervation of the skin.

The motor responses (▶ Fig. 2.13) of the individual nerves are as follows:

- Suprascapular nerve: abduction and external rotation of the shoulder (supraspinatus and infraspinatus muscles)
- Musculocutaneous nerve: elbow flexion (biceps brachii muscle)
- Median nerve: palmar flexion at the wrist, pronation of the forearm, flexion of the middle phalanges of the fingers, flexion of the distal phalanges of D II and D III, flexion of the thumb
- Ulnar nerve: ulnar duction and flexion of the wrist, flexion of the proximal phalanges of D III–V, adduction of the thumb
- Radial nerve: extension of the elbow (triceps muscle), extension (and radial abduction) of the wrist, supination of the forearm and hand, extension of the fingers

## 2.4 Historical Overview—Upper Limb

▶ **Intraneural techniques.** After the introduction of cocaine in 1884, Halsted injected the diluted local anesthetic directly intraneurally in the same year, after surgical exposure of the nerve roots of the brachial plexus. Although only 0.5 mL of the diluted local anesthetic was needed for each nerve root, complete anesthesia of the upper limb was achieved. The obvious disadvantage of the method was that the exposure of the nerve roots involved a greater surgical procedure than the planned operation itself. In a similar manner, Crile (1897) surgically exposed the brachial plexus behind the sternocleidomastoid to apply the local anesthetic intraneurally under visual control.

▶ **Transcutaneous techniques.** Transcutaneous techniques for brachial plexus block were first described in 1911. Hirschel reported on the axillary approach (Hirschel 1911) and Kulenkampff on the supraclavicular approach for brachial plexus block (Kulenkampff 1928).

Although the axillary approach was associated with fewer complications than the supraclavicular technique and numerous variations have been described, the axillary technique was not made popular until 1958 by Burnham (1959). Burnham was the first to point out the firm connective-tissue sheath around vessels and nerves, to identify the correct needle position for performing an axillary plexus block. He spoke of a characteristic "click" when the needle penetrated the fascia. This meant it was no longer necessary to find and identify the nerves with the help of paresthesia. Burnham reported over 42 cases of complete anesthesia of the arm using this technique, in which 8 mL was injected above and 8 mL below the artery.

De Jong (1961), however, found based on anatomical studies that a volume of at least 40 to 50 mL was needed to achieve a sufficient block of all large nerves in the axillary region supplying the arm. De Jong also injected above and below the axillary artery and recommended inducing paresthesia to ensure the correct position of the needle.

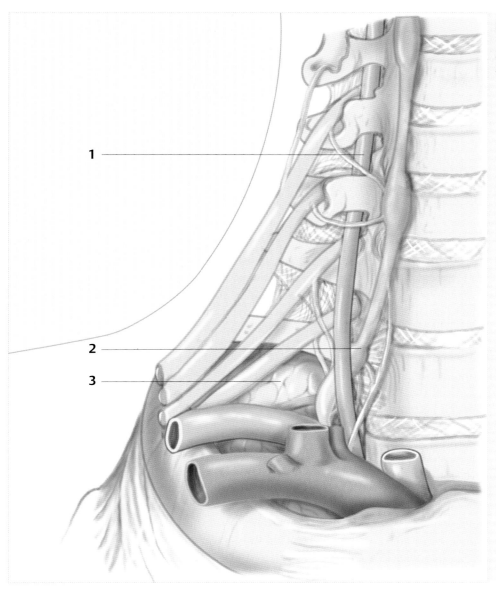

**Fig. 2.11** Anatomy of the interscalene region.
1 Vertebral artery
2 Stellate ganglion
3 Dome of the pleura

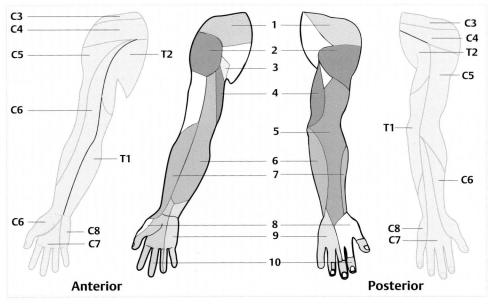

**Fig. 2.12** Sensory supply of the upper limb.
1 Supraclavicular nerve
2 Axillary nerve (lateral cutaneous nerve of the arm)
3 Intercostobrachial nerve
4 Medial cutaneous nerve of arm
5 Dorsal cutaneous nerve of forearm (radial nerve)
6 Medial cutaneous nerve of forearm
7 Lateral cutaneous nerve of forearm (musculocutaneous nerve)
8 Radial nerve
9 Ulnar nerve
10 Median nerve

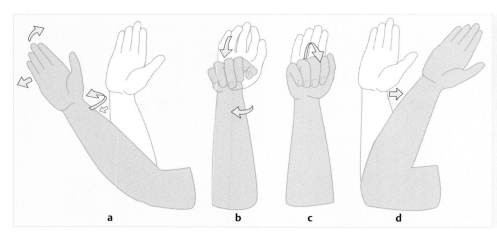

**Fig. 2.13** Motor stimulus response of the individual nerves of the upper limb.
**a** Radial nerve
**b** Median nerve
**c** Ulnar nerve
**d** Musculocutaneous nerve

> **Note**
>
> The simplicity of this type of axillary plexus block meant that there were no more obstacles to its wide dissemination.

▶ **Single-injection technique.** Eriksson (1979) and Winnie (Winnie and Collins 1964) were the first to recommend a single injection into the neurovascular sheath on the basis of the anatomical insight that a common neurovascular sheath is present.

Despite the apparent success of a single injection, the discussion of a single neurovascular sheath that allows the local anesthetic to spread unhindered persists up to the present. This is due primarily to the failure rate of approximately 5 to 20% that we find in nearly all techniques for axillary plexus anesthesia.

Thompson and Rorie (1983) concluded based on anatomical studies that there is septation within the axillary neurovascular sheath that prevents the even spread of the local anesthetic, thus making the single-injection technique illogical and worthless.

However, this is in complete contradiction to the success rates of 80 to 95% for the single-injection technique.

Partridge et al (1987) challenged the studies made by Thomson and Rorie and concluded on the basis of their own studies that septa do exist within the neurovascular sheath, but they are functionally incomplete and do not generally have an effect on the even spread of the local anesthetic.

> **Note**
>
> The single-injection technique has the advantage of being fast and easy to apply without the need to induce paresthesia, but its particular benefit is that the single-injection technique forms the basis for continuous regional block.

▶ **Continuous regional block.** As early as 1946, Ansbro described a technique in which the needle was stabilized in the supraclavicular region with a cork so that repeated injections could be made (Ansbro 1946). However, this method was not proven to work as part of the regular routine.

▶ **Multi-injection technique.** This method has again gained interest in recent years due to the use of the nerve stimulator

and ultrasound. In 1994, Dupré described the "bloc du plexus brachial au canal huméral" (Dupré 1994), which in English literature is incorrectly called the "midhumeral approach." In fact, it is a technique that is conducted at the junction of the proximal and middle thirds of the upper arm.

> **Note**
>
> Many variations of the multi-injection technique have been described. One advantage of the techniques is based on the short onset time, but a continuous block is not possible.

▶ **Percutaneous supraclavicular technique.** In addition to the axillary block, there is hardly a site along the brachial plexus where a needle approach has not been described. The percutaneous supraclavicular technique for brachial plexus block as described in 1911 by Kulenkampff is a single-injection technique. Kulenkampff discovered that the nerves here also lie close to each other, enclosed in a connective-tissue sheath. The technique remains to the present day, but a major disadvantage is the not-to-be-underestimated risk of pneumothorax because the medial, dorsal, and caudal puncture direction is directly above the clavicle toward the first rib.

▶ **Supraclavicular perivascular block.** Alternatively, Winnie and Collins (1964) described the supraclavicular perivascular block, which can also be used for a continuous block. Brown et al (1993) showed the supraclavicular technique (called "plumb-bob technique") perpendicular to the bed as an alternative. Using this technique, Ashley et al (1995) also succeeded in conducting a continuous block by inserting a flexible catheter.

> **Note**
>
> Due to the increased use of ultrasound in regional anesthesia, the supraclavicular techniques for brachial plexus block have regained significance in recent years. The use of ultrasound requires modifications of the originally described techniques, but continuous methods are also possible.

▶ **Infraclavicular plexus anesthesia.** Infraclavicular plexus anesthesia was first described by Bazy in 1917 (Bazy 1917). In 1973, the infraclavicular method was again described by Raj (Raj et al 1973), and modified in 1977 by Sims (Sims 1977) and in 1981 by Whiffler (Whiffler 1981). The disadvantage of all variations was that the anatomical landmarks were defined only very imprecisely. However, there was a notable tendency to prefer single injections to multiple injections, to use thinner, less traumatic needles, and to use a nerve stimulator.

In 1995, Kilka, Geiger, and Merkens from Ulm described an infraclavicular plexus anesthesia as a "vertical infraclavicular plexus block" (VIB), featuring simple anatomical landmarks.

Originally introduced as a single-injection technique, this technique can also be used as a continuous method. However, application under ultrasound requires modifications of the technique. The Raj technique modified by Borgeat or the approach described by Klaastad et al (1999) allows an infraclavicular brachial plexus block to be performed under ultrasound guidance.

▶ **Interscalene plexus block.** The interscalene plexus block described in 1970 by Winnie (Winnie 1970) is especially suited for procedures in the shoulders. Winnie was thus the first to describe an interscalene single-injection approach.

The problem with this approach is that the needle is directed toward risk structures (vertebral artery, spinal canal, lungs, pleura). In this technique, the interscalene groove is punctured at the level of the cricoid cartilage so that the needle is advanced perpendicular to the skin toward the transverse process of C6.

| Note |
| --- |
| Winnie already conceded that the perpendicular position of the needle to the nerve plexus makes it difficult to advance an indwelling catheter for continuous anesthesia. |

Hempel et al (1981) describe a technique in which an indwelling catheter is advanced from the supraclavicular region along the interscalene groove toward the nerve roots—in a "retrograde" direction. A continuous interscalene block was also possible using this method. The potential risk of puncturing the vertebral artery also remained here as a disadvantage of this technique.

▶ **Anterior interscalene technique.** The anterior interscalene technique described by Meier et al (1997) is considerably safer because of the lateral injection direction and also makes it possible to insert an indwelling catheter for a continuous block.

▶ **Posterior interscalene technique.** In addition to the anterior approach to the interscalene brachial plexus, a posterior approach was described as early as the start of the 20th century. Pippa et al (1990) revived this technique. The posterior approach can also be used as a continuous method.

▶ **Individual peripheral nerve blocks.** Individual peripheral nerve blocks of the arm and hand can be conducted for completing incomplete brachial plexus blocks near the trunk using technical aids (nerve stimulator, ultrasound; Büttner and Meier 2011). While a block of an already partially anesthetized arm is associated with the potential risk of nerve damage without the use of these aids, the nerve stimulator or ultrasound indicate the correct position of the needle, at least for the larger nerves carrying motor fibers, even in a partially anesthetized arm. The selective placement of peripheral catheters for specific postoperative pain therapy of individual nerves is another development based on this technique.

▶ **Suprascapular nerve block.** The blockade of the suprascapular nerve was used by Bonica back in 1958 for the treatment of shoulder pain (Bonica 1958). Meier et al have described a continuous technique for this as well (Meier et al 2002) that, depending on the indication, can be considered to be an alternative to the interscalene plexus block.

# References

Ansbro FP. A method of continuous brachial plexus block. Am J Surg 1946; 71: 716–722

Ashley S, Wood L, Antoine LJM, Wooten D. A comparison of single shot versus continuous supraclavicular nerve block using the "plumb bob" approach. Reg Anesth Pain Med 1995; 20: 133(abstract)

Bazy. L. L'anesthesie du plexus brachial. In: Pauchet V, Sourdat P, Labouré J, eds. L'Anesthesie Regionale. Paris: Doin; 1917: 222–225

Bonica JJ. Diagnostic and therapeutic blocks, a reappraisal based on 15 years' experience. Anesth Analg 1958; 37: 58–68

Brown DL, Cahill DR, Bridenbaugh LD. Supraclavicular nerve block: anatomic analysis of a method to prevent pneumothorax. Anesth Analg 1993; 76: 530–534

Büttner J, Meier G. Memorix AINS—Periphere Regionalanästhesie. Stuttgart: Thieme; 2011

Burnham PJ. Simple regional nerve block for surgery of the hand and forearm. J Am Med Assoc 1959; 169: 941–943

Crile GW. Anesthesia of nerve roots with cocaine. Cleve Med J 1897; 2: 355

De Jong RH. Axillary block of the brachial plexus. Anesthesiology 1961; 22: 215–225

Dupré LJ. Brachial plexus block through humeral approach. [Article in French] Cah Anesthesiol 1994; 42: 767–769

Eriksson E. Illustrated Handbook in Local Anaesthesia. 2nd ed. Copenhagen: Schultz; 1979: 82–83

Hempel V, van Finck M, Baumgärtner E. A longitudinal supraclavicular approach to the brachial plexus for the insertion of plastic cannulas. Anesth Analg 1981; 60: 352–355

Hirschel G (1911) Die Anästhesierung des Plexus brachialis bei Operationen an der Oberen Extremität. Münch Med Wochenschr 29:1555–1556

Klaastad O, Lilleås FG, Røtnes JS, Breivik H, Fosse E. Magnetic resonance imaging demonstrates lack of precision in needle placement by the infraclavicular brachial plexus block described by Raj et al. Anesth Analg 1999; 88: 593–598

Kohli S, Yadav N, Prasad A, Banerjee SS. Anatomic variation of subclavian artery visualized on ultrasound-guided supraclavicular brachial plexus block. Case Rep Med 2014; 2014: 394920

Kulenkampff D. Brachial plexus anaesthesia. Its indications, technique, and dangers. Ann Surg 1928; 87: 883–891

Meier G, Bauereis C, Maurer H et al. Interscalene brachial plexus catheter for anesthesia and postoperative pain therapy. Experience with a modified technique. [Article in German] Anaesthesist 1997; 46: 715–719

Meier G, Bauereis C, Maurer H. The modified technique of continuous suprascapular nerve block. A safe technique in the treatment of shoulder pain. [Article in German] Anaesthesist 2002; 51: 747–753

Partridge BL, Katz J, Benirschke K. Functional anatomy of the brachial plexus sheath: implications for anesthesia. Anesthesiology 1987; 66: 743–747

Pippa P, Cominelli E, Marinelle C, Aito S. Brachial plexus block using the posterior approach. Eur J Anaesthesiol 1990; 7: 411–420

Raj P, Montgomery SJ, Nettles D, Jenkins MT. Infraclavicular brachial plexus block—a new approach. Anesth Analg 1973; 52: 897–904

Selander D. Catheter technique in axillary plexus block. Presentation of a new method. Acta Anaesthesiol Scand 1977; 21: 324–329

Sims JK. A modification of landmarks for infraclavicular approach to brachial plexus block. Anesth Analg 1977; 56: 554–555

Thompson GE, Rorie DK. Functional anatomy of the brachial plexus sheaths. Anesthesiology 1983; 59: 117–122

Whiffler K. Coracoid block—a safe and easy technique. Br J Anaesth 1981; 53: 845–848

Winnie AP, Collins VJ. The subclavian perivascular technique of brachial plexus anesthesia. Anesthesiology 1964; 25: 353–363

Winnie AP. Interscalene brachial plexus block. Anesth Analg 1970; 49: 455–466

# 3 Interscalene Techniques of Brachial Plexus Block

## 3.1 Anatomy

The brachial plexus is formed by the anterior rami of spinal nerves C5–C8 and T1, and it sometimes receives contributions from C4 and T2. The roots of the spinal nerves exit from the spinal canal behind the vertebral artery and cross the transverse process of the corresponding vertebral body. They then combine to form three trunks and run together toward the most lateral convexity of the body of the first rib (▶ Fig. 3.1).

- The upper trunk is formed by the junction of the roots of C5/6, and the suprascapular nerve arises immediately as a lateral branch from the upper trunk.

- The middle trunk is formed by root C7.
- The lower trunk is formed by roots C8/T1.

The trunks, which here lie on top of one another, cross the (posterior) interscalene groove between the scalenus anterior and scalenus medius muscles. Just above the clavicle, the trunks each split into an anterior and a posterior division (▶ Fig. 3.2).

- The three posterior divisions unite to form the posterior cord.
- The anterior divisions of the upper trunk and middle trunk form the lateral cord.
- The medial cord is the continuation of the anterior division of the lower trunk.

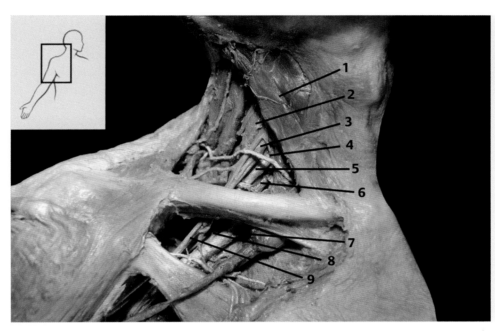

**Fig. 3.1** Anatomy of the brachial plexus.
1 Sternocleidomastoid
2 Scalenus medius
3 Upper trunk
4 Phrenic nerve
5 Middle trunk
6 Lower trunk
7 Subclavian artery
8 Posterior cord
9 Lateral cord

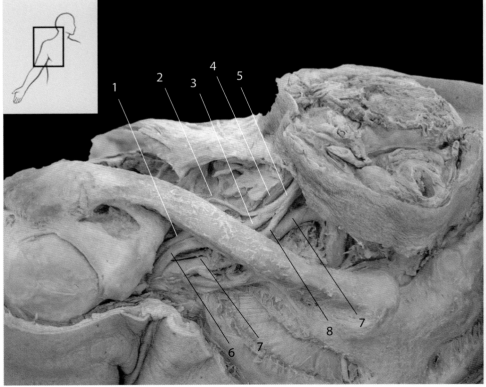

**Fig. 3.2** Anatomy of the brachial plexus.
1 Posterior cord
2 Suprascapular nerve
3 Upper trunk, posterior division
4 Scalenus medius
5 Upper trunk
6 Lateral cord
7 Subclavian artery
8 Upper trunk, anterior division

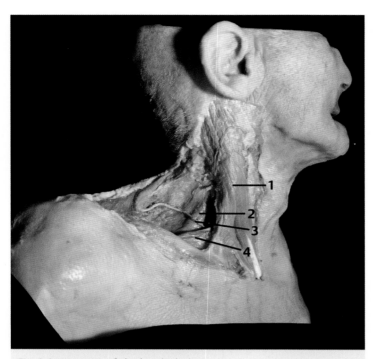

**Fig. 3.3** Anatomy of the brachial plexus (neurovascular sheath).
1 Sternocleidomastoid
2 Neurovascular bundle under the prevertebral fascia
3 Transverse cervical artery
4 Omohyoid muscle with middle cervical fascia

In the interscalene region, we thus first have the trunks, dividing in the immediate supraclavicular and infraclavicular region, and then the cords.

The lower trunk lies deepest and can be reached by an interscalene block only with difficulty (see ► Fig. 3.1). At the caudal end of the (posterior) interscalene groove just behind and above the clavicle, the subclavian artery, generally located directly in front of the lower trunk, passes with the brachial plexus through the interscalene groove, while the subclavian vein joins them only after they pass through the anterior interscalene groove. Anteriorly, the posterior interscalene groove is crossed by the omohyoid muscle, which can usually be easily palpated.

The phrenic nerve (C3–C5) runs on the belly of the anterior scalene muscle, enclosed in the prevertebral fascia covering the muscle. The cervical and thoracocervical sympathetic ganglia and the recurrent laryngeal nerve are in the immediate vicinity of the brachial plexus, but always medial to the interscalene grooves. The vertebral artery lies anterior to the exit of the cervical spinal nerves through the intervertebral foramina. The cervical epidural and subarachnoid space can be reached or punctured accidentally through the intervertebral foramina. Cervical epidural or high spinal anesthesia can occur (► Fig. 3.8).

From where it passes through the interscalene groove as far as the axillary region, the entire brachial plexus is surrounded by a firm connective-tissue sheath (► Fig. 3.3 and ► Fig. 3.4). There is connective-tissue septation within this neurovascular sheath. However, in the majority of people, it does not appear to impede an even spread of local anesthetic.

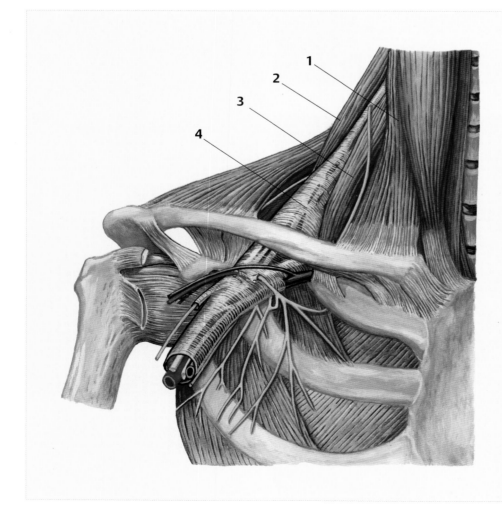

**Fig. 3.4** Anatomy of the brachial plexus (neurovascular sheath).
1 Sternocleidomastoid
2 Scalenus medius
3 Scalenus anterior with phrenic nerve
4 Neurovascular sheath (brachial plexus)

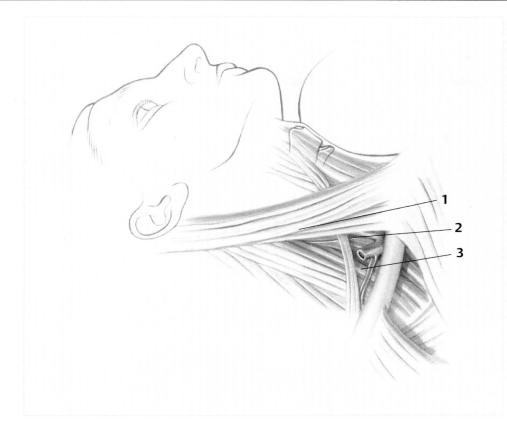

**Fig. 3.5** Anatomy for orientation in interscalene plexus anesthesia.
1 Sternocleidomastoid
2 Scalenus anterior (with phrenic nerve)
3 Interscalene groove (with upper trunk and middle trunk)

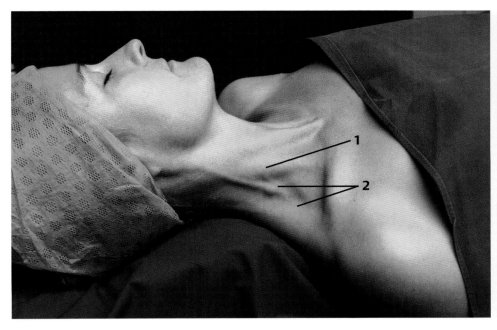

**Fig. 3.6** Orientation in interscalene plexus anesthesia: Lifting the head that is turned to the opposite side makes the sternocleidomastoid muscle stand out clearly, and in slim patients the scalene groove can be visualized on deep inspiration.
1 Sternocleidomastoid
2 Interscalene groove

The posterior border of the sternocleidomastoid muscle is used for orientation. It becomes prominent when the head is elevated ("sniffing position," ▸ Fig. 3.5 and ▸ Fig. 3.6). In very thin patients, the posterior interscalene groove can be palpated easily and it sometimes even becomes visible on deep inspiration.

## 3.2 Meier Approach ▸

The classical technique by Winnie was oriented directly toward the transverse process of C6 (▸ Fig. 3.7) with the risk of puncture near the spinal cord or of the vertebral artery (▸ Fig. 3.8, see also historical overview, p33).

The modification (Meier et al 1997: anterior–lateral) of the "classical" technique (▸ Fig. 3.9) makes it possible to insert an indwelling catheter for a continuous block because of the medial to lateral direction of the needle and the lateral direction of the needle makes it safer (Hofmann-Kiefer et al 2009).

### 3.2.1 Positioning

The patient's head is turned to the opposite side and the needle direction corresponds to the course of the interscalene groove (lateral, caudal, dorsal). The target is the distal end of the interscalene groove lateral to the subclavian artery (▸ Fig. 3.10 and ▸ Fig. 3.11). (Note: an oxygen mask prevents the sterile drape from lying on the patient's mouth and nose!)

The needle normally first reaches the brachial plexus (▸ Fig. 3.12).

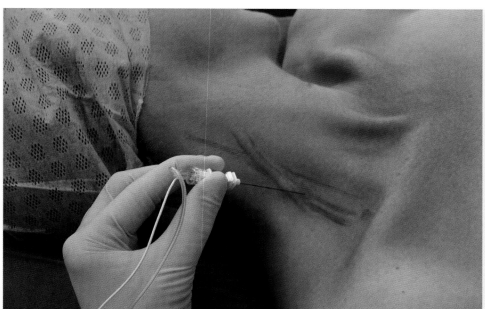

**Fig. 3.7** Interscalene block, Winnie approach.

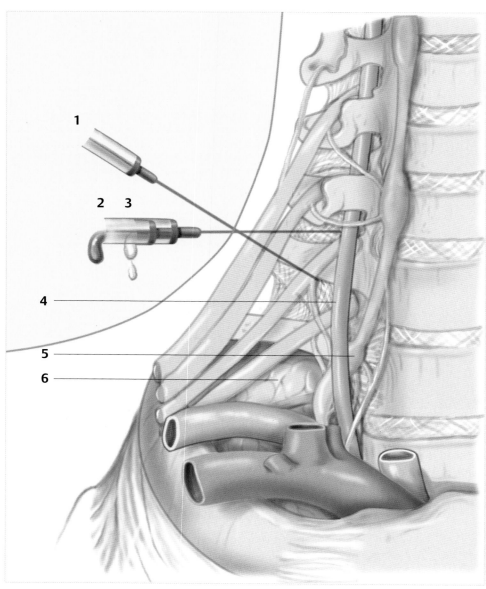

**Fig. 3.8** Interscalene block, Winnie approach. Note 1) A needle insertion direction perpendicular to the brachial plexus makes it difficult to advance the indwelling catheter. 2) The vertebral artery can be punctured. 3) The epidural or spinal space can be punctured!
1 Direction of the needle (Winnie approach)
2 Accidental puncture of the vertebral artery
3 Accidental subarachnoid (spinal) puncture
4 Vertebral artery
5 Stellate ganglion
6 Dome of the pleura

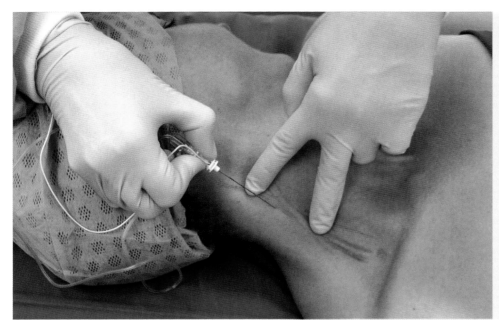

**Fig. 3.9** Interscalene block, Meier approach.

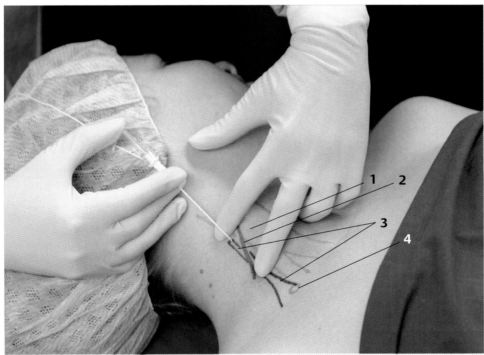

**Fig. 3.10** Interscalene plexus anesthesia. Position, site of injection, direction of needle.
1 Sternocleidomastoid
2 External jugular vein
3 Interscalene groove
4 Subclavian artery (medial border of the interscalene groove)

Note the phrenic nerve, which runs on the scalenus anterior muscle medial to the brachial plexus (▶ Fig. 3.13). If this is stimulated (response: hiccup), the needle must be corrected in the lateral and dorsal direction. The suprascapular nerve is variable and can leave the upper trunk very far proximally (▶ Fig. 3.13). If there is a motor response (abduction and external rotation in the shoulder region), the needle must be corrected in the medial and anterior direction.

The patient lies supine with the head turned slightly to the opposite side. The *posterior border of the sternocleidomastoid muscle* serves for orientation. It becomes prominent when the patient elevates the head slightly ("sniffing" position). The scalenus anterior muscle can be palpated behind the sternocleidomastoid and the fingers slide laterally over the scalenus anterior muscle into the posterior interscalene groove, which is formed by the scalenus anterior and medius muscles.

The *posterior interscalene groove* can usually be palpated easily; it runs posterolaterally from the sternocleidomastoid muscle in a slightly lateral direction. The subclavian artery is palpable directly above the clavicle and marks the caudal end of the interscalene groove. The artery can also be imaged using a vascular Doppler probe. The posterior interscalene groove feels like the gap between two fingers lying lightly next to one another. On deep inspiration, it sometimes becomes more visible.

In the caudal region, the posterior interscalene groove is crossed by the omohyoid muscle, which is usually easy to palpate. If the interscalene groove cannot be palpated, a horizontal line 3 cm long can be drawn at the level of the annular cartilage (C6) from the middle of the sternocleidomastoid muscle laterally (▶ Fig. 3.14 and ▶ Fig. 3.15). The end of this line marks the interscalene groove (Meier et al 2001).

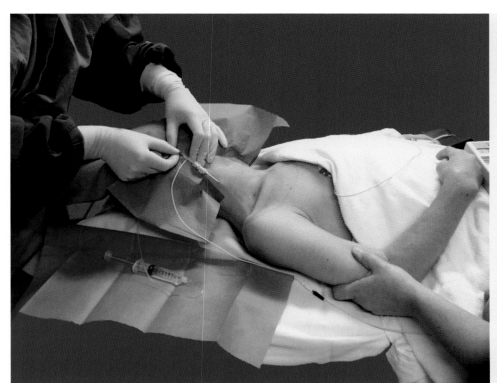

**Fig. 3.11** Position, site of injection, and direction of needle in interscalene plexus anesthesia (traction on the upper arm facilitates anatomical orientation).

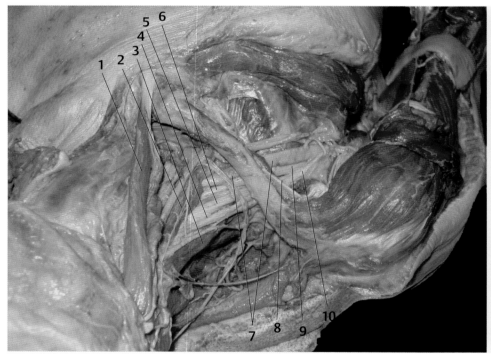

**Fig. 3.12** Anatomy of the interscalene region as seen by the person performing the block.
1 Sternocleidomastoid (clavicular head removed)
2 Scalenus anterior
3 Scalenus medius
4 Upper trunk
5 Middle trunk
6 Lower trunk
7 Subclavian artery
8 Posterior cord
9 Medial cord
10 Lateral cord

The intersection of a horizontal line about 2 cm above the annular cartilage marks the needle insertion site, and this is therefore further cranial than the classical insertion site with the Winnie technique (Winnie 1970).

## 3.2.2 Needle Approach

The interscalene groove is palpated: the upper finger of the palpating hand slides cranially in the posterior interscalene groove until it disappears under the sternocleidomastoid (▶ Fig. 3.10). The posterior border of the sternocleidomastoid is pushed slightly cranially, while the lower finger lies further caudally in the interscalene groove.

The insertion site is as far cranial as possible, usually directly beneath the cranially palpating finger. The needle approach is performed along the plexus in the direction of the interscalene groove, that is, in the direction of the medial border of the "Mohrenheim fossa" (▶ Fig. 3.15). Depending on the angle of needle insertion (approx. 30° to the skin) the brachial plexus is reached after about 2.5 cm to a maximum of 5 cm. A pronounced click is often felt on penetration of the prevertebral fascia (▶ Fig. 3.16, ▶ Fig. 3.17, ▶ Fig. 3.18, ▶ Fig. 3.19).

The use of a nerve stimulator and/or ultrasound (Chapter 3.2.3) is mandatory while performing this technique.

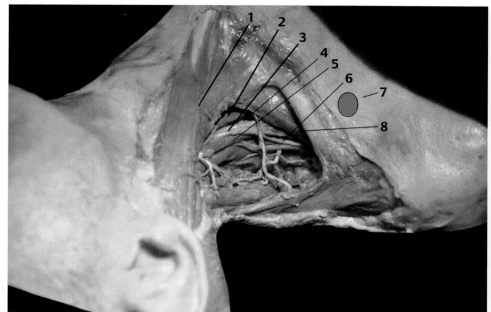

**Fig. 3.13** Anatomy of the interscalene region as seen by the person performing the block.
1 Sternocleidomastoid
2 Scalenus anterior with phrenic nerve
3 Brachial plexus, upper trunk
4 Brachial plexus, middle trunk
5 Scalenus medius
6 Suprascapular nerve
7 Injection site for vertical infraclavicular plexus anesthesia
8 Omohyoid muscle

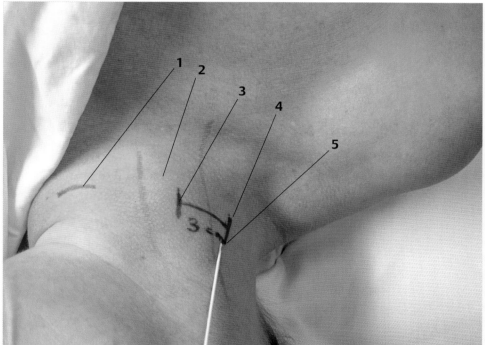

**Fig. 3.14** Interscalene plexus anesthesia (Meier approach): aids to orientation.
1 Cricoid cartilage
2 Sternocleidomastoid
3 Middle of the sternocleidomastoid belly
4 Line following the interscalene groove
5 Site of insertion

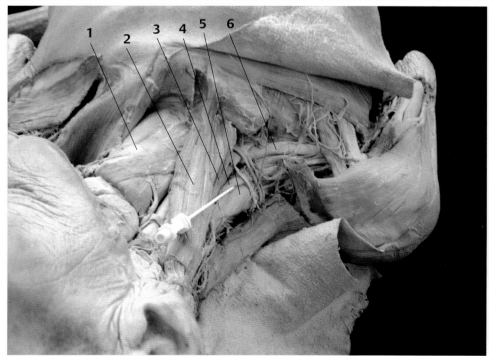

**Fig. 3.15** Interscalene plexus anesthesia (Meier approach): anatomy (clavicle partially removed).
1 Cricoid cartilage
2 Sternocleidomastoid
3 Scalenus anterior
4 Brachial plexus
5 Scalenus medius
6 Subclavian artery

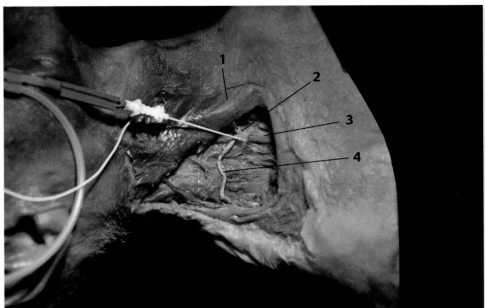

**Fig. 3.16** Right interscalene groove viewed from cranial direction.
1 Sternocleidomastoid
2 Prevertebral fascia
3 Brachial plexus
4 Transverse cervical artery

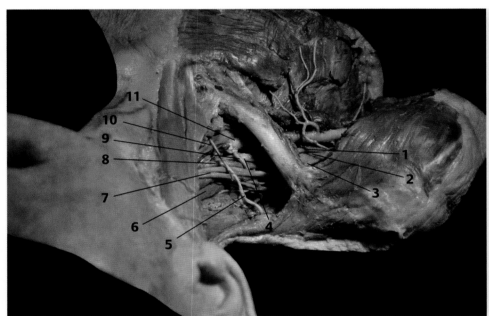

**Fig. 3.17** Right interscalene groove viewed from cranial direction.
1 Medial cord
2 Posterior cord
3 Lateral cord
4 Lower trunk
5 Superficial cervical artery
6 Scalenus medius
7 Upper trunk
8 Middle trunk
9 Dorsal scapular artery
10 Scalenus anterior
11 Subclavian artery

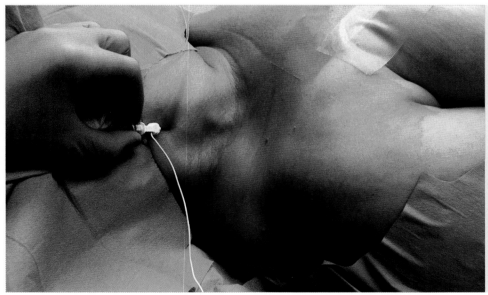

**Fig. 3.18** Interscalene plexus anesthesia (Meier approach) posterior interscalene groove, lateral orientation of the needle.

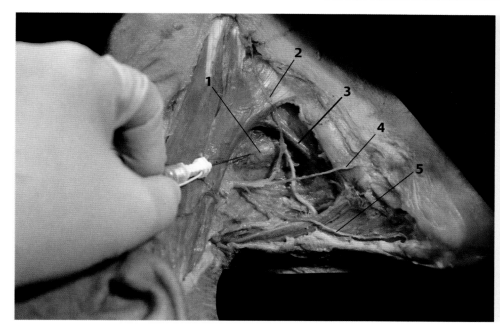

Fig. 3.19 Region viewed from cranial direction: needle is advanced beneath the prevertebral fascia.
1 Prevertebral fascia
2 Medial supraclavicular nerve
3 Omohyoid
4 Intermediate supraclavicular nerve
5 Lateral supraclavicular nerve

▶ **Motor response.** The motor response usually arises through stimulation of the upper trunk (deltoid, biceps brachii, or triceps muscle). This response is adequate (Silverstein et al 2000, Urmey 2000).

If there is a motor response of the phrenic nerve (twitching of the diaphragm, "hiccup") the needle is too far medially and forward, and it must be corrected laterally and backward.

If there is a motor response of the suprascapular nerve (supraspinatus and infraspinatus: external rotation and abduction of the shoulder), the needle is at the outer border of the brachial plexus and correction in the medial and anterior direction may be necessary. A motor response in the hand region should not be striven for.

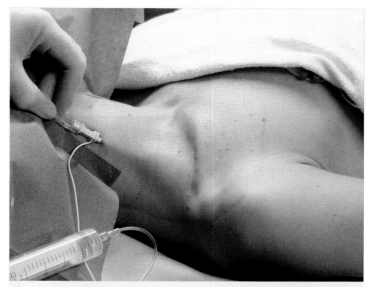

Fig. 3.20 Interscalene plexus anesthesia (Meier approach) after injection of local anesthetic (note the triangular swelling of the prevertebral fascia).

> **Note**
>
> This technique can be performed as a "single-shot" or as a continuous technique (▶ Fig. 3.20).

## Material

- Single injection: needle 5 to 6 cm
- Continuous technique: 6-cm needle with "pencil-point" tip and lateral opening

- Orientation is made much easier in obese patients using an adhesive dressing to pull the muscle and fat tissue downward (▶ Fig. 3.21).
- The technique should always be performed with a nerve stimulator and/or ultrasound.
- The motor response usually occurs due to stimulation of the upper trunk (deltoid, biceps brachii, or triceps). This response is sufficient and should be striven for (Silverstein et al 2000, Urmey 2000).
- If there is a motor response of the phrenic nerve (twitching of the diaphragm, "hiccup"), the needle is too far medially and forward and must be corrected laterally and backward.
- If there is a motor response of the suprascapular nerve (supraspinatus and infraspinatus: external rotation and abduction in the shoulder), the needle is at the outer border of the brachial plexus and correction medially and forward may be necessary.
- A motor response in the region of the hand does not have to be striven for.
- If performed correctly, the risk of injuring the pleura (pneumothorax) is slight.
- Orientation aid for finding the posterior interscalene groove (see ▶ Fig. 3.14 and ▶ Fig. 3.15). At the level of the cricoid cartilage, a 3-cm long horizontal line is drawn laterally from the middle of the belly of the sternocleidomastoid; the end of the line marks the interscalene groove. The injection site is approximately 2 cm further cranially at the intersection of the posterior interscalene groove and the posterior border of the sternocleidomastoid.
- The needle is advanced under stimulation to the medial border of the "Mohrenheim fossa" until a response in the region of the upper trunk is produced. An adequate response is contraction of the biceps brachii, deltoid, or triceps. Depending on the puncture angle and patient's constitution, the plexus is reached after 2.5 to 5 cm.
- Under ultrasound guidance, the nerve structures can be readily visualized (Chapter 3.2.3). With sufficient experience in this technique, ultrasound can be very helpful for difficult anatomical conditions.
- When the needle is in the correct position, a volume of 20 to 30 mL is injected.
- In slender patients, a triangular swelling in the prevertebral fascia is visible in the region of the interscalene groove (▶ Fig. 3.20).

▶ **Continuous technique**

With the continuous technique, a pencil-point needle with lateral opening should be used. The opening must point in the anterolateral direction after successful stimulation and injection of some of the local anesthetic, so that the catheter can be advanced readily (see ▶ Fig. 3.16). The catheter usually slides along the upper trunk. If the lateral direction is not observed, there is the danger of an epidural or intrathecal position of the catheter (Walter et al 2005, Yanovski et al 2012).

- The catheter tip should be advanced no more than 3 to 4 cm past the tip of the needle, or infraclavicular parts of the plexus may be reached. The skin level of the catheter is usually 7 to 8 cm. The frequency of dislocation is extremely low. If it is advanced too far, especially if the direction of the needle indicated above for the Meier technique is not followed, there is a risk of an epidural or intrathecal position, which could be fatal if anesthetic is accidentally injected (Yanovski et al 2012).
- Before the patient is transferred to the normal ward, a sufficient dose of local anesthetic should be administered via the catheter so an unintentional epidural or intrathecal position of the catheter can be ruled out or detected while the patient is still under close anesthesiology monitoring!

## Local Anesthetics

Initially: 20 to 30 mL of 1% mepivacaine or 1% prilocaine, alternatively: 20 to 30 mL of 0.75% (7.5 mg/mL) ropivacaine or 0.5% (5 mg/mL) bupivacaine.

Continuous: 0.2 to 0.375% (2–3.75 mg/mL) of ropivacaine or 0.25% (2.5 mg/mL) bupivacaine 6 to 8 mL/h.

With a suitable needle, a catheter can be introduced without difficulty. The catheter is advanced in the line of the plexus. During the puncture, the person injecting is located at the patient's head end.

If the catheter is advanced too far, the local anesthetic spreads in the infraclavicular region. This results in complete anesthesia in the region of the arm and hand, while the shoulder region (especially the suprascapular nerve) may be insufficiently anesthetized. The catheter should then be withdrawn. Depending on the depth of penetration of the puncture needle, the catheter is then advanced approximately 3 to 4 cm beyond the tip of the needle (6–8 cm skin level).

## 3.2.3 Interscalene Brachial Plexus Block with Ultrasound

Linear transducer: 10 to 12 MHz
Needle: 6 cm

## Finding the brachial plexus in the interscalene region (trace-back method)

The brachial plexus should first be located distally in the supraclavicular region as it is usually easy to identify there.

The transducer is positioned directly above the clavicle and pointed below the clavicle. The subclavian artery is visualized in the short axis (circular, pulsating); laterally and somewhat in front of it is the brachial plexus, visible here as a dense bundle of hypoechoic round structures (junction from the trunks to the cords; ▶ Fig. 3.22; see also Chapter 1). Following these structures in the image, the ultrasound plane is first tilted cranially, then moved until the typical image of the three roots of C5, C6, and C7 lying over one another becomes visible (▶ Fig. 3.22). This is the target area for the puncture (▶ Fig. 3.23).

## Needle Approach

The needle is usually inserted using the out-of-plane technique as in the Meier approach. To do this, the plexus is placed in the center of the image in the short axis and the needle is inserted about 2 to 3 cm cranial and at a right angle to the transducer in the laterocaudal direction of the needle described above.

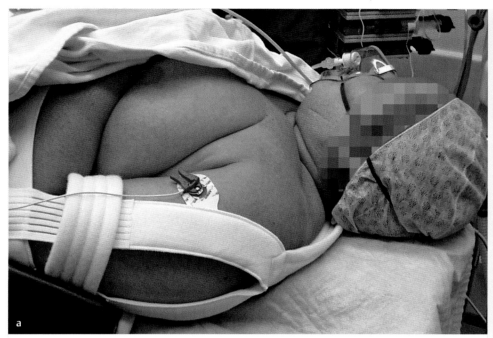

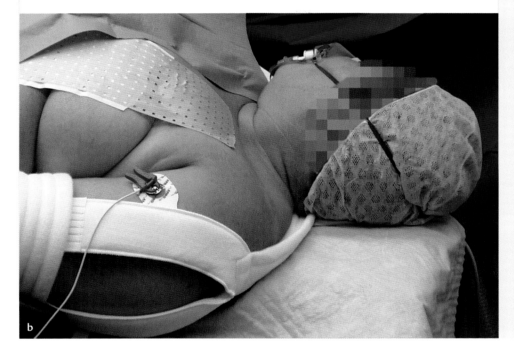

**Fig. 3.21** Obese patient.
**a** Difficult conditions for performing the block.
**b** Improved conditions by using an adhesive strip to pull tissue away.

It is often observed that the prevertebral fascia is first depressed before it is penetrated. A small "test dose" of 2 to 3 mL of fluid (e.g., local anesthetic, 0.9% saline solution, or 5% glucose) indicates whether there is spread beneath the prevertebral fascia in the region of the nerve roots or trunks. If this does not occur, the needle position must be corrected. The needle can be placed between the scalenus anterior muscle and nerve roots C5, C6, C7, or between the nerve roots and the scalenus medius muscle.

> **Note**
>
> Theoretically, to prevent paresis of the phrenic nerve (the phrenic nerve runs along the scalenus anterior muscle) it may be more useful to locate the space between the nerve roots and the scalenus medius muscle.

The local anesthetic should spread in a circle around the nerve roots; the mass of connective tissue containing the brachial plexus is usually preserved (▶ Fig. 3.24).

## Catheter Placement

The catheter is placed using the same technique (visualization of the short axis, out-of-plane needle insertion). The tip of the catheter or the local anesthetic emerging from the tip can generally be visualized in the supraclavicular region. Ultrasound-guided catheter placement has been proven to be qualitatively equal to the technique using the nerve stimulator but faster (Fredrickson et al 2009).

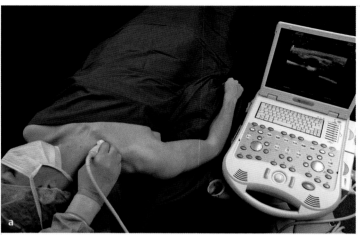

**Fig. 3.22  a–i** Locating the interscalene brachial plexus (trace-back method).
1 First rib
2 Subclavian artery
3 Brachial plexus
4 Pleura
5 Scalenus anterior
6 Scalenus medius
7 Sternocleidomastoid
8 Internal jugular vein

**a–c** Supraclavicular view:
**a** Position image.

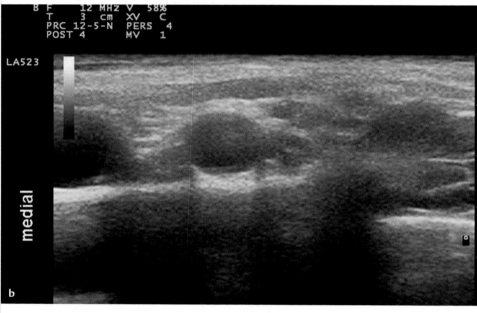

**b** Ultrasound (unlabeled).

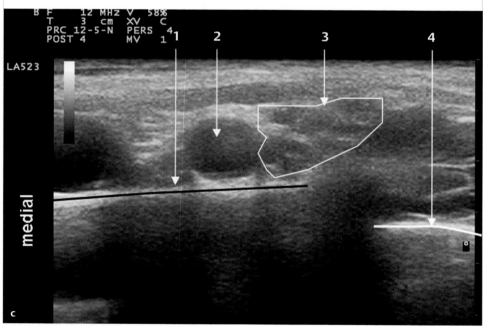

**c** Ultrasound (labeled).

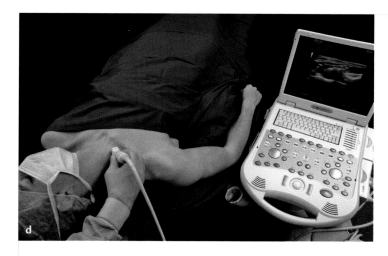

d

**Fig. 3.22 a–i (continued)**
**d–f** Transducer advanced cranially:
**d** Position image.

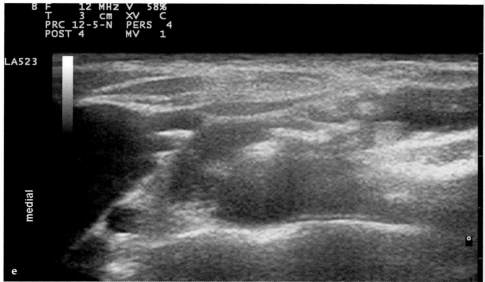

e

e Ultrasound (unlabeled).

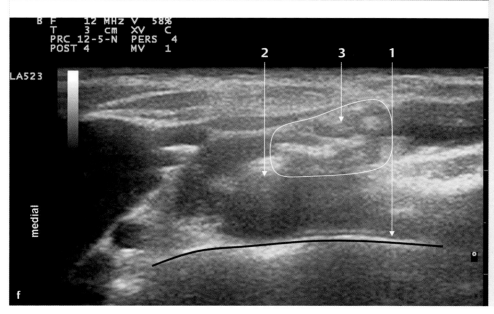

f

f Ultrasound (labeled).

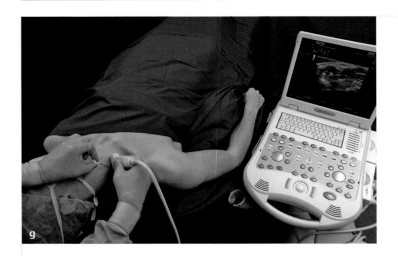

**Fig. 3.22 a–i (continued)**
**g–i** Final position of the transducer:
**g** Position image.

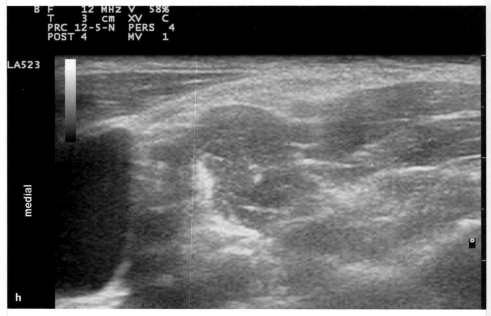

**h** Ultrasound (unlabeled).

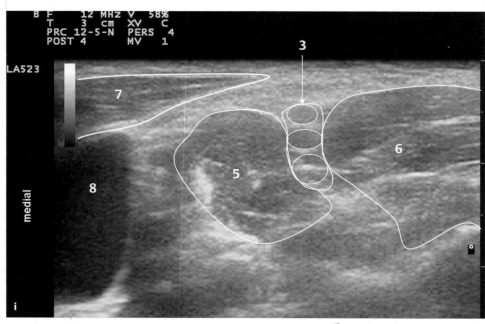

**i** Ultrasound (labeled).

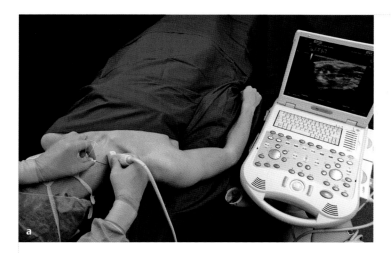

**Fig. 3.23 a–c** Nerve roots of C5, C6, C7 as target region for the interscalene block with ultrasound (visualization in the short axis).
1 C5, C6, C7
2 Sternocleidomastoid
3 Scalenus anterior
4 Scalenus medius
**a** Clinical setting.

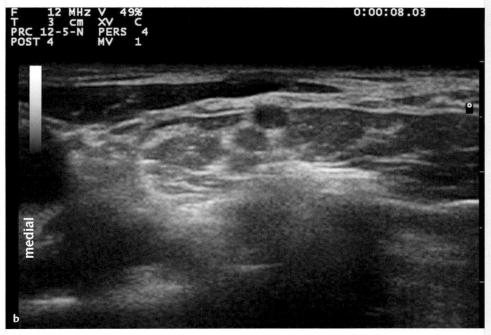

**b** Visualization in ultrasound (unlabeled).

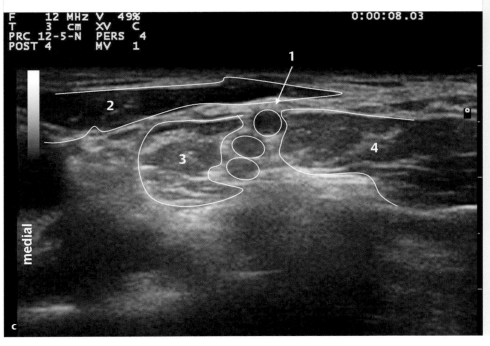

**c** Visualization in ultrasound (labeled).

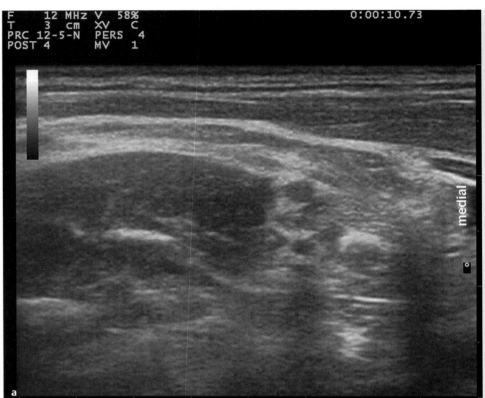

Fig. 3.24 **a–d** Interscalene plexus anesthesia, left side.
1 Scalenus medius
2 Plexus
3 Scalenus anterior
4 Space filled with local anesthetic
**a** Before injecting local anesthetic (unlabeled).

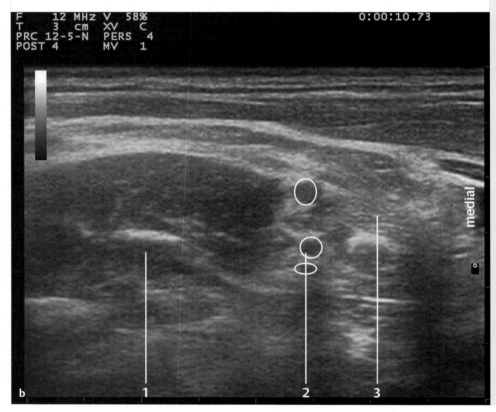

**b** As **a**, but labeled.

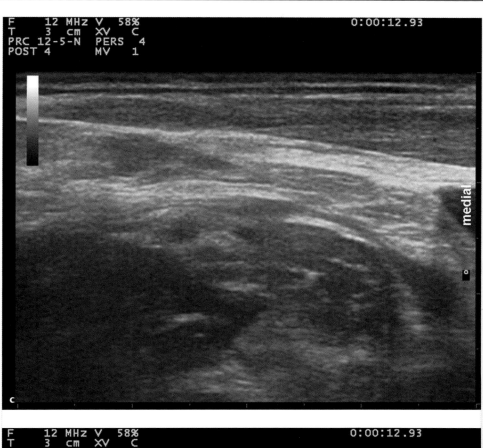

Fig. 3.24 a–d (continued)
c After injecting local anesthetic (unlabeled).

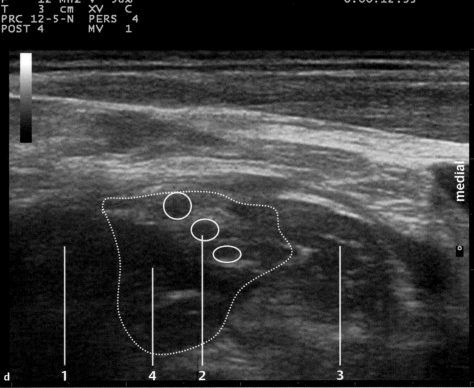

d As c, but labeled.

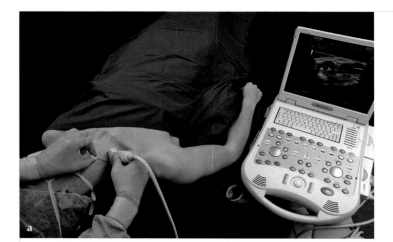

**Fig. 3.25 a–c** Anatomy of the brachial plexus at the level of the cricoid cartilage: note the immediate vicinity of the phrenic nerve to root C5.

1 Cricoid cartilage (lamina)
2 Right common carotid artery
3 Vagus nerve (X)
4 Scalenus anterior
5 Prevertebral fascia
6 Sternocleidomastoid
7 C5
8 Phrenic nerve
9 C6
10 C7
**a** Clinical setting.

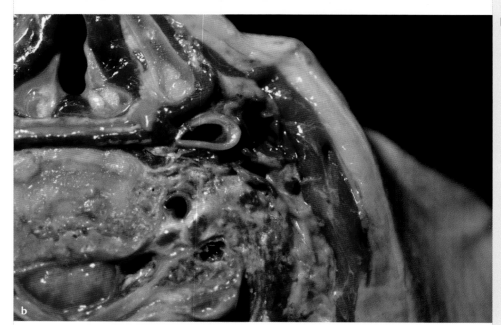

**b** Anatomical section (unlabeled).

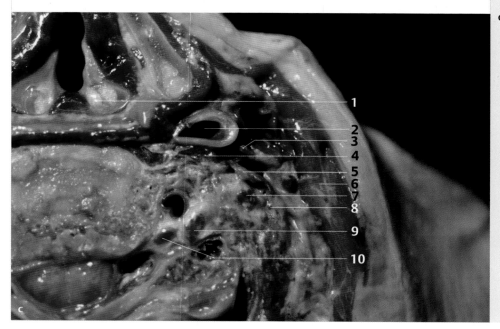

**c** Anatomical section (labeled).

- The superficial cervical artery runs across the scalenus muscles and the brachial plexus in the target region. It can sometimes be visualized by ultrasound, but is usually not an obstacle in practice. In general, for all hypoechoic structures that cannot be clearly identified as nerves, compression and/ or color Doppler should be used to determine whether it is a vessel.
- The vertebral artery does not become visible until below the transverse process of C6 anterior to the transverse process of C7.
- To prevent a phrenic nerve block, it is advisable not to place the block at the level of the cricoid cartilage, but further caudally (Renes et al 2009), as the phrenic nerve is in the immediate vicinity of root C5 at the level of the cricoid cartilage (▶ Fig. 3.25), but is further from the brachial plexus at the level of the transverse process at C7 (▶ Fig. 3.26) (Kessler et al 2008).
- For a puncture at the level of the cricoid cartilage, reducing the volume from 20 mL to 10 mL yields no advantage with respect to preventing a phrenic nerve block (Sinha et al 2011). For a block at the level of the root of C7, 10 mL of local anesthetic is sufficient for a block while preserving diaphragm function in 93% of patients (Renes et al 2009).
- Anatomical variations are possible; in particular, root C5 occasionally passes through the scalenus anterior muscle. In this case, it can be located there under ultrasound guidance and also blocked.

# 3.3 Pippa Approach

A posterior approach was described as early as the start of the 20th century. In 1990, this technique by Pippa et al (1990) was brought back into use. It can also be performed as a continuous procedure.

## 3.3.1 Posterior Approach (▶ Fig. 3.27, ▶ Fig. 3.28, ▶ Fig. 3.29)

### Positioning

The patient is in sitting position or lying on his or her side. The head should be in the axis of the body and the cervical spine should be flexed forward as far as possible (▶ Fig. 3.30). The landmark is the spinous process of C7 (vertebra prominens), which is usually easily palpable. With maximum head flexion, the spinous process of C6 can also be palpated above the spinous process of C7.

### Needle Insertion

A horizontal line is drawn from midway between the two spinous processes (C6/C7), 3 cm laterally to the side to be blocked. This is the insertion site.

The insertion of the needle is performed with a 10-cm needle strictly in the sagittal plane perpendicular to the skin (▶ Fig. 3.31), aiming roughly at the level of the cricoid cartilage. Deviation in the medial direction must be strictly avoided.

After 4 to 7 cm the transverse process of C7 is reached. After slight correction, the needle is pushed cranially over the transverse process a further 1 to 2 cm until the brachial plexus is reached.

## Material

Needle: 6 to 12 cm; catheter technique is possible

The technique must always be performed using a nerve stimulator and/or ultrasound (Chapter 3.3.2). Otherwise, major complications such as puncture of larger vessels (vertebral artery, carotid artery), puncture close to the spinal cord (Voermans et al 2006), or pneumothorax cannot safely be ruled out.

## 3.3.2 Interscalene Block of the Brachial Plexus Using Ultrasound (Pippa Approach)

Linear transducer: 10 to 12 MHz
Needle: 10 to 12 cm

### Locating the brachial plexus in the interscalene region

The brachial plexus is located by ultrasound using the method described in Chapter 3.2.3.

### Needle insertion

The needle insertion is performed as described in Chapter 3.3.1. The patient is in lateral position with the side to be punctured on top. In this case, the ultrasound-guided method is an in-plane

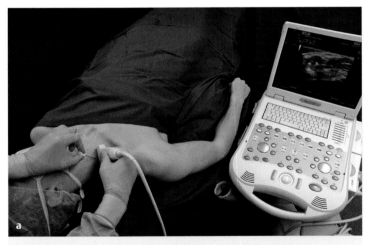

**Fig. 3.26 a–f** Interscalene block at level C7: "sonoanatomy."
1 Carotid artery
2 Sternocleidomastoid
3 Vertebral artery
4 Scalenus anterior
5 Phrenic nerve
6 C7
7 C6
8 C5
9 Scalenus medius
a Clinical setting.

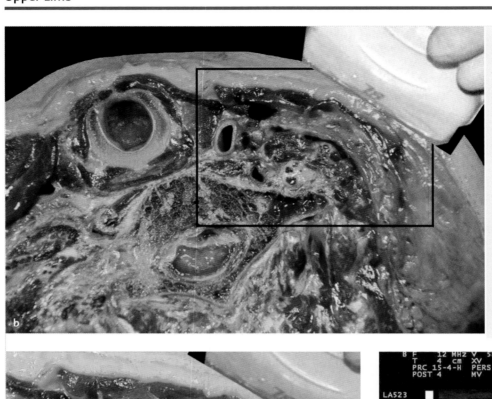

**Fig. 3.26 a–f (continued)**
**b** Overview image.
**c** Detail of **b**.
**d** Detail of **b** in ultrasound.
**e** Detail of b (labeled).
**f** Detail of **b** (ultrasound, labeled).

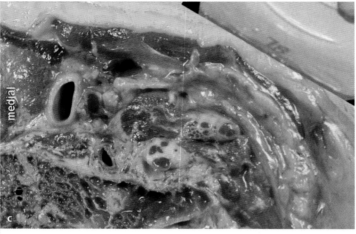

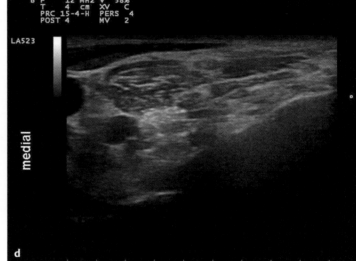

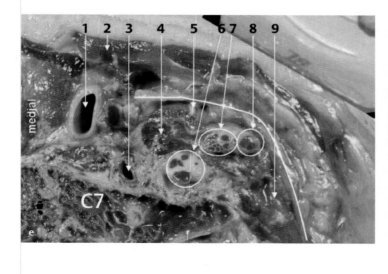

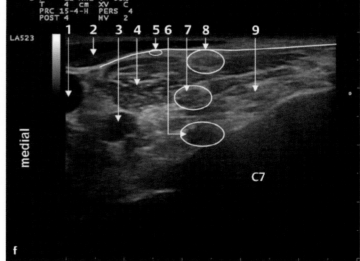

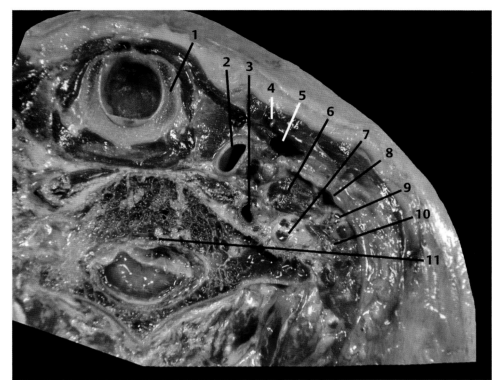

**Fig. 3.27** Neck region at level of the cricoid cartilage in supine position, cranial view.
1 Cricoid cartilage
2 Right common carotid artery
3 Right vertebral artery
4 Sternocleidomastoid
5 Right internal jugular vein
6 Scalenus anterior
7 Segment C6
8 Prevertebral fascia
9 Segments C6 and C5
10 Scalenus medius
11 Body of C7 vertebra

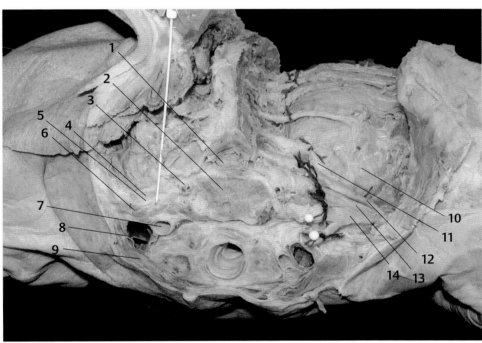

**Fig. 3.28** Direction of needle in the Pippa approach.
1 Spinal cord
2 Body of C7 vertebra
3 Vertebral artery
4 Scalenus medius
5 Brachial plexus
6 Scalenus anterior
7 Common carotid artery
8 Internal jugular vein
9 Sternocleidomastoid
10 Dome of the pleura
11 Subclavian artery
12 Lower trunk
13 Middle trunk
14 Upper trunk

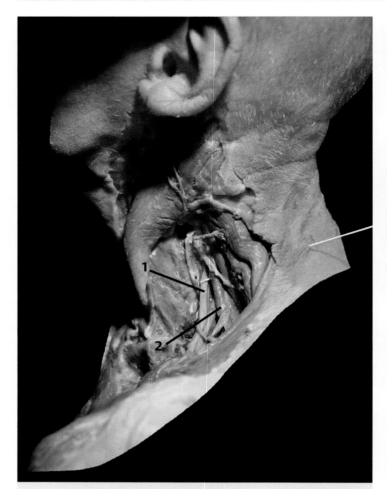

**Fig. 3.29** Direction of needle in Pippa approach, inserted 3 cm lateral to midline between the spinous processes of C6/7.
1 Upper trunk
2 Scalenus medius

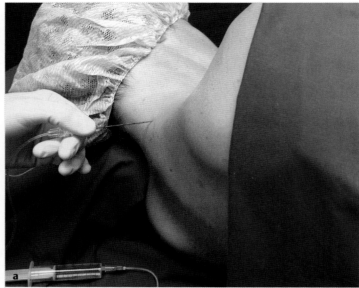

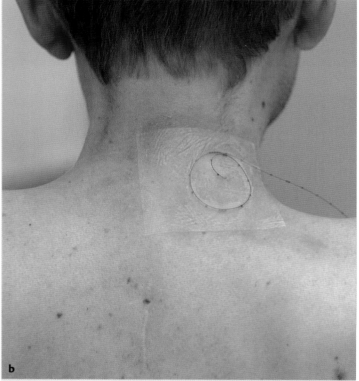

**Fig. 3.31** Approach according to Pippa.
**a** Lateral position.
**b** Continuous technique of dorsal interscalene plexus anesthesia.

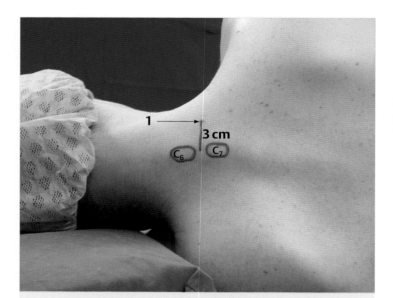

**Fig. 3.30** Interscalene plexus block, Pippa approach: posterior needle insertion in lateral position, anatomical landmarks.
1 Site of puncture

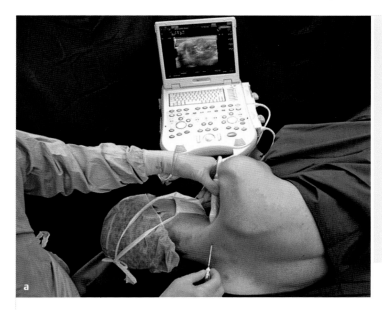

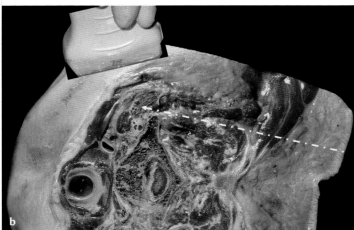

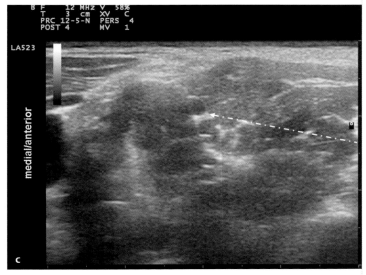

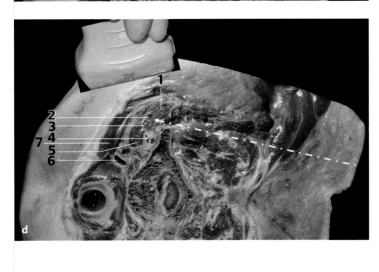

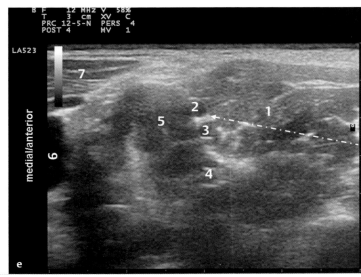

**Fig. 3.32** Pippa approach with ultrasound.
**a** Clinical setting.
**b** Anatomical section (unlabeled).
**c** Ultrasound image of **b**.
**d** As **b**, labeled.
**e** As **c**, labeled.
1 Scalenus medius
2 C5
3 C6
4 C7
5 Scalenus anterior
6 Right internal jugular vein
7 Sternocleidomastoid
--- Direction of needle

technique; the nerve roots are visualized in the short axis (▶ Fig. 3.32).

## Catheter Placement

A catheter can be placed using this technique (visualization in the short axis, in-plane puncture; Antonakakis et al 2009, Mariano et al 2009a, 2009b), but the results are poorer in comparison with catheter placement using the anterolateral technique (Chapter 3.2; Fredrickson et al 2011).

### Tips and Tricks

This technique should be used only by practitioners experienced in using ultrasound because of the high risk of serious complications if catheter placement is incorrect.

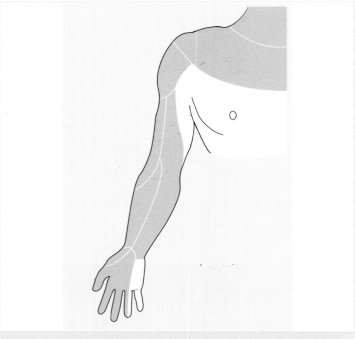

Fig. 3.33 Sensory effects of complete interscalene plexus anesthesia.

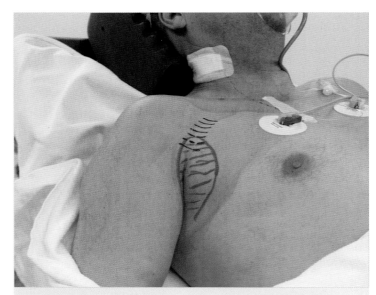

Fig. 3.34 Problematic regions in open shoulder surgery under interscalene plexus anesthesia. Black: Innervation area of the supraclavicular nerves (cervical plexus). Red: Innervation territory of T2.

## 3.4 Sensory and Motor Effects

There is generally sensory loss in segments C5–C7 (upper and middle trunk), while segments C8 and T1 are usually spared. A sensation of numbness in the thumb and the index and middle fingers is typical, while the ring and little fingers are often spared or are anesthetized after a delay (▶ Fig. 3.33). If the incision in shoulder operations is in the anterior axillary line, the supraclavicular nerves (cervical plexus) may also have to be blocked by subcutaneous infiltration below the clavicle if the operation is to be performed under regional anesthesia alone (▶ Fig. 3.34). Segments T2 and T3 are not included in the interscalene block. There is motor block of the axillary nerve (C5/6) and musculocutaneous nerve (C5/6), and often also a partial block of the radial nerve and median nerve (C6/7).

Evidence that the block is adequate for an operation is provided by the "deltoid sign" (abduction of the arm [axillary nerve] is no longer possible; Wiener and Speer 1994) and the "money sign" (Brown and Ragukonis 1996), when the thumb and middle finger can no longer be rubbed together.

## 3.5 Indications and Contraindications

### 3.5.1 Indications

Indications are:
- Anesthesia and analgesia for arthroscopic and open procedures on the shoulder and proximal upper arm region
- Reduction of shoulder dislocation (▶ Fig. 3.35)
- Physiotherapy treatment in the shoulder region postoperatively or in frozen shoulder
- Therapy of pain syndromes (CRPS, sympathetic block)

### 3.5.2 Contraindications

Besides the general contraindications to peripheral nerve blocks, the following special contraindications must be noted in the case of interscalene block:
- Contralateral phrenic nerve paresis
- Contralateral recurrent nerve paresis (Kempen et al 2000)
- COPD/bronchial asthma (relative contraindication)

## 3.6 Supraclavicular Nerve Block (Cervical Plexus)

In open shoulder surgery, certain regions are not anesthetized even with well-positioned interscalene plexus block. These regions are innervated by the T2 segment or by the supraclavicular nerves, which derive from the cervical plexus. While an additional regional block (paravertebral T2) is difficult to carry out in the former, the supraclavicular nerves can be anesthetized easily using subcutaneous infiltration below the clavicle (▶ Fig. 3.36, ▶ Fig. 3.37, ▶ Fig. 3.38, ▶ Fig. 3.39).

## 3.7 Complications, Side Effects, Method-Specific Problems

Intravascular injection (vertebral artery), high spinal or epidural anesthesia, cervical spine injury, or pneumothorax can be prevented by the correct performance of the Meier approach.

Incorrect intrathecal positions of an interscalene plexus catheter have been described (Dutton et al 1994, Walter et al 2005, Yanovski et al 2012); one case had a fatal outcome due to the unnoticed intrathecal application of 10 mL of bupivacaine

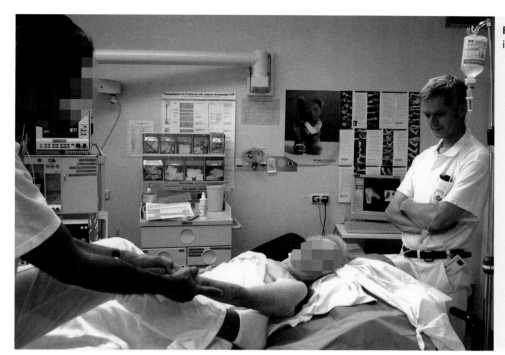

**Fig. 3.35** Reducing a shoulder dislocation after interscalene plexus block.

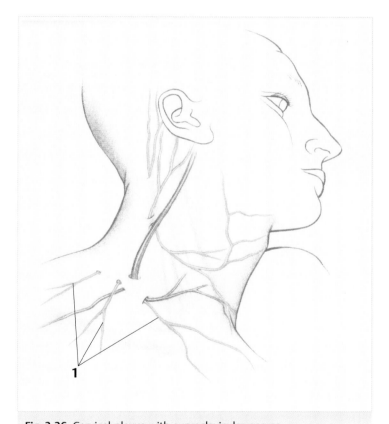

**Fig. 3.36** Cervical plexus with supraclavicular nerves.
1 Supraclavicular nerves from the cervical plexus

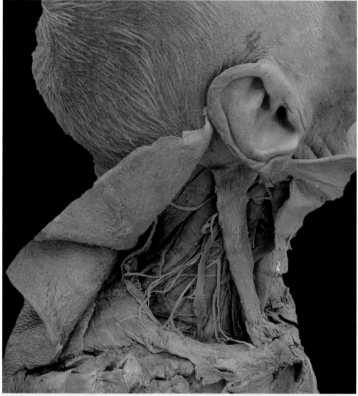

**Fig. 3.37** Cervical plexus with supraclavicular nerves.
See Fig. 3.36.

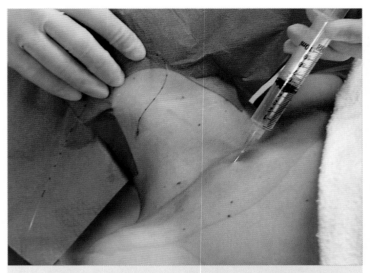

Fig. 3.38 Block of the supraclavicular nerves (cervical plexus) by subcutaneous infiltration along the clavicle.

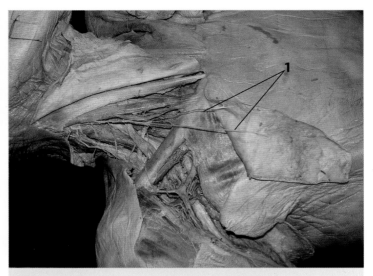

Fig. 3.39 Cervical plexus. Note: the supraclavicular nerves extend to the infraclavicular region.
1 Supraclavicular nerves from the cervical plexus

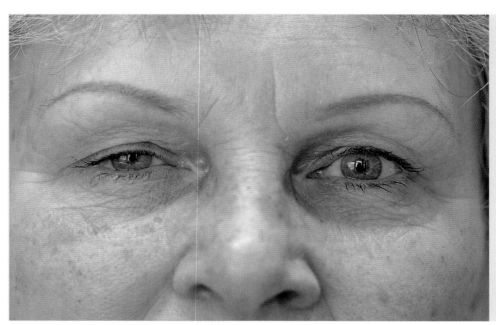

Fig. 3.40 Side effects of interscalene plexus anesthesia: Horner syndrome on patient's right (miosis, ptosis, enophthalmos).

(Yanovski et al 2012). The following points should be noted:
- Maintain lateral needle direction.
- Never advance the catheter more than 2 to 3 cm beyond the tip of the needle.
- Inject a test dose through the catheter to rule out an intrathecal position.

### 3.7.1 Neurological Complications after Shoulder Surgery in Interscalene Plexus Anesthesia

Neurological complications caused by an interscalene plexus block are rare and the prognosis is usually favorable. In 50% of cases, they are sequelae of the surgical procedure itself (Candido et al 2005), although it is not always possible to clearly determine the cause (Tetzlaff et al 1997, Besmer et al 2005).

In case reports, high spinal or epidural anesthesia (Aramideh et al 2002, Walter et al 2005, Gomez and Mendes 2006), phrenic nerve paresis (Robaux et al 2001) and permanent paralysis of the upper limb have been reported after posterior injection (Voermans et al 2006). The extent to which ultrasound contributes to preventing complications when it is performed is not yet known. Nerve stimulation and ultrasound are thus considered equally useful techniques (Quabach et al 2010).

### 3.7.2 Side Effects Intrinsic to the Method

- Horner syndrome: miosis, ptosis, enophthalmos (▶ Fig. 3.40). The reported incidence varies between 12.5% and 75%.
- Hearing loss: A reversible impairment of hearing can occur, also caused by sympathetic block (Rosenberg et al 1995).
- Bronchospasm: The upper thoracic sympathetic ganglia supply the smooth muscles of the bronchi. Bronchospasm produced by sympathetic block in the course of an interscalene block has been described (Lim 1979, Thiagarajah et al 1984) but appears to be an extremely rare event, so that the risk and benefit should be weighed carefully.

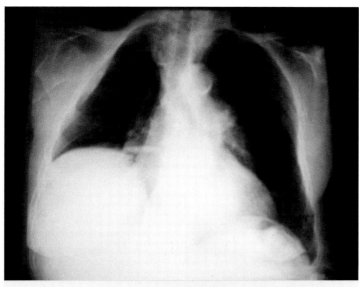

**Fig. 3.41** Side effects of interscalene plexus anesthesia: Phrenic paresis on patient's right with elevated diaphragm.

- Recurrent nerve paresis: In 6 to 8% of cases, ipsilateral recurrent nerve paresis has to be expected (hoarseness). Simultaneously existing contralateral recurrent nerve paresis can cause an acute respiratory distress syndrome that necessitates immediate intubation (Kempen et al 2000).
- Phrenic nerve paresis: Phrenic nerve paresis (▶ Fig. 3.41) in association with interscalene plexus block is described in up to

100% of cases (Urmey et al 1991), sometimes presenting as severe postoperative dyspnea (Jariwala 2014). In the case of interscalene block performed according to the Meier approach (Meier et al 1997, 2001), clinical signs of phrenic nerve paresis occurred in only 7% of patients and clinically relevant respiratory insufficiency was not observed.

- Bezold–Jarisch reflex: A fall in blood pressure associated with bradycardia was observed in about 10% of patients after they were placed in the "beach chair position" (▶ Fig. 3.42). The event occurred on average about 60 minutes after performing the block (Roch and Sharrock 1991, D'Alessio et al 1995, Liguori et al 1998). Cardiocirculatory arrest requiring resuscitation can occur. Treatment consists of administration of an adrenergic stimulating drug (e.g., ephedrine), and possibly lowering the patient's head and volume administration. Prophylactic administration of metoprolol is recommended (D'Alessio et al 1995, Liguori et al 1998). This phenomenon was not described and was not observed during continuous administration of local anesthetic for postoperative pain therapy.

In this connection, the necessity of continuous monitoring of the patients during an operative procedure should be stressed; capnometric monitoring of spontaneous respiration has proved useful. Transcutaneous $CO_2$ measurement (TOSCA) or EEG monitoring (BIS, Narcotrend; see Chapter 21.2.3) are also possible. The patient should always be given $O_2$ through a mask. A transparent dressing allows the injection site to be inspected daily without changing the dressing.

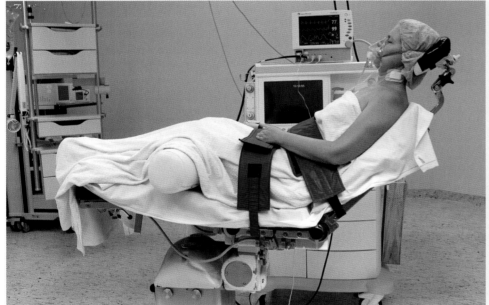

**Fig. 3.42** Beach chair position in shoulder surgery.

# References

Antonakakis JG, Sites BD, Shiffrin J. Ultrasound-guided posterior approach for the placement of a continuous interscalene catheter. Reg Anesth Pain Med 2009; 34: 64–68

Aramideh M, van den Oever HL, Walstra GJ, Dzoljic M. Spinal anesthesia as a complication of brachial plexus block using the posterior approach. Anesth Analg 2002; 94: 1338–1339

Benumof JL. Permanent loss of cervical spinal cord function associated with interscalene block performed under general anesthesia. Anesthesiology 2000; 93: 1541–1544

Besmer I, Schüpfer G, Schleppers A. Neurologische Komplikationen nach Schulterchirurgie in Interskalenusblockade. Anästh Intensivmed 2005; 46: 139–143

Brown AR, Ragukonis TP. Early sign of successful bupivacaine interscalene block: the "money sign." Reg Anesth 1996; 21: 166–167

Candido KD, Sukhani R, Doty R, Jr et al. Neurologic sequelae after interscalene brachial plexus block for shoulder/upper arm surgery: the association of patient, anesthetic, and surgical factors to the incidence and clinical course. Anesth Analg 2005; 100: 1489–1495

Cook L B. Unsuspected extradural catheterization in an interscalene block. Br J Anaesth 1991; 67: 473–475

D'Alessio JG, Weller RS, Rosenblum M. Activation of the Bezold-Jarisch reflex in the sitting position for shoulder arthroscopy using interscalene block. Anesth Analg 1995; 80: 1158–1162

Dutton RP, Eckhardt WF, III, Sunder N. Total spinal anesthesia after interscalene blockade of the brachial plexus. Anesthesiology 1994; 80: 939–941

Fredrickson MJ, Ball CM, Dalgleish AJ, Stewart AW, Short TG. A prospective randomized comparison of ultrasound and neurostimulation as needle end points for interscalene catheter placement. Anesth Analg 2009; 108: 1695–1700

Fredrickson MJ, Ball CM, Dalgleish AJ. Posterior versus anterolateral approach interscalene catheter placement: a prospective randomized trial. Reg Anesth Pain Med 2011; 36: 125–133

Gomez RS, Mendes TC. Epidural anaesthesia as a complication of attempted brachial plexus blockade using the posterior approach. Anaesthesia 2006; 61: 591–592

Hofmann-Kiefer K, Jacob M, Rehm M, Lang P. Options and limits of interscalene nerve blocks. [Article in German] Anasthesio l Intensivmed Notfallmed Schmerzther 2009; 44: 522–529

Jariwala A, Kumar BC, Coventry DM. Sudden severe postoperative dyspnea following shoulder surgery: Remember inadvertent phrenic nerve block due to interscalene brachial plexus block. Int J Shoulder Surg 2014; 8: 51–54

Kempen PM, O'Donnell J, Lawler R, Mantha V. Acute respiratory insufficiency during interscalene plexus block. Anesth Analg 2000; 90: 1415–1416

Kessler J, Schafhalter-Zoppoth I, Gray AT. An ultrasound study of the phrenic nerve in the posterior cervical triangle: implications for the interscalene brachial plexus block. Reg Anesth Pain Med 2008; 33: 545–550

Liguori GA, Kahn RL, Gordon J, Gordon MA, Urban MK. The use of metoprolol and glycopyrrolate to prevent hypotensive/bradycardic events during shoulder arthroscopy in the sitting position under interscalene block. Anesth Analg 1998; 87: 1320–1325

Lim EK. Inter-scalene brachial plexus block in the asthmatic patient. Anaesthesia 1979; 34: 370

Mariano ER, Afra R, Loland VJ et al. Continuous interscalene brachial plexus block via an ultrasound-guided posterior approach: a randomized, triple-masked, placebo-controlled study. Anesth Analg 2009a; 108: 1688–1694

Mariano ER, Loland VJ, Ilfeld BM. Interscalene perineural catheter placement using an ultrasound-guided posterior approach. Reg Anesth Pain Med 2009b; 34: 60–63

Meier G, Bauereis C, Heinrich C. Interscalene brachial plexus catheter for anesthesia and postoperative pain therapy. Experience with a modified technique. [Article in German] Anaesthesist 1997; 6: 715–719

Meier G, Bauereis C, Maurer H. Interscalene plexus block. Anatomic requirements—anesthesiologic and operative aspects. [Article in German] Anaesthesist 2001; 50: 333–341

Pippa P, Cominelli E, Marinelle C, Aito S. Brachial plexus block using the posterior approach. Eur J Anaesthesiol 1990; 7: 411–420

Quabach R, Adam C, Standl T. Neurologische Komplikationen in der Anästhesie. Anästh Notfallmed Schmerzther 2010; 45: 534–542

Renes SH, Rettig HC, Gielen MJ, Wilder-Smith OH, van Geffen GJ. Ultrasound-guided low-dose interscalene brachial plexus block reduces the incidence of hemidiaphragmatic paresis. Reg Anesth Pain Med 2009; 34: 498–502

Robaux S, Bouaziz H, Boisseau N, Raucoules-Aimé M, Laxenaire MC S.O.S. Regional Hot Line Service. Persistent phrenic nerve paralysis following interscalene brachial plexus block. Anesthesiology 2001; 95: 1519–1521

Roch J, Sharrok NE. Hypotension during shoulder arthroscopy in the sitting position under interscalene block. Reg Anesth 1991; 64: 64

Rosenberg PH, Lamberg TS, Tarkkila P, Marttila T, Björkenheim JM, Tuominen M. Auditory disturbance associated with interscalene brachial plexus block. Br J Anaesth 1995; 74: 89–91

Silverstein WB, Saiyed MU, Brown AR. Interscalene block with a nerve stimulator: a deltoid motor response is a satisfactory endpoint for successful block. Reg Anesth Pain Med 2000; 25: 356–359

Sinha SK, Abrams JH, Barnett JT et al. Decreasing the local anesthetic volume from 20 to 10 mL for ultrasound-guided interscalene block at the cricoid level does not reduce the incidence of hemidiaphragmatic paresis. Reg Anesth Pain Med 2011; 36: 17–20

Tetzlaff JE, Dilger J, Yap E, Brems J. Idiopathic brachial plexitis after total shoulder replacement with interscalene brachial plexus block. Anesth Analg 1997; 85: 644–646

Thiagarajah S, Lear E, Azar I, Salzer J, Zeiligsohn E. Bronchospasm following interscalene brachial plexus block. Anesthesiology 1984; 61: 759–761

Urmey WF, Talts KH, Sharrock NE. One hundred percent incidence of hemidiaphragmatic paresis associated with interscalene brachial plexus anesthesia as diagnosed by ultrasonography. Anesth Analg 1991; 72: 498–503

Urmey WF. Interscalene block: the truth about twitches. Reg Anesth Pain Med 2000; 25: 340–342

Voermans NC, Crul BJ, de Bondt B, Zwarts MJ, van Engelen BG. Permanent loss of cervical spinal cord function associated with the posterior approach. Anesth Analg 2006; 102: 330–331

Walter M, Rogalla P, Spies C, Kox WJ, Volk T. Intrathecal misplacement of an interscalene plexus catheter. [Article in German] Anaesthesist 2005; 54: 215–219

Wiener DN, Speer KP. The deltoid sign. Anesth Analg 1994; 79: 192

Winnie AP. Interscalene brachial plexus block. Anesth Analg 1970; 49: 455–466

Yanovski B, Gaitini L, Volodarski D, Ben-David B. Catastrophic complication of an interscalene catheter for continuous peripheral nerve block analgesia. Anaesthesia 2012; 67: 1166–1169

# 4 Supraclavicular and Infraclavicular Techniques of Brachial Plexus Block

## 4.1 Anatomy

Just above the clavicle, each of the trunks splits into an anterior and a posterior division:

- The three posterior divisions combine to form the *posterior cord.*
- The anterior divisions of the upper and middle trunks form the *lateral cord.*

- The *medial cord* is the continuation of the anterior division of the lower trunk (▶ Fig. 4.1 and ▶ Fig. 4.4).

The cords are located very close to one another in the infraclavicular region (▶ Fig. 4.2, ▶ Fig. 4.3, ▶ Fig. 4.4, ▶ Fig. 4.5, ▶ Fig. 4.6, ▶ Fig. 4.7, ▶ Fig. 4.8).

- The *lateral cord* lies most superficially (lateral to and in front of the subclavian artery).

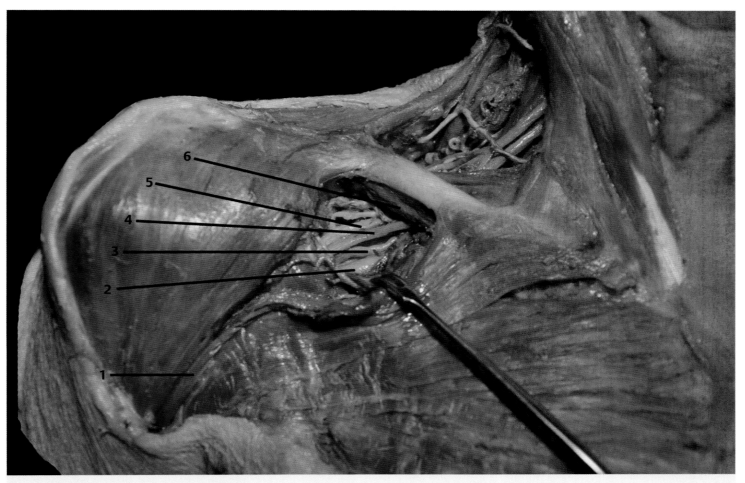

**Fig. 4.1** Brachial plexus, infraclavicular region.
1 Cephalic vein
2 Subclavian artery
3 Medial cord
4 Lateral cord
5 Posterior cord
6 Subclavian muscle

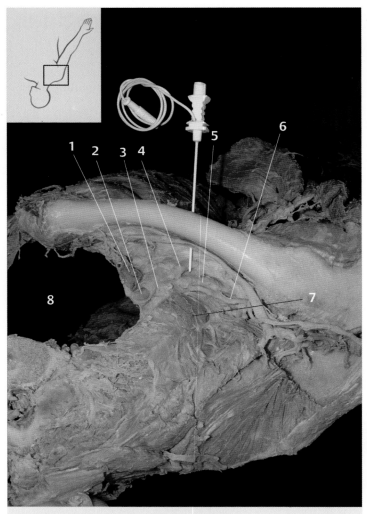

**Fig. 4.2** Anatomy of the infraclavicular region, seen from cranial aspect.
1 Scalenus anterior
2 Subclavian artery
3 Medial cord
4 Lateral cord
5 Posterior cord
6 Suprascapular nerve
7 Scalenus medius
8 Pleural cavity

- The *posterior cord* is found a little deeper and slightly lateral to the lateral (!) cord (lateral to and behind the subclavian artery).
- The *medial cord* lies deep (behind the subclavian artery, see ► Fig. 4.3 and ► Fig. 4.4).

The subclavian artery and the brachial plexus run medial to the coracoid process to the axilla.

> **Note**
>
> Note the 90° rotation of the cords around the subclavian artery from the infraclavicular to the axillary region. While the posterior cord lies furthest lateral (but deeper) compared with the lateral cord in the infraclavicular region, the designations of the cords reflect their actual positions in the axillary region.

The medial cord passes below the artery and then lies medial to the artery, giving off a medial root that joins the lateral root of the lateral cord to form the median nerve.

# 4.2 Supraclavicular Block Techniques

The supraclavicular block of the brachial plexus, similarly to the infraclavicular block, has the advantage that the nerves supplying the arm are bundled very compactly in the area where the trunks separate into the cords. However, the classical supraclavicular block techniques by Kulenkampff (Kulenkampff 1911) and later Winnie and Collins (1964) have been used less than the infraclavicular block in recent decades due to the increased risk of pneumothorax. The introduction of ultrasound-guided techniques has, at least theoretically, the advantage of minimizing the risk of pneumothorax, although a pneumothorax cannot be completely precluded even with ultrasound (Bhatia et al 2010).

Sensory and motor effects, indications and contraindications, and complications, side effects, and method-specific problems are, unless specified otherwise, similar to those of the infraclavicular block techniques (Chapter 3.2.3).

> **Note**
>
> The supraclavicular plexus block should be performed only under ultrasound guidance and possibly with a nerve stimulator as well.

## 4.2.1 Ultrasound-Guided Supraclavicular Block of the Brachial Plexus

Linear transducer: 10 to 12 MHz
Needle: 6 to 10 cm

### Visualization of the Brachial Plexus Using Ultrasound

As already described for the trace-back method for locating the interscalene brachial plexus (Chapter 3.2.3), the transducer is placed immediately above and parallel to the clavicle in the supraclavicular fossa and the beam is directed obliquely under the clavicle toward the thorax (not perpendicularly; ► Fig. 4.9).

First the subclavian artery (round, pulsating, hypoechoic structure) is visualized. If the finding is unclear, color Doppler can be used to clarify the situation. Lateral and slightly anterior to the subclavian artery is the brachial plexus, visible as a bundle of small, hypoechoic circles (grapelike structure; ► Fig. 4.9)

### Needle Approach

The in-plane needle approach from lateral to medial is preferred to avoid a pneumothorax (► Fig. 4.10). The needle is inserted at the lateral end of the transducer and advanced in the beam strictly along the transducer axis up to the desired structures. As in the interscalene block, a slight loss of resistance is felt when the fascia surrounding the plexus (prevertebral fascia) is penetrated. This phenomenon is also visible in the ultrasound image as a slight depression of the fascia followed by recoil (loss of resistance).

A few milliliters are injected to check whether the local anesthetic spreads in the correct compartment. It is crucial that the local anesthetic also spreads into the deep nerve structures in the

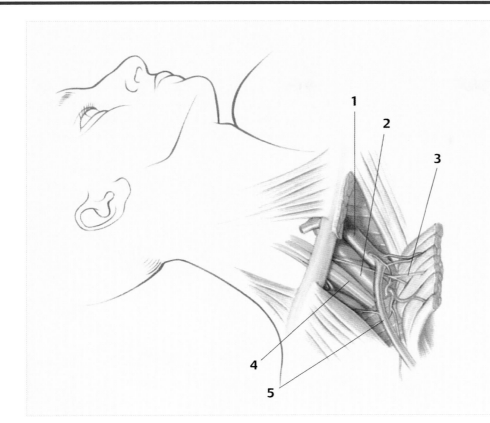

**Fig. 4.3** Brachial plexus, infraclavicular region.
1 Subclavian vein
2 Subclavian artery
3 Pectoral nerves
4 Brachial plexus
5 Cephalic vein

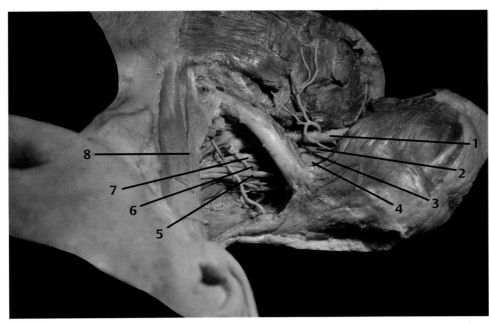

**Fig. 4.4** Anatomy of the brachial plexus.
1 Subclavian artery
2 Medial cord
3 Posterior cord
4 Lateral cord
5 Upper trunk
6 Middle trunk
7 Lower trunk
8 Sternocleidomastoid

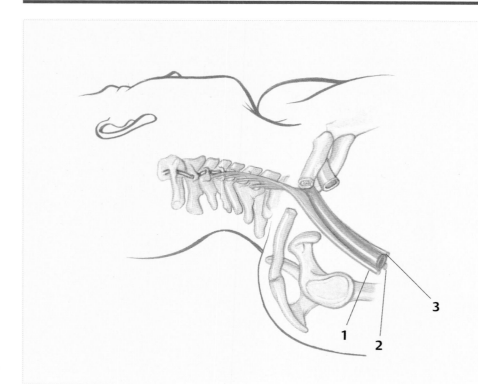

**Fig. 4.5** Brachial plexus in relation to the sub-clavian (axillary) artery. Note that the cords rotate 90° around the subclavian artery from the infraclavicular region to the axillary region. While the posterior cord is furthest laterally (but deeper) compared to the lateral cord in the infraclavicular region, in the axillary region the names of the cords correspond to their actual positions relative to one another.
1 Lateral cord
2 Posterior cord
3 Medial cord

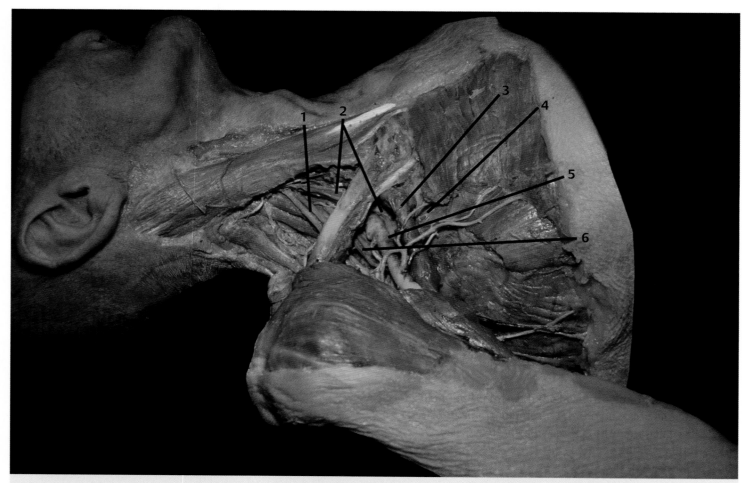

**Fig. 4.6** Lateral aspect of the interscalene groove with the shoulder raised.
1 Upper trunk
2 Scalenus anterior with phrenic nerve
3 Subclavian vein
4 First rib
5 Subclavian artery
6 Lower trunk

angle between the first rib and the subclavian artery (corner pocket; ▸ Fig. 4.9), as there may otherwise be an incomplete block in the region of the ulnar nerve (▸ Fig. 4.10). Information on the required volume of local anesthetic to be applied fluctuates between 15 mL (Soares et al 2007) and 30 mL (Fredrickson et al 2009, Perlas et al 2009).

## Catheter Placement

A catheter can be placed using the technique described here, but is less successful than infraclavicular catheter placement with respect to postoperative analgesia (Mariano et al 2011). The reason for this is the unfavorable angle between the needle and the course of the brachial plexus for advancing the catheter.

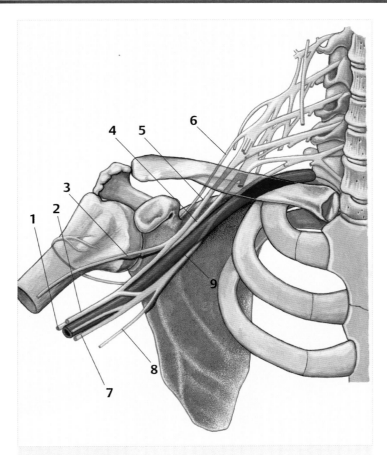

**Fig. 4.7** Anatomy of the brachial plexus.
1 Radial nerve
2 Median nerve
3 Musculocutaneous nerve
4 Posterior cord
5 Lateral cord
6 Suprascapular nerve
7 Ulnar nerve
8 Medial cutaneous nerve of the forearm
9 Medial cord

### Tips and Tricks

- The ultrasound-guided supraclavicular block can be performed in combination with nerve stimulation. As described above, a response in the hand should be striven for. Note: After administration of local anesthetic and/or normal saline, the function of the nerve stimulator is impaired! Use dextrose 5% if necessary.
- The targeted application of the local anesthetic in the corner pocket between the first rib and the subclavian artery should lead to a very reliable block with rapid onset (Soares et al 2007, Tran et al 2006). However, a comparative study of this method with the "in plane" infraclavicular plexus anesthesia showed a better block in the region of the ulnar nerve with the same onset time (30 min; Fredrickson et al 2009) in favor of the infraclavicular block.
- In the same visualization of the supraclavicular brachial plexus as described above (in the short axis), an out-of-plane puncture similar to the perivascular supraclavicular block described by Winnie and Collins (Tran et al 2008) is also possible. The angle to the transducer should be as steep as possible. Using continuous small movements (local tissue movement, see Chapter 1), the practitioner can determine the position of the tip of the needle. The risk of a pneumothorax may be greater than in the in-plane technique. A catheter is easier to place.

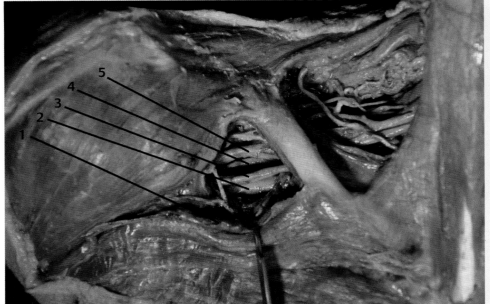

**Fig. 4.8** Anatomy of the infraclavicular region.
1 Cephalic vein
2 Subclavian artery
3 Lateral cord
4 Medial cord
5 Posterior cord

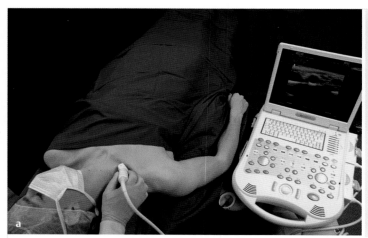

**Fig. 4.9** Visualization of the right supraclavicular plexus using ultrasound ("sonoanatomy"). Note the angle between the subclavian artery and the first rib (corner pocket). Here are segments of the brachial plexus (marked with an *), from which the medial cord and the ulnar nerve are formed.
**a** Clinical setting.
**b** Ultrasound image (unlabeled).
**c** Anatomy (section in the acoustic window).
**d** Ultrasound image (labeled).
**e** Anatomy (section in the acoustic window with markings).
1 First rib
2 Subclavian artery
3 Brachial plexus
4 Pleura

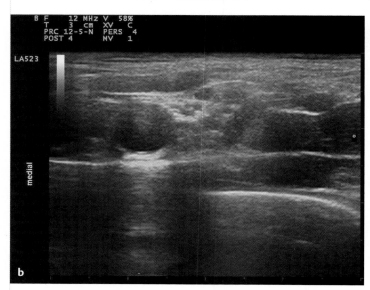

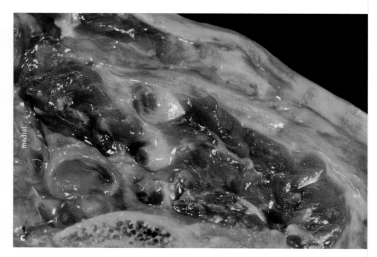

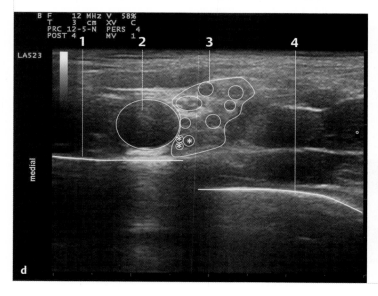

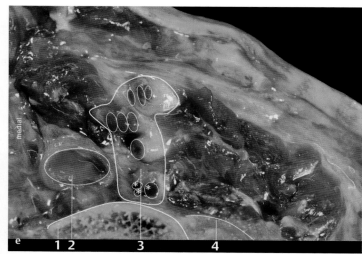

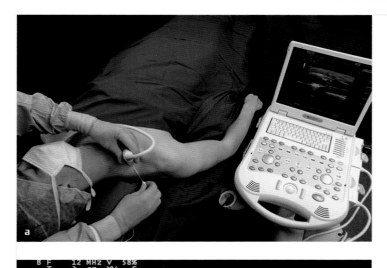

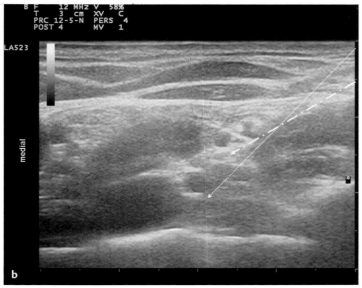

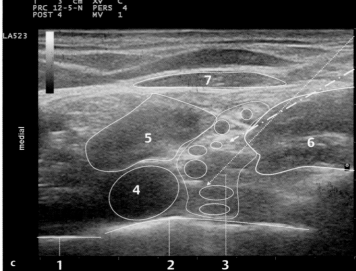

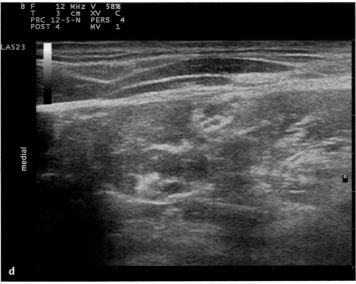

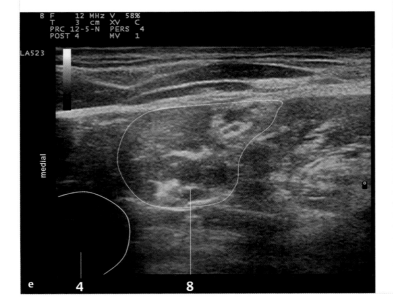

**Fig. 4.10** Supraclavicular plexus block, ultrasound-guided in-plane puncture.

Arrow (dash-dot line): needle direction. Arrow (dotted line): correction possibly needed if local anesthetic does not reach corner pocket (as in **d**, **e**).

**a** Patient position.
**b** Before injection of the local anesthetic.
**c** With structures marked.
**d** After injection of the local anesthetic.
**e** With structures marked.

| | |
|---|---|
| 1 Pleura | 6 Scalenus medius |
| 2 First rib | 7 Omohyoid |
| 3 Brachial plexus | 8 Brachial plexus (after injection |
| 4 Subclavian artery | of the local anesthetic) |
| 5 Scalenus anterior | |

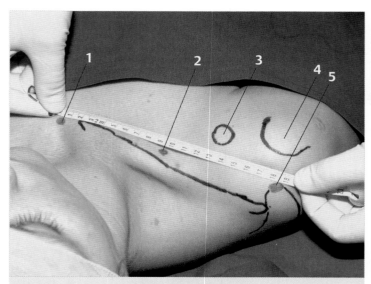

**Fig. 4.11** Orientation points for vertical infraclavicular plexus anesthesia. (The puncture site is half way between the middle of the jugular notch and the anterior part of the acromion.)
1 Middle of the jugular notch
2 Puncture site
3 Coracoid process
4 Head of humerus
5 Anterior part of the acromion

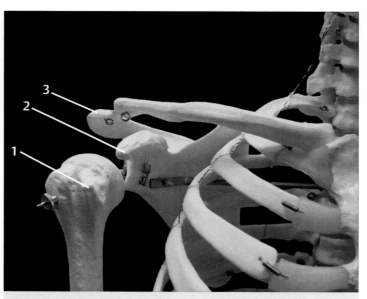

**Fig. 4.12** Overview of the bony structures for performing vertical infraclavicular plexus anesthesia.
1 Head of humerus
2 Coracoid process
3 Anterior part of the acromion

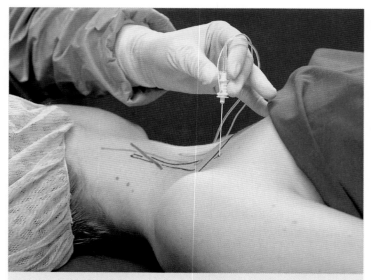

**Fig. 4.13** VIB puncture site: vertical to surface on the horizontal supine patient. Note the relation to the supraclavicular region.

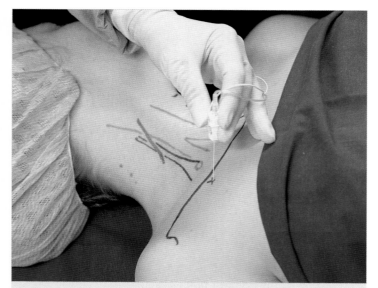

**Fig. 4.14** VIB puncture site: vertical to surface on the horizontal supine patient. Note the relation to the supraclavicular region.

## 4.3 Vertical Infraclavicular Block According to Kilka, Geiger, and Mehrkens ▶

In contrast to the other infraclavicular techniques, the vertical infraclavicular block (VIB) described by Kilka et al (1995) has clear landmarks.

These landmarks are the anterior end of the acromion and the middle of the jugular notch. The midpoint of the line connecting these two points marks the injection site, which here lies just below the clavicle (▶ Fig. 4.11 and ▶ Fig. 4.12).

## 4.3.1 Positioning

The patient lies supine; special positioning of the arm is not necessary. If possible, the patient's hand should lie comfortably on his or her abdomen (▶ Fig. 4.13).

## 4.3.2 Needle Approach

The needle approach is performed just below the clavicle strictly vertical (perpendicular) to the surface the patient is lying on (▶ Fig. 4.14 and ▶ Fig. 4.15).

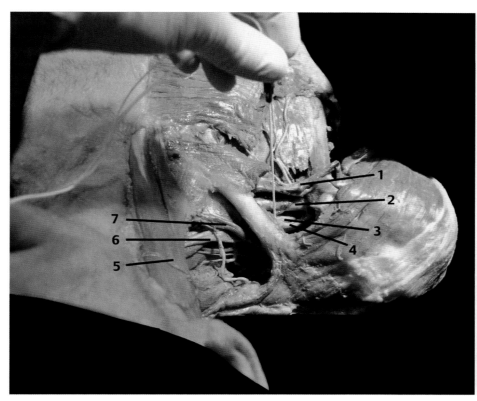

**Fig. 4.15** Anatomy of the infraclavicular region, view from above.
1 Cephalic vein
2 Subclavian artery
3 Lateral cord
4 Posterior cord
5 Sternocleidomastoid
6 Upper trunk
7 Omohyoid with medial cervical fascia

After penetrating clavipectoral fascia, which is often very tough, there is a stimulus response after 2.5 to 4 cm. Peripheral muscle contractions in the fingers are striven for as a response indicating success (posterior cord/radial nerve, lateral cord/median nerve, medial cord/ulnar nerve). Stimulation of the lateral cord only, which leads to contraction of the biceps muscle and/or pronator teres, may result in an incomplete block. In order to obtain a successful response, the needle in this case must be withdrawn to a subcutaneous position, and after moving the skin slightly more laterally (0.5 to 1.0 cm) it should be advanced again vertically to the underlying surface. The desired response is about 0.5 cm deeper and is then usually in the region of the posterior cord, which here lies laterally (care !) and deeper than the lateral cord.

▶ **Needle.** A 4 to 6 cm long insulated needle is used; a catheter technique is possible. The needle is inserted just below the clavicle strictly vertical (perpendicular) to the surface the patient is lying on.

### Tips and Tricks

- Because of the potential danger of a pneumothorax, a medial needle direction, a puncture site too far medially, and excessively deep puncture should be avoided at all costs (▶ Fig. 4.16). The depth of puncture must never be more than 6 cm even in large patients. In slim patients where the distance between the acromion and the jugular notch is short (< 20 cm), the risk of a pneumothorax is increased, as the plexus is sometimes located at a depth of < 3 cm (Neuburger et al 2001). Even when all the rules are followed, a pneumothorax cannot always be avoided (Neuburger et al 2000).
- When the distance from the acromion to the jugular notch is < 20 cm it is advisable to move the puncture site further laterally by 0.3 cm for each centimeter by which the distance falls

below 20 cm (e.g., jugular-acromion distance 17 cm; puncture site not 8.5 cm but 7.6 cm from the anterior end of the acromion or 9.4 cm from the middle of the jugular notch on the J–A line; Neuburger et al 2003).

- The injection point is largely identical with the medial boundary of the "infraclavicular fossa" (clavipectoral trigone or Mohrenheim fossa). The plexus emerges under the clavicle exactly at the lateral margin of the superficial part of pectoralis major. The so-called "finger point" (▶ Fig. 4.17) acts as an additional orientation and thus provides certainty that the correct injection site has been defined. The anesthetist's index finger (right index finger when the right limb is to be blocked, left index finger when the left limb is to be blocked) is placed in the gap between the deltoid and pectoralis major muscles and pressed laterally on the coracoid process. The tip of this finger encounters the clavicle and its ulnar border marks the medial margin of the infraclavicular fossa (deltopectoral groove) and thus the puncture site (Neuburger et al 2003).

▶ **Anterior part of the acromion.** Identification of the anterior end of the acromion is often difficult. It is advisable to look for the lateral margin of the spine of the scapula, called the acromial angle, from behind (▶ Fig. 4.18). This is where the lateral boundary of the acromion commences, and it passes forward at a right angle to the spine of the scapula. If one feels forward along the lateral boundary, one comes automatically to the anterior end of the acromion. If the acromion is now followed over the "vertex" (= anterior end), the acromioclavicular joint is reached, which is medial and slightly dorsal to the anterior end. On no account should the anterior end be confused with the head of the humerus or coracoid process. The humerus moves under the palpating finger during rotation of the arm and so can be well demarcated from the acromion

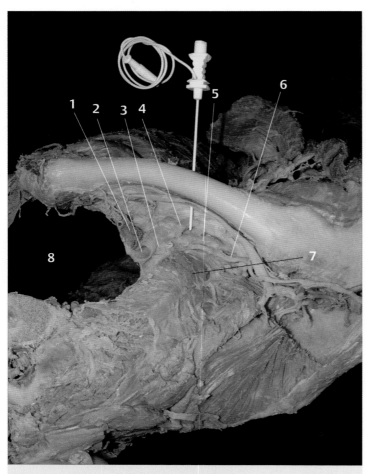

**Fig. 4.16** Anatomy of the infraclavicular region, view from above.
1 Scalenus anterior
2 Subclavian artery
3 Medial cord
4 Lateral cord
5 Posterior cord
6 Suprascapular nerve
7 Scalenus medius
8 Pleural cavity

▶ **Catheter.** Contrary to expectations, a catheter can often be introduced here, although the opening of the needle is relatively vertical to the brachial plexus (▶ Fig. 4.19).

The loss of resistance when the clavipectoral fascia is penetrated does not indicate that the needle is in the correct position, so that this technique is not a "loss-of-resistance" method.

▶ **Puncture site.** Vascular puncture occurs relatively frequently (10–30%; Kilka et al 1995; Neuburger et al 1998). Usually it is not the subclavian artery that is punctured but the cephalic vein or branches of the thoracoacromial trunk that arise from the subclavian artery, which can cross the puncture site in this region (▶ Fig. 4.20). Vascular puncture indicates that the puncture site is too medial.

If there is a response in the pectoralis major muscle, the puncture site is likewise too far medial (the pectoral nerves run medial to the cords) and local contractions of the infraclavicular muscles should not be interpreted as a correct stimulus response.

## 4.3.3 Local Anesthetics, Dosages

Initially: 30 to 50 mL of a short/medium-acting (e.g., mepivacaine 1%, prilocaine 1% [10 mg/mL]) or long-acting (e.g., ropivacaine 0.5–0.75% [5–7.5 mg/mL]) local anesthetic. Complete block of all nerves supplying the arm is usually achieved with this volume (▶ Fig. 4.21). The success rate is reported at 88% and 94.8% for surgical anesthesia.

Continuous block: 5 to 10 mL/h of ropivacaine 0.2 to 0.375% (2–3.75 mg/mL).

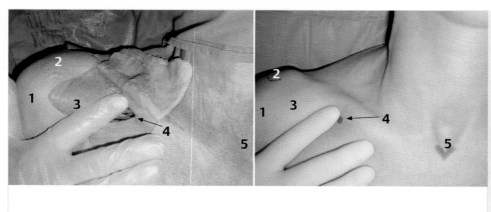

**Fig. 4.17** The so-called "finger point" is helpful in finding the puncture site for vertical infraclavicular plexus anesthesia. To do this, the index finger of the person administering the plexus anesthesia (right index finger with plexus anesthesia on the right) is placed in the patient's infraclavicular fossa. The puncture site determined this way is usually on the ulnar side of this finger. If there are greater deviations, the measurement must be repeated.
1 Head of humerus
2 Acromion
3 Coracoid process
4 Brachial plexus (puncture site)
5 Jugular notch

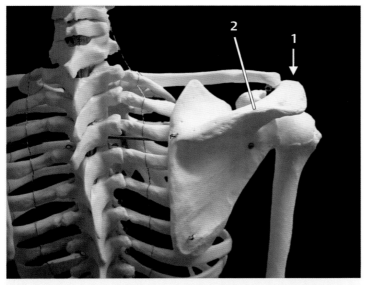

Fig. 4.18 Scapula, orientation to the anterior part of the acromion over the spine of the scapula.
1 Anterior part of the acromion
2 Spine of the scapula

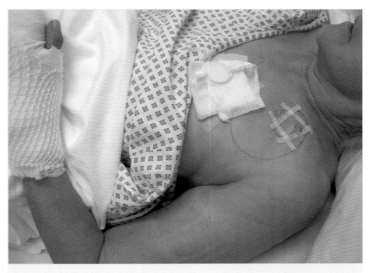

Fig. 4.19 Indwelling infraclavicular plexus catheter in place.

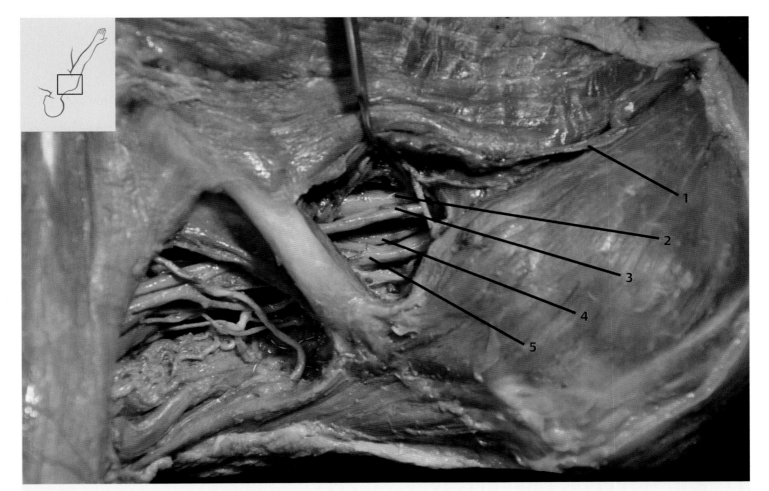

Fig. 4.20 Anatomy of the infraclavicular region, view from above.
1 Cephalic vein
2 Subclavian artery
3 Lateral cord
4 Medial cord
5 Posterior cord

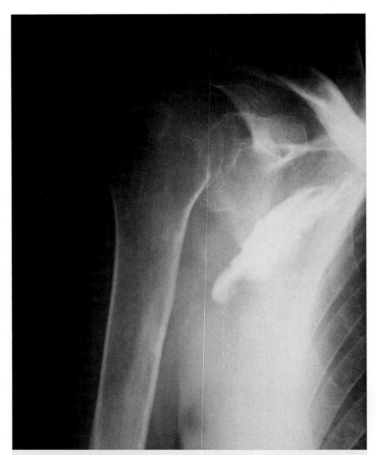

Fig. 4.21 Contrast medium visualization of the infraclavicular region in vertical infraclavicular plexus anesthesia.

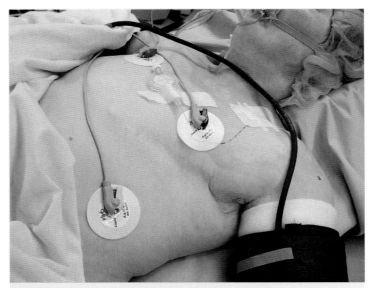

Fig. 4.22 Differential indication for infraclavicular plexus block versus axillary plexus block: previous mastectomy with axillary lymph node clearance.

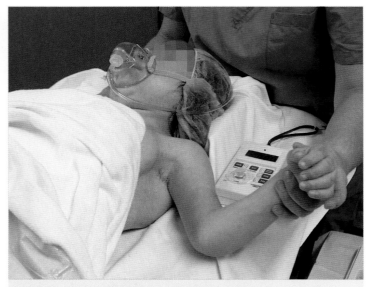

Fig. 4.23 Differential indication for infraclavicular plexus block versus axillary plexus block: frozen shoulder with inability to abduct the arm.

### 4.3.4 Comparison of the Vertical Infraclavicular Technique with the Axillary Technique

The range of indications for the two approaches to the brachial plexus is largely identical. With complex injuries of the arm, abduction can be very painful. If there has been previous surgery (breast surgery with axillary lymph node clearance; ▶ Fig. 4.22) or frozen shoulder (▶ Fig. 4.23), axillary blockade is not feasible. In this case, techniques close to the clavicle, which can be performed without abduction of the arm, are of benefit (vertical infraclavicular plexus anesthesia or supraclavicular techniques). The vertical infraclavicular technique is characterized by a faster onset of effect and a greater success rate, particularly compared to the perivascular axillary technique (Neuburger et al 1998). Ultrasound guidance is not possible in the vertical infraclavicular technique.

## 4.4 Raj Technique, Modified by Borgeat ▶

The technique described by Raj et al (1973) was modified by Borgeat et al (2001). The modified technique is also suitable for

placing a catheter (continuous technique due to the lateral needle direction).

### 4.4.1 Positioning

The patient lies supine with the head turned to the opposite side. The puncture site is identical with the puncture site for vertical infraclavicular plexus anesthesia. The injection point is half way between the anterior part of the acromion and the middle of the jugular notch about 1 cm below the clavicle (▶ Fig. 4.24 and ▶ Fig. 4.25).

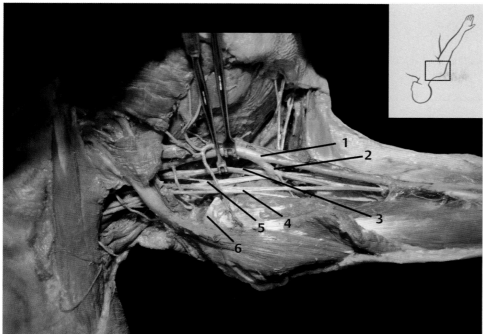

**Fig. 4.24** Anatomy of the infraclavicular region: Raj technique (view from above).
1 Axillary artery
2 Deep brachial artery with branch of the posterior circumflex humeral artery
3 Middle cord
4 Lateral cord
5 Posterior cord
6 Coracoid process

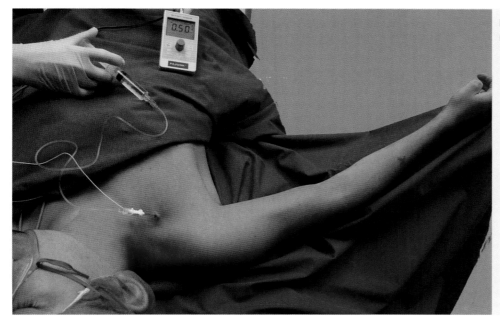

**Fig. 4.25** Infraclavicular plexus anesthesia, modified Raj technique.

## 4.4.2 Needle Approach

The injection point is determined with the arm adducted. For needle insertion, the arm is abducted 90° and elevated about 30°. The needle is directed laterally to the most proximal point at which the axillary artery can still just be palpated in the axilla (▶ Fig. 4.26, ▶ Fig. 4.27, ▶ Fig. 4.28, ▶ Fig. 4.29). The angle to the skin is approximately 45 to 60°. After about 3 to 8 cm a response is obtained in the arm, wrist, or hand. In order to obtain a satisfactory success rate, a distal response in the hand or fingers should be striven for (Minville et al 2007).

## 4.4.3 Material

Needle: 6 to 10 cm; a continuous technique is possible.

> **Practical Notes**
>
> Because of the lateral direction of the needle, the danger of pneumothorax is lower. Needle insertion under ultrasound guidance allows an especially good anatomical overview (Chapter 4.4.5).

Vascular puncture (usually venous, cephalic vein) is observed.

Because of the tangential approach to the plexus, a catheter can be advanced readily (▶ Fig. 4.29). Using ultrasound, the infraclavicular block can be performed using the Klaastad method (Klaastad et al 2004, Sauter et al 2006). A catheter can also be easily advanced using this method (▶ Fig. 4.30).

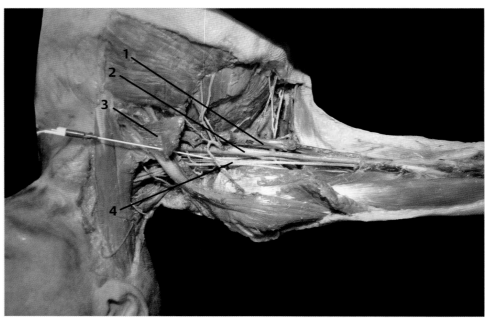

**Fig. 4.26** Anatomy of the infraclavicular region, Raj technique.
1 Subclavian vein
2 Subclavian artery
3 Pectoralis major
4 Lateral cord

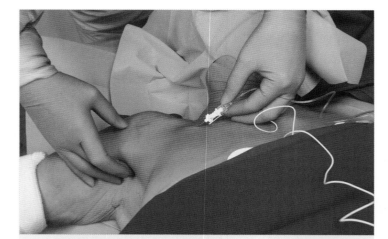

**Fig. 4.27** Needle direction. The needle is directed to the most proximal point where the axillary artery can still be palpated in the axilla.

### 4.4.4 Local Anesthetics, Dosages

Initially: 30 to 50 mL of a short/medium-acting (e.g., mepivacaine 1% [10 mg/mL], prilocaine 1% [10 mg/mL]) or long-acting (e.g., ropivacaine 0.5–0.75% [5–7.5 mg/mL]) local anesthetic. This volume usually results in adequate block of all nerves supplying the arm (▶ Fig. 4.31 and ▶ Fig. 4.32).

Continuous block: Ropivacaine 0.2 to 0.375% (2–3.75 mg/mL), 5 to 10 mL/h.

## 4.5 Infraclavicular Brachial Plexus Block Using Ultrasound ▶

Linear transducer: 7.5 to 10 MHz (alternatively curved array 2–6 MHz)
Needle: 6 to 10 cm

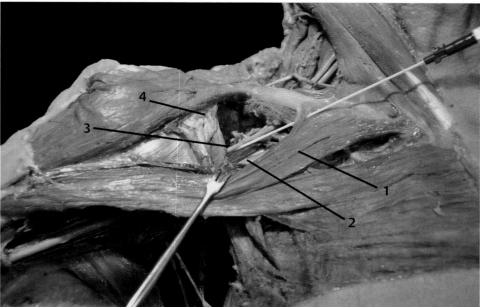

**Fig. 4.28** Raj technique, needle direction.
1 Pectoralis major
2 Subclavian artery
3 Lateral cord
4 Coracoid process

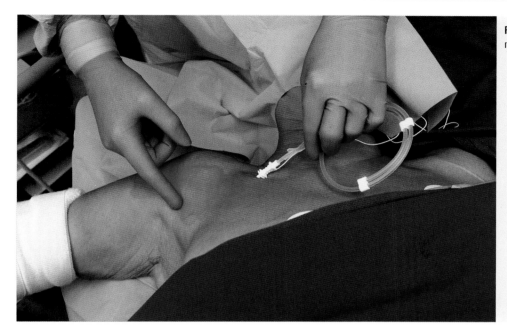

Fig. 4.29 Placing a catheter (Raj technique, modified by Borgeat).

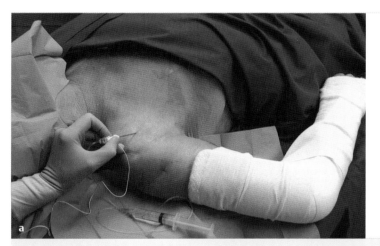

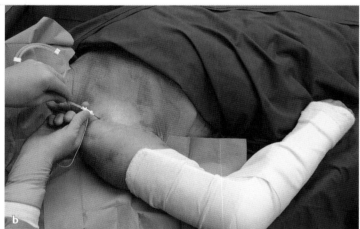

Fig. 4.30 Infraclavicular plexus blocks (here according to Klaastad) should be performed under ultrasound guidance.
a Needle direction.
b Advancing a catheter.

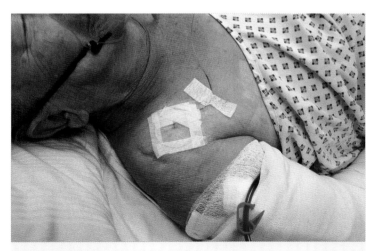

Fig. 4.31 Infraclavicular plexus catheter.

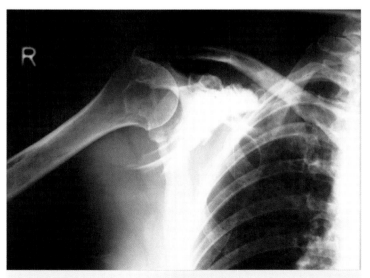

Fig. 4.32 Infraclavicular plexus block, Raj technique; spread of contrast medium.

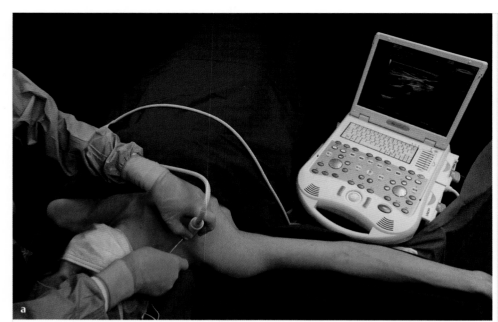

**Fig. 4.33** Infraclavicular plexus anesthesia, "sonoanatomy," see also ► Fig. 4.34 (enlarged section).
Line (dash-dot): course of needle in the in-plane technique.
**a** Clinical setting.
**b** Anatomical section (unlabeled).
**c** Anatomical section (labeled).
1 Pectoralis major
2 Pectoralis minor
3 Rib
4 Axillary vein
5 Axillary artery
6 Scapula
7 Medial cord
8 Posterior cord
9 Lateral cord
10 Clavicle

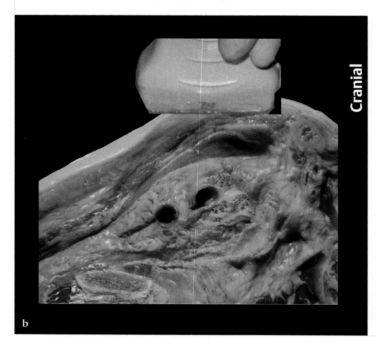

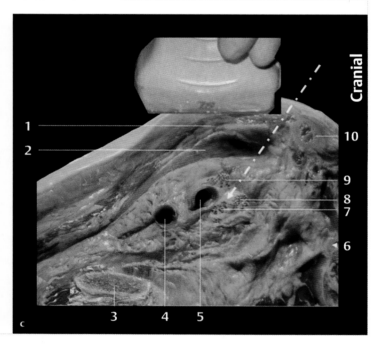

## 4.5.1 Ultrasound Visualization of the Brachial Plexus

The vertical infraclavicular plexus anesthesia described in Chapter 4.3 cannot be performed as an ultrasound-guided block, because the position of the transducer makes a vertical puncture impossible. The plexus also lies in the "shadow" of the clavicle.

For an ultrasound guided infraclavicular puncture, the brachial plexus is found somewhat further laterally in the infraclavicular fossa (Mohrenheim fossa) using the infraclavicular Raj technique described in Chapter 4.4. A comparable method was also described by Klaastad et al (2004). In this region, the cords were shown to be in the immediate vicinity of the axillary artery (Sauter et al 2006). The position of the cords relative to the artery changes within a few centimeters from proximal to peripheral direction. In the proximal infraclavicular region, the posterior cord is located furthest laterally; the lateral cord anterior to it is

somewhat further medially (► Fig. 4.33 and ► Fig. 4.34; see Chapter 4.3). Somewhat further distally (laterally), the posterior cord lies below the axillary artery, the lateral cord lateral to, and the medial cord medial to, the axillary artery (► Fig. 4.36).

The transducer is placed medial to the coracoid process in the sagittal plane. The arm can be adducted.

> **Practical Note**
>
> Abducting the arm by 90° improves visualization of the structures: The cords are bundled more and closer to the surface of the body.

Orientation is primarily along the axillary artery, which in this technique appears as a circular, echo-free structure (pulsating). In this region, the cords are very difficult to differentiate from the surrounding tissue (► Fig. 4.34 and ► Fig. 4.35), often only after a

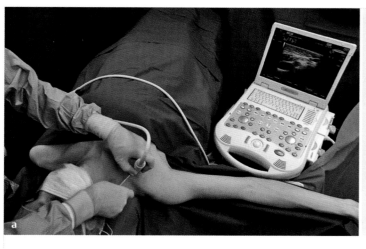

**Fig. 4.34** Infraclavicular plexus anesthesia: "sonoanatomy" (section from ► Fig. 4.33).
1 Pectoralis major
2 Pectoralis minor
3 Axillary vein
4 Axillary artery
5 Cords
a Clinical setting.
b Ultrasound finding (unlabeled).
c Corresponding anatomical section (unlabeled).
d Ultrasound finding (labeled).
e Corresponding anatomical section (labeled).

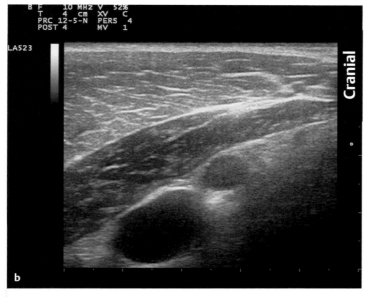

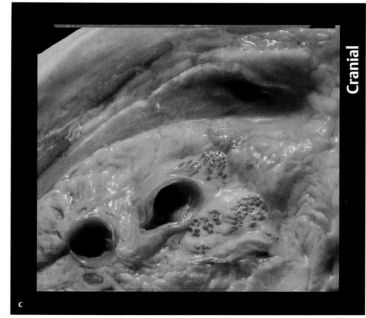

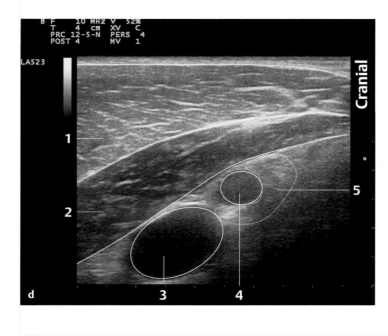

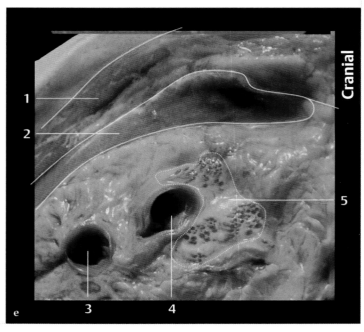

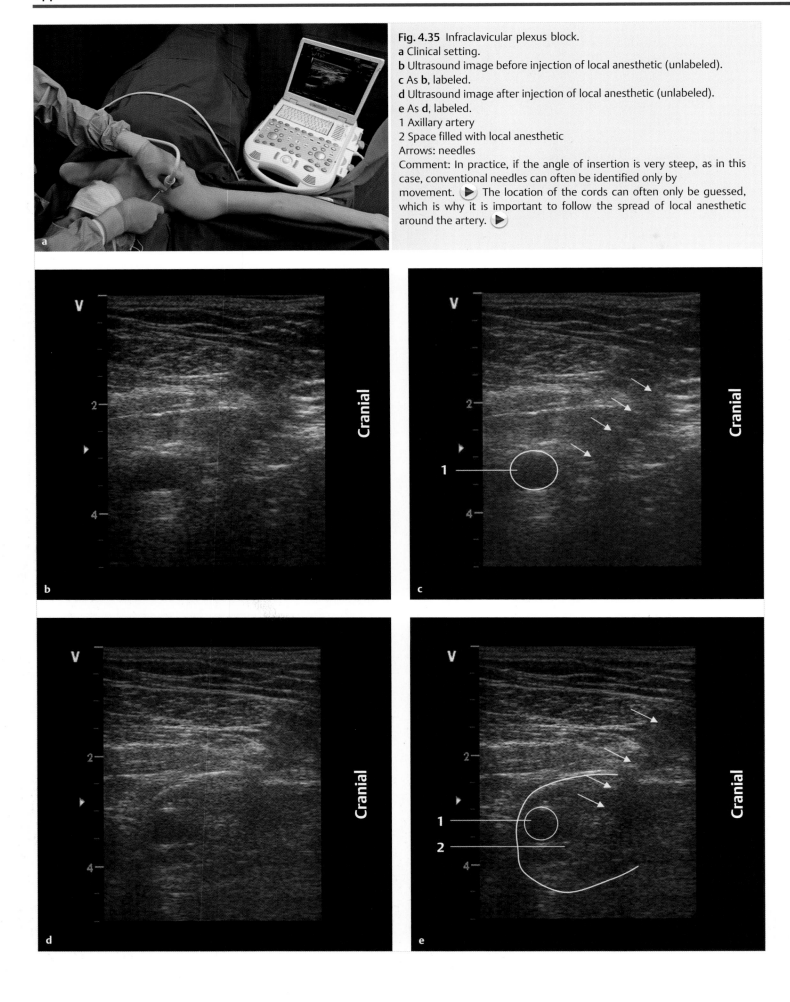

**Fig. 4.35** Infraclavicular plexus block.
**a** Clinical setting.
**b** Ultrasound image before injection of local anesthetic (unlabeled).
**c** As **b**, labeled.
**d** Ultrasound image after injection of local anesthetic (unlabeled).
**e** As **d**, labeled.
1 Axillary artery
2 Space filled with local anesthetic
Arrows: needles
Comment: In practice, if the angle of insertion is very steep, as in this case, conventional needles can often be identified only by movement. ▶ The location of the cords can often only be guessed, which is why it is important to follow the spread of local anesthetic around the artery. ▶

fluid is injected (e.g., local anesthetic). When the cords become visible, they are hyperechoic (light) in this region, in contrast to the supraclavicular region (▶ Fig. 4.36). This is explained by the increasing amount of connective tissue in relation to the axons (see also Chapter 1). The axillary artery with the cords in its immediate vicinity lies at an average depth of 3 to 4 cm. When the transducer is angled medially for orientation, the rib and pleura can be visualized.

## 4.5.2 Needle Approach

▶ **In-plane approach.** The needle is inserted "in-plane" from cranial to caudal (see ▶ Fig. 4.33, ▶ Fig. 4.34, ▶ Fig. 4.35, ▶ Fig. 4.36) at an angle of 45 to 60° below the clavicle until the tip of the needle is immediately posterior to the axillary artery. After the resistance felt when penetrating the clavipectoral fascia there is sometimes a second perceptible loss of resistance on penetration of the septum, which runs posterior and lateral to the axillary artery and can prevent even spread to all three cords

(Morimoto et al 2007, Lévesque et al 2008). This septum must be overcome to achieve a reliable block. A U-shaped (below and at both sides of the artery; Dingemans et al 2007) or circular spread around the axillary artery (▶ Fig. 4.35 and ▶ Fig. 4.36) is striven for. In particular it should be noted that the local anesthetic spreads posterior to the axillary artery in order to reach the posterior cord (▶ Fig. 4.36).

▶ **Out-of-plane approach.** An out-of-plane approach using the modified Raj technique (see Chapter 4.4) is possible. Placement and positioning of the transducer are the same as in the in-plane approach; the axillary artery is set at the center of the image. The direction of insertion is vertical to the transducer from medial to lateral. The angle of the needle should be relatively steep (puncture ca. 2 cm medial to the transducer). The tip of the needle should come to a stop below the axillary artery; spread should be circular or U-shaped around the axillary artery (▶ Fig. 4.37). The out-of-plane technique has an increased risk of puncturing a vessel.

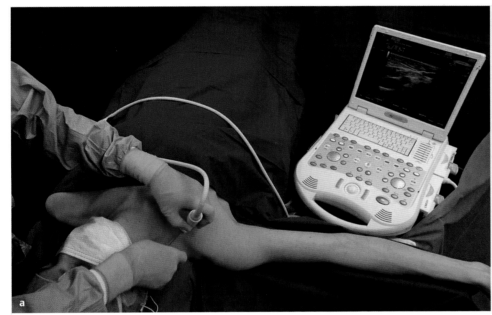

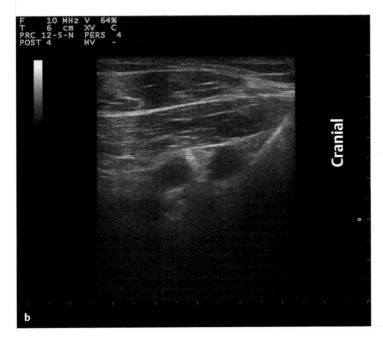

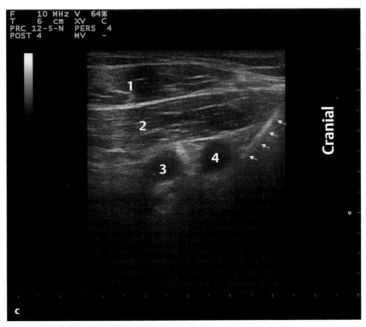

**Fig. 4.36 a–g** Infraclavicular block with ultrasound "in plane," visualization in the short axis.
**a** Clinical setting.
**b** Before injection of local anesthetic (unlabeled).
**c** As **b**, unlabeled.
Comment: In **b**, the cords cannot be definitely identified; the posterior cord in particular can be hidden by the axillary artery in the acoustic enhancement. In **d**, the posterior cord is prominent; it can be clearly distinguished from the posterior acoustic enhancement and appears to be displaced posteriorly. In **f**, the local anesthetic is clearly visualized as a hypoechoic area. The lateral cord cannot be definitely identified. Note: the special "ultrasound needle" is clearly more visible here than in ▶ Fig. 4.35, despite the steep insertion angle.

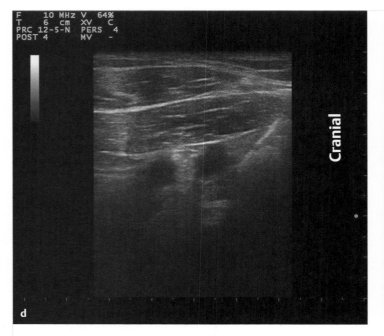

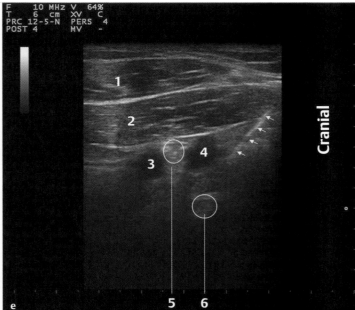

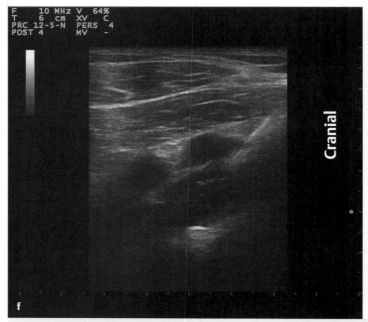

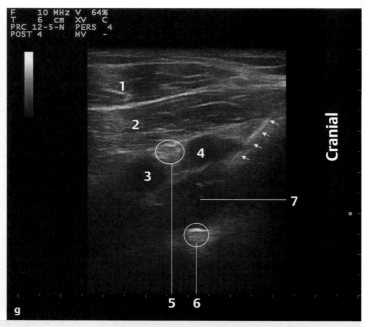

**Fig.4.36 a–g (continued)**
**d** After injection of a few milliliters of local anesthetic (unlabeled).
**e** As **d**, labeled.
**f** After injection of 15 mL of local anesthetic (unlabeled).
**g** As **f**, labeled.

1 Pectoralis major
2 Pectoralis minor
3 Axillary vein
4 Axillary artery
5 Medial cord
6 Posterior cord
7 Local anesthetic
Arrows: Needle (SonoPlex needle, Pajunk GmbH)

## 4.5.3 Catheter Placement

A catheter can be placed using the same technique; the catheter should not be advanced too far (approx. 3 cm; Dhir and Ganapathy 2008). Experience shows the catheter can also be readily placed using the in-plane technique.

---

**Tips and Tricks**

- Combination with nerve stimulation is possible, but has no extra advantage (Gürkan et al 2010).
- Since the cords are difficult to identify in this region, orientation is primarily using the axillary artery (Dingemans et al 2007, Koscielniak-Nielsen et al 2009, Fredrickson et al 2010).
- The tip of the needle should come to a stop posterior to the axillary artery; a circular or U-shaped spread around the axillary artery should be striven for; the axillary artery should displace anteriorly when the injection is made (▶ Fig. 4.36).
- The puncture angle is unexpectedly steep (> 45°, often 60°), thus the visualization of the needle is difficult if conventional needles are used (▶ Fig. 4.35; see also Chapter 1).
- The volume required for the block is reported to be 30 to 40 mL.
- The onset time is 20 to 30 minutes.
- Tran et al describe the "double bubble sign" to verify the correct position of the needle posterior to the axillary artery (Tran et al 2006). After definitive positioning of the needle, 2 mL of local anesthetic are injected. If the needle location is correct, two bubbles, one over the other, can be seen: the axillary artery is the top bubble and the depot of the local anesthetic is the lower bubble (slightly visible in ▶ Fig. 4.36). If this image is not seen, the needle position must be corrected.
- A "multi-injection technique" has no advantage compared with the single injection under the axillary artery (Tran et al 2008, Fredrickson et al 2010).

---

## 4.6 Sensory and Motor Effects

In the region of the clavicle, the divisions and cords of the brachial plexus lie very close together so that profound sensory and motor block of all the nerves supplying the arm can be expected here. The nerves that leave the plexus further cranially (e.g., suprascapular nerve) are not included. An interscalene block should be performed for anesthesia and analgesia in the region of the shoulder and proximal upper arm. Because of the similar indications for axillary and infraclavicular brachial plexus block, the risks and benefits of these techniques must be weighed against one another.

## 4.7 Indications and Contraindications

### 4.7.1 Indications

Anesthesia or analgesia and sympathetic block in the distal upper arm, elbow, forearm, and hand. An increase in skin temperature (see Chapter 21.3.3) as a sign of sympathetic block after applying infraclavicular plexus anesthesia was proven by Minville et al (2009).

### 4.7.2 Contraindications

▶ **Contralateral phrenic nerve paresis.** While a varying incidence of phrenic nerve paresis is reported with supraclavicular blocks (Neal et al 1998), this complication is less likely with infraclavicular block (Rodriguez et al 1998) but can occur (Stadlmeyer et al 2000). For this reason, contralateral phrenic nerve paresis should be regarded as a contraindication to infraclavicular plexus anesthesia also, particularly in the case of the vertical technique.

▶ **Contralateral recurrent nerve paresis.** Similarly to phrenic nerve paresis, potential recurrent nerve paresis can be expected because of the anatomical proximity in both supraclavicular and infraclavicular block, although there have been no reports of this in association with the infraclavicular technique.

▶ **Respiratory insufficiency.** Marked respiratory insufficiency is regarded as a relative contraindication.

▶ **Other contraindications.** Chest deformities and clavicular fractures that have healed with dislocation make anatomical orientation difficult, so the risk of a pneumothorax is increased.

A *bilateral block* is also regarded as contraindicated due to the risk of pneumothorax, as it is in the case of an existing contralateral pneumothorax, or status after contralateral pneumonectomy.

## 4.8 Complications, Side Effects, Method-Specific Problems

### 4.8.1 Horner Syndrome

An incidence between 1% and 6.9% is reported with the infraclavicular vertical technique (Kilka et al 1995, Neuburger et al 1998).

Hoarseness and a foreign body sensation in the throat are presumably caused by block of the recurrent laryngeal nerve.

Horner syndrome and hoarseness are side effects rather than complications. These phenomena are usually of shorter duration than the actual block effect and are rarely observed to be lasting with a continuous block.

### 4.8.2 Phrenic Nerve Paresis

Impairment of diaphragm mobility was shown by Rettig et al (2005). There have been reports of acute respiratory insufficiency in association with vertical infraclavicular block, due to unilateral phrenic nerve paresis (Stadlmeyer et al 2000, Gentili et al 2002, Heid et al 2002).

For this reason, marked respiratory insufficiency is regarded as a relative contraindication for vertical infraclavicular block. The modified technique according to Raj was not reported to adversely affect diaphragmatic function (Dullenkopf et al 2004).

### 4.8.3 Pneumothorax

*Pneumothorax* is a feared complication of all blocks performed close to the clavicle. The reported incidence varies between 0.06% and 6% (Neuburger et al 1998, Jankovic et al 2000, Gauss et al 2014), depending on the block technique. This complication must

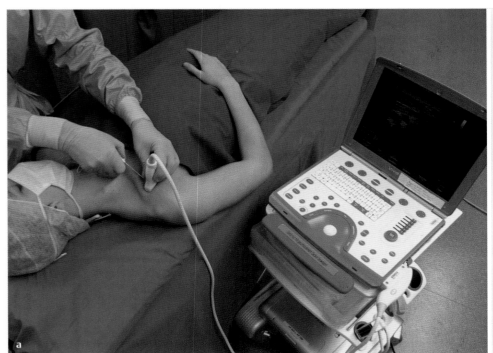

**Fig. 4.37** Infraclavicular out-of-plane block.
1 Axillary vein
2 Axillary artery
3 Tip of needle (optimal position)
4 Cord
5 Pectoralis minor
6 Pectoralis major
Comment: The position of the tip of the needle can be clearly identified only in a moving image. The point was determined using the video image.
**a** Clinical setting.
**b** Ultrasound image (unlabeled).
**c** Ultrasound image (labeled).

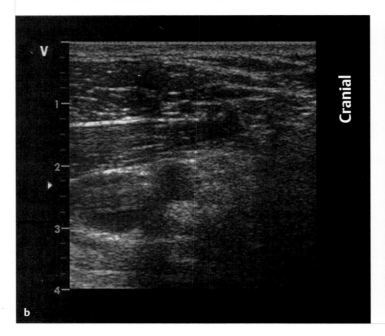

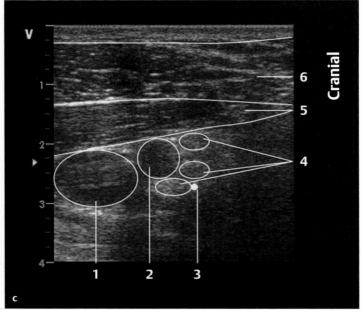

always be anticipated and the patient must be informed accordingly. Particularly in conjunction with general anesthesia with positive-pressure ventilation (e.g., incomplete block for operation with subsequent intubation), the development of a life-threatening tension pneumothorax must be considered. A unilateral decrease in breath sounds after the block is given must be distinguished in the differential diagnosis from ipsilateral phrenic nerve paresis. Particularly because of the danger of pneumothorax, ambulant regional anesthesia in this region is regarded as a relative contraindication and requires special informed consent.

# References

Bhatia A, Lai J, Chan VW, Brull R. Case report: pneumothorax as a complication of the ultrasound-guided supraclavicular approach for brachial plexus block. Anesth Analg 2010; 111: 817–819

Borgeat A, Ekatodramis G, Dumont C. An evaluation of the infraclavicular block via a modified approach of the Raj technique. Anesth Analg 2001; 93: 436–441

Dhir S, Ganapathy S. Comparative evaluation of ultrasound-guided continuous infraclavicular brachial plexus block with stimulating catheter and traditional technique: a prospective-randomized trial. Acta Anaesthesiol Scand 2008; 52: 1158–1166

Dingemans E, Williams SR, Arcand G et al. Neurostimulation in ultrasound-guided infraclavicular block: a prospective randomized trial. Anesth Analg 2007; 104: 1275–1280

Dullenkopf A, Blumenthal S, Theodorou P, Roos J, Perschak H, Borgeat A. Diaphragmatic excursion and respiratory function after the modified Raj technique of the infraclavicular plexus block. Reg Anesth Pain Med 2004; 29: 110–114

Fredrickson MJ, Patel A, Young S, Chinchanwala S. Speed of onset of "corner pocket supraclavicular" and infraclavicular ultrasound guided brachial plexus block: a randomised observer-blinded comparison. Anaesthesia 2009; 64: 738–744

Fredrickson MJ, Wolstencroft P, Kejriwal R, Yoon A, Boland MR, Chinchanwala S. Single versus triple injection ultrasound-guided infraclavicular block: confirmation of the effectiveness of the single injection technique. Anesth Analg 2010; 111: 1325–1327

Gauss A, Tugtekin I, Georgieff M, Dinse-Lambracht A, Keipke D, Gorsewski G. Incidence of clinically symptomatic pneumothorax in ultrasound-guided infraclavicular and supraclavicular brachial plexus block. Anaesthesia 2014; 69: 327–336

Gentili ME, Deleuze A, Estèbe JP, Lebourg M, Ecoffey C. Severe respiratory failure after infraclavicular block with 0.75% ropivacaine: a case report. J Clin Anesth 2002; 14: 459–461

Gürkan Y, Tekin M, Acar S, Solak M, Toker K. Is nerve stimulation needed during an ultrasound-guided lateral sagittal infraclavicular block? Acta Anaesthesiol Scand 2010; 54: 403–407

Heid FM, Kern T, Brambrink AM. Transient respiratory compromise after infraclavicular vertical brachial plexus blockade. Eur J Anaesthesiol 2002; 19: 693–694

Jankovic D. Regionalblockaden in Klinik und Praxis. 2nd ed. Berlin: Blackwell; 2000: 58–86

Kilka HG, Geiger P, Mehrkens HH. Infraclavicular vertical brachial plexus blockade. A new method for anesthesia of the upper extremity. An anatomical and clinical study. [Article in German] Anaesthesist 1995; 44: 339–344

Klaastad Ø, Smith HJ, Smedby O et al. A novel infraclavicular brachial plexus block: the lateral and sagittal technique, developed by magnetic resonance imaging studies. Anesth Analg 2004; 98: 252–256

Koscielniak-Nielsen ZJ, Frederiksen BS, Rasmussen H, Hesselbjerg L. A comparison of ultrasound-guided supraclavicular and infraclavicular blocks for upper extremity surgery. Acta Anaesthesiol Scand 2009; 53: 620–626

Kulenkampff D. Die Anästhesierung des Plexus brachialis. Zentralbl Chir 1911; 38: 1337

Lévesque S, Dion N, Desgagné MC. Endpoint for successful, ultrasound-guided infraclavicular brachial plexus block. Can J Anaesth 2008; 55: 308–309, author reply 308–309

Mariano ER, Sandhu NS, Loland VJ et al. A randomized comparison of infraclavicular and supraclavicular continuous peripheral nerve blocks for postoperative analgesia. Reg Anesth Pain Med 2011; 36: 26–31

Minville V, Fourcade O, Bourdet B et al. The optimal motor response for infraclavicular brachial plexus block. Anesth Analg 2007; 104: 448–451

Minville V, Gendre A, Hirsch J et al. The efficacy of skin temperature for block assessment after infraclavicular brachial plexus block. Anesth Analg 2009; 108: 1034–1036

Morimoto M, Popovic J, Kim JT, Kiamzon H, Rosenberg AD. Case series: Septa can influence local anesthetic spread during infraclavicular brachial plexus blocks. Can J Anaesth 2007; 54: 1006–1010

Neal JM, Moore JM, Kopacz DJ, Liu SS, Kramer DJ, Plorde JJ. Quantitative analysis of respiratory, motor, and sensory function after supraclavicular block. Anesth Analg 1998; 86: 1239–1244

Neuburger M, Kaiser H, Rembold-Schuster I. Vertical infraclavicular brachial-plexus blockade. A clinical study of reliability of a new method for plexus anesthesia of the upper extremity. [Article in German] Anaesthesist 1998; 47: 595–599

Neuburger M, Landes H, Kaiser H. Pneumothorax in vertical infraclavicular block of the brachial plexus. Review of a rare complication. [Article in German] Anaesthesist 2000; 49: 901–904

Neuburger M, Kaiser H, Uhl M. Biometric data on risk of pneumothorax from vertical infraclavicular brachial plexus block. A magnetic resonance imaging study. [Article in German] Anaesthesist 2001; 50: 511–516

Neuburger M, Kaiser H, Åss B, Franke C, Maurer H. Vertical infraclavicular blockade of the brachial plexus (VIP). A modified method to verify the puncture point under consideration of the risk of pneumothorax. Anaesthesist 2003; 52: 619–624

Perlas A, Lobo G, Lo N, Brull R, Chan VW, Karkhanis R. Ultrasound-guided supraclavicular block: outcome of 510 consecutive cases. Reg Anesth Pain Med 2009; 34: 171–176

Raj PP, Montgomery SJ, Nettles D, Jenkins MT. Infraclavicular brachial plexus block—a new approach. Anesth Analg 1973; 52: 897–904

Rettig HC, Gielen MJ, Boersma E, Klein J, Groen GJ. Vertical infraclavicular block of the brachial plexus: effects on hemidiaphragmatic movement and ventilatory function. Reg Anesth Pain Med 2005; 30: 529–535

Rodríguez J, Bárcena M, Rodríguez V, Aneiros F, Alvarez J. Infraclavicular brachial plexus block effects on respiratory function and extent of the block. Reg Anesth Pain Med 1998; 23: 564–568

Sauter AR, Smith HJ, Stubhaug A, Dodgson MS, Klaastad Ø. Use of magnetic resonance imaging to define the anatomical location closest to all three cords of the infraclavicular brachial plexus. Anesth Analg 2006; 103: 1574–1576

Soares LG, Brull R, Lai J, Chan VW. Eight ball, corner pocket: the optimal needle position for ultrasound-guided supraclavicular block. Reg Anesth Pain Med 2007; 32: 94–95

Stadlmeyer D, Neubauer J, Finkl RO, Groh J. Unilateral phrenic nerve paralysis after vertical infraclavicular plexus block. [Article in German] Anaesthesist 2000; 49: 1030–1033

Tran QH, Charghi R, Finlayson RJ. The "double bubble" sign for successful infraclavicular brachial plexus blockade. Anesth Analg 2006; 103: 1048–1049

Tran QH, Clemente A, Tran DQ, Finlayson RJ. A comparison between ultrasound-guided infraclavicular block using the "double bubble" sign and neurostimulation-guided axillary block. Anesth Analg 2008; 107: 1075–1078

Tran QH, Munoz L, Russo G, Finlayson RJ. A trick shot to the corner pocket. Reg Anesth Pain Med 2008; 33: 503–504, author reply 504

Winnie AP, Collins VJ. The subclavian perivascular technique of brachial plexus anesthesia. Anesthesiology 1964; 25: 353–363

# 5 Suprascapular Nerve Block

## 5.1 Anatomy

The upper trunk is formed by the roots of C5/C6. The suprascapular nerve branches from the brachial plexus in the region of the upper trunk (▶ Fig. 5.1 and ▶ Fig. 5.2). It continues along the lateral border of the brachial plexus in the supraclavicular fossa as far as the scapular notch. After passing through the notch, which is bordered by the sometimes calcified superior transverse scapular ligament, it reaches the supraspinous fossa (▶ Fig. 5.3).

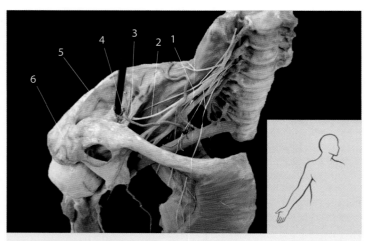

**Fig. 5.1** Course of the suprascapular nerve.
1 Upper trunk
2 Suprascapular nerve
3 Transverse ligament
4 Suprascapular artery
5 Spine of scapula
6 Acromion

The supraspinous fossa is shaped like a tub. On the floor of this "tub," the nerve runs laterally and then passes along the posterior branch of the neck of the scapula to reach the infraspinous fossa and shoulder. It divides into a motor branch to the supraspinatus and infraspinatus muscles and gives off a sensory branch to the shoulder (▶ Fig. 5.4, ▶ Fig. 5.5, ▶ Fig. 5.6).

## 5.2 Meier Approach ▶

Meier et al (2002) were able to show from anatomical studies that dye, when injected on the floor of the supraspinous fossa, drains out through the notch and thus definitely reaches the suprascapular nerve (▶ Fig. 5.7). Dangoisse et al (1994) and Feigl et al (2007) also arrived at similar results.

### 5.2.1 Procedure

The patient is in sitting position with the head bent slightly forward. A line is drawn from the medial end of the spine of the scapula to the lateral posterior border of the acromion. Half way along this line, the injection site is established 2 cm medial and 2 cm cranial from this point (▶ Fig. 5.8 and ▶ Fig. 5.9).

A 6-cm needle is advanced in a lateral direction on the floor of the supraspinous fossa at an angle of 75° to the skin surface. The needle should be directed roughly toward the head of the humerus (▶ Fig. 5.10). For a continuous technique, the catheter is advanced 2 to 3 cm ahead (▶ Fig. 5.11 and ▶ Fig. 5.12).

### Material

Needle: 6 cm

Continuous technique: pencil-point needle (catheter-through-needle technique)

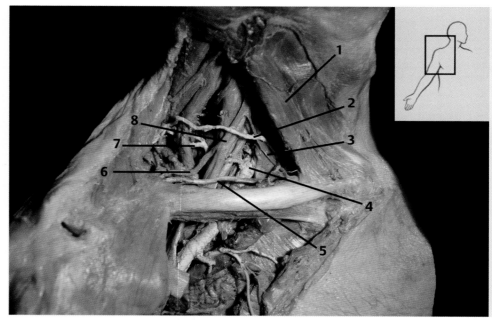

**Fig. 5.2** Suprascapular nerve, origin from upper trunk.
1 Sternocleidomastoid
2 Superficial cervical artery
3 Scalenus anterior muscle with phrenic nerve
4 Subclavian artery
5 Suprascapular artery
6 Suprascapular nerve
7 Dorsal scapular artery
8 Upper trunk

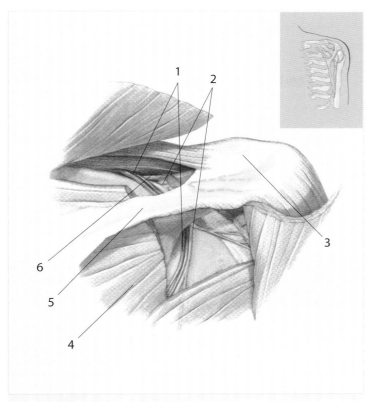

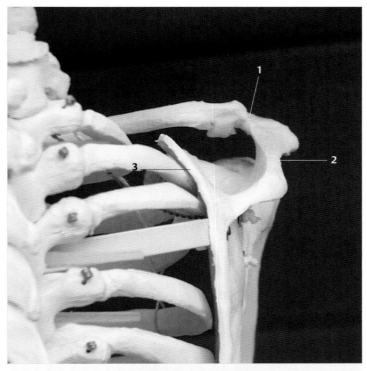

**Fig. 5.3** Scapula, seen from behind.
1 Suprascapular artery and vein
2 Suprascapular nerve
3 Acromion
4 Infraspinatus
5 Spine of the scapula
6 Transverse ligament

**Fig. 5.4** Scapula, seen obliquely from behind. Note "tub" shape between the scapula and the spine of the scapula (supraspinous fossa).
1 Acromion
2 Spine of the scapula
3 Scapula

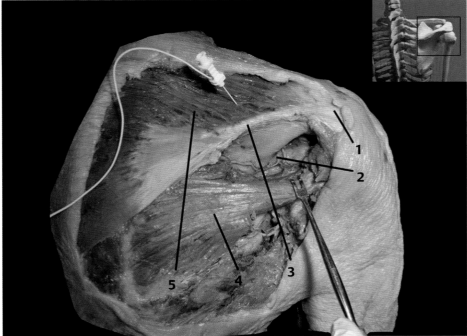

**Fig. 5.5** Suprascapular nerve block, Meier approach (view from behind).
1 Acromion
2 Suprascapular nerve
3 Spine of the scapula
4 Infraspinatus
5 Trapezius

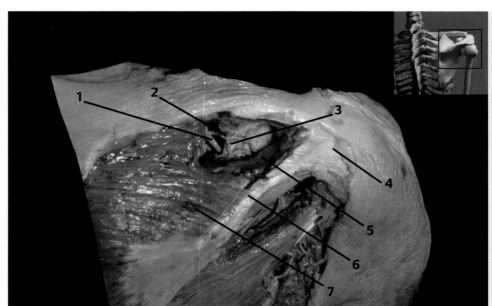

**Fig. 5.6** Suprascapular nerve block, Meier approach (view from behind).
1 Suprascapular nerve
2 Suprascapular artery
3 Superior transverse scapular ligament
4 Acromion
5 Supraspinatus
6 Spine of the scapula
7 Trapezius

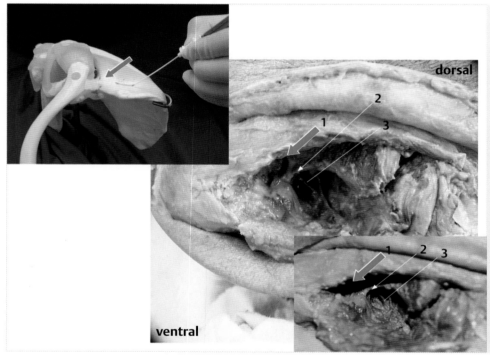

**Fig. 5.7** Right shoulder region, seen from above after injection of dye into the supraspinous fossa. Note the passage of the dye through the scapular notch with staining of the suprascapular nerve. Dissection in prone position.
1 Dye in the supraspinous fossa
2 Transverse ligament with scapular notch
3 Suprascapular nerve before its passage through the scapular notch, bathed in dye

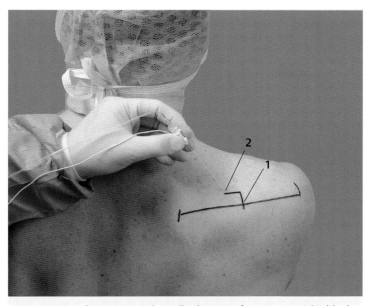

**Fig. 5.8** Site of injection and needle direction for suprascapular block, Meier approach.
1 Middle of spine of the scapula
2 Injection site (2 cm cranial and 2 cm medial to the middle of the spine of the scapula)

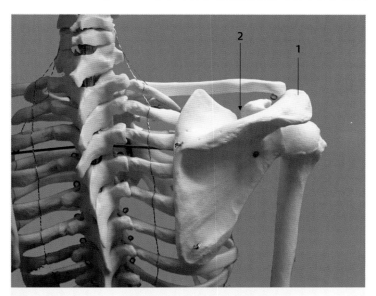

**Fig. 5.9** Scapula, seen from behind. Note "tub" shape.
1 Acromion
2 Scapular notch

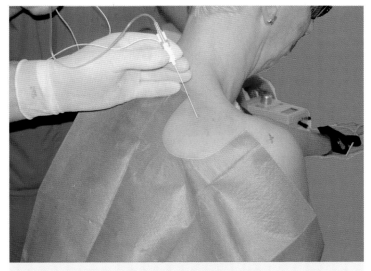

**Fig. 5.10** Suprascapular nerve block, Meier approach: needle direction.

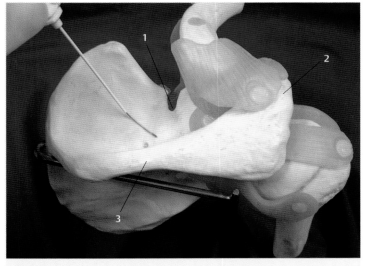

**Fig. 5.11** Supraspinous fossa, seen from above: position of indwelling catheter.
1 Scapular notch
2 Acromion
3 Spine of the scapula

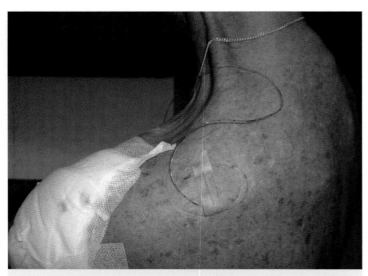

**Fig. 5.12** Suprascapular nerve catheter for postoperative pain therapy. Alternative when an interscalene plexus catheter is not possible.

---

**Tips and Tricks**

- The block can be performed with or without a nerve stimulator. The presence of a motor response at 0.5 mA and 0.1 ms shows that the needle is in the correct position. If no nerve stimulator is used, bone contact is found and the needle is then withdrawn somewhat.
- A catheter can be advanced without difficulty using a pencil-point needle with lateral opening that should be facing laterally.
- The block technique takes advantage of the fact that the blade of the scapula forms a "tub" with the spine of the scapula that can be filled with local anesthetic. Local anesthetic thus reaches the suprascapular nerve through the scapular notch. There is practically no danger of causing pneumothorax (Büttner and Meier 2006).
- An ultrasound-guided block is possible and easy to perform (Chan and Peng 2011).

---

### Local Anesthetics

Initially: In adults, 10 mL of a medium-acting local anesthetic (e.g., mepivacaine 1% [10 mg/mL], for diagnostic purposes or a long-acting local anesthetic (e.g., ropivacaine 0.5–0.75% [5–75 mg/mL] or bupivacaine 0.5% [5 mg/mL]) for pain therapy is administered. According to anatomical studies by Feigl et al (2007), 5 mL is sufficient for an adequate block.

Continuous block: 0.2 to 0.375% (2–3.75 mg/mL) ropivacaine or 0.25% (2.5 mg/mL) bupivacaine, 6 to 8 mL/h.

## 5.2.2 Suprascapular Nerve Block with Ultrasound

- Linear transducer: 10 MHz
- Penetration depth: 5 cm
- Needle: 6 cm

### Ultrasound Orientation

The suprascapular nerve runs on the floor of the supraspinous fossa under the trapezius and supraspinatus muscles between the scapular notch and the spinoglenoidal notch.

It can be visualized here using ultrasound in the short axis. The transducer is placed in the coronal plane at a right angle to the line connecting the coracoid process and the spine of the scapula and tilted slightly anteriorly. A hyperechoic structure can be visualized here on the floor of the supraspinous fossa that includes the suprascapular nerve (▶ Fig. 5.13; Chan and Peng 2011).

### Puncture

The puncture is made in plane ( ▶ ) or out of plane.
Volume: 5 mL

## 5.3 Sensory and Motor Effects

The suprascapular nerve is responsible for about 70% of the sensory innervation of the shoulder (Ritchie et al 1997). As it does not innervate any area of skin, this block on its own is inadequate for operative purposes. In pain therapy it is an alternative to the interscalene technique. The motor effect is impairment in the shoulder region (abduction, external rotation).

## 5.4 Indications and Contraindications

### 5.4.1 Indications

For diagnostic purposes to investigate shoulder pain; also pain therapy for shoulder pain of any cause and status post shoulder trauma and/or surgery (▶ Fig. 5.14).

### 5.4.2 Contraindications

No special contraindications.

## 5.5 Complications, Side Effects, Method-Specific Problems

The risk profile of the technique described is much better than that of the classical technique (Bonica 1958) of suprascapular nerve block. In particular, there is a low risk of pneumothorax. The problem of difficulty in inserting an indwelling catheter, with the risk of a bottleneck syndrome in the region of the scapular notch, does not exist with this technique.

The catheter should not be advanced more than 3 cm. The catheter direction laterally is also the optimal anatomical direction and the end point corresponds with the results of anatomical studies by Feigl et al (2007).

The puncture site described in Chapter 5.2 is necessary to place a catheter because otherwise it cannot be advanced or possibly will not reach the shoulder joint.

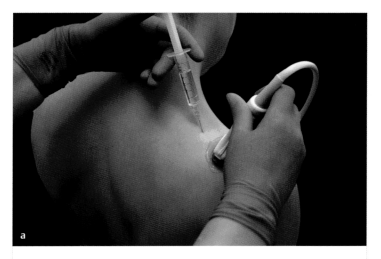

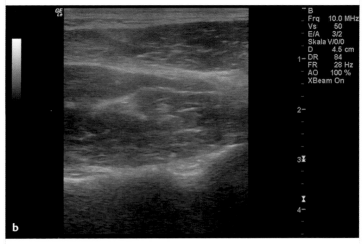

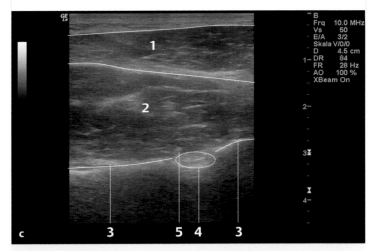

Fig. 5.13 Suprascapular nerve blockade using ultrasound (out of plane, short axis).
a Clinical setting.
b Ultrasound image, unlabeled.
c Ultrasound image, labeled.
1 Trapezius muscle
2 Supraspinatus muscle
3 Floor of the supraspinous fossa
4 Suprascapular nerve
5 Tip of needle

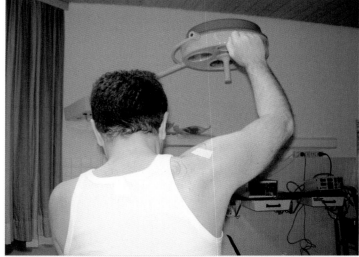

Fig. 5.14 Successful suprascapular nerve block for pain therapy for frozen shoulder.

For a single injection, the insertion point can also be selected in the middle or somewhat further laterally and the needle direction can be vertical. The distance of 2 cm above the spine of the scapula must be maintained because the bony protrusion of the spine can be relatively wide.

Compared to interscalene block there is no motor impairment in the arm and hand with the exception of the muscles innervated by the suprascapular nerve.

The suprascapular block has proved very effective for perioperative pain therapy in conjunction with general anesthesia (Ritchie et al 1997). Numerous articles confirm its effectiveness in pain syndromes due to trauma (Breen and Haigh 1990), in shoulder pain and restriction of movement of rheumatic origin (Brown et al 1988, Emery et al 1989, Gado and Emery 1993, Vecchio et al 1993), and in shoulder pain associated with hemiplegia (Lee and Khunadorn 1986, Hecht 1992, Jeon et al 2014).

In direct contrast, however, interscalene block for immediate postoperative pain therapy after shoulder operations is markedly superior to suprascapular block (Lhotel et al 2001). Both blocks were significantly more effective than intra-articular injection of local anesthetics or systemic intravenous pain therapy (Lee and Khunadorn 1986).

# References

Bonica JJ. Diagnostic and therapeutic blocks, a reappraisal based on 15 years' experience. Anesth Analg 1958; 37: 58–68

Breen TW, Haigh JD. Continuous suprascapular nerve block for analgesia of scapular fracture. Can J Anaesth 1990; 37: 786–788

Brown DE, James DC, Roy S. Pain relief by suprascapular nerve block in glenohumeral arthritis. Scand J Rheumatol 1988; 17: 411–415

Büttner J, Meier G. Zugangswege zum Plexus brachialis. Anasthesiol Intensivmed Notfallmed Schmerzther 2006; 7: 491–497

Chan CW, Peng PWH. Suprascapular nerve block: a narrative review. Reg Anesth Pain Med 2011; 36: 358–373

Dangoisse MJ, Wilson DJ, Glynn CJ. MRI and clinical study of an easy and safe technique of suprascapular nerve blockade. Acta Anaesthesiol Belg 1994; 45: 49–54

Emery P, Bowman S, Wedderburn L, Grahame R. Suprascapular nerve block for chronic shoulder pain in rheumatoid arthritis. BMJ 1989; 299: 1079–1080

Feigl GC, Anderhuber F, Dorn C, Pipam W, Rosmarin W, Likar R. Modified lateral block of the suprascapular nerve: a safe approach and how much to inject? A morphological study. Reg Anesth Pain Med 2007; 32: 488–494

Gado K, Emery P. Modified suprascapular nerve block with bupivacaine alone effectively controls chronic shoulder pain in patients with rheumatoid arthritis. Ann Rheum Dis 1993; 52: 215–218

Hecht JS. Subscapular nerve block in the painful hemiplegic shoulder. Arch Phys Med Rehabil 1992; 73: 1036–1039

Jeon WH, Park GW, Jeong HJ, Sim YJ. The comparison of effects of suprascapular nerve block, intra-articular steroid injection, and a combination therapy on hemiplegic shoulder pain: pilot study. Ann Rehabil Med 2014; 38: 167–173

Lee KH, Khunadorn F. Painful shoulder in hemiplegic patients: a study of the suprascapular nerve. Arch Phys Med Rehabil 1986; 67: 818–820

Lhotel L, Fabre B, Okais I, Singelyn F. Postoperative analgesia after arthroscopic shoulder surgery: suprascapular nerve block, intraarticular analgesia or interscalene brachialplexus block. Reg Anesth Pain Med 2001; 26 Suppl: 34

Meier G, Bauereis C, Maurer H. The modified technique of continuous suprascapular nerve block. A safe technique in the treatment of shoulder pain. [Article in German] Anaesthesist 2002; 51: 747–753

Ritchie ED, Tong D, Chung F, Norris AM, Miniaci A, Vairavanathan SD. Suprascapular nerve block for postoperative pain relief in arthroscopic shoulder surgery: a new modality? Anesth Analg 1997; 84: 1306–1312

Vecchio PC, Adebajo AO, Hazleman BL. Suprascapular nerve block for persistent rotator cuff lesions. J Rheumatol 1993; 20: 453–455

# 6 Axillary Block

## 6.1 Anatomy

In the axilla the cords are located medially, laterally, and posteriorly, corresponding to their names (▶ Fig. 6.1).

- The ulnar nerve, the cutaneous nerve of the arm, the medial nerve of the forearm, and also part of the median nerve arise from the medial cord.
- After the musculocutaneous nerve has arisen from the lateral cord, it forms a lateral root that unites with the medial root of the medial cord to form the median nerve.
- The posterior cord separates into the axillary nerve and radial nerve (▶ Fig. 6.2 and ▶ Fig. 6.3).

▶ **Deep axillary fascia and deep axillary space.** From where it passes through the posterior interscalene space as far as the axillary region, the entire brachial plexus is surrounded by a connective-tissue sheath, which is called the deep axillary fascia in the region of the axillary fossa. The space lying under this is called the deep axillary space, which extends proximally to the infraclavicular region up to the interscalene space and further medially.

Besides the nerves, this space also contains the blood vessels (axillary artery and vein; ▶ Fig. 6.4 and ▶ Fig. 6.5). There are connective-tissue septa within this so-called neurovascular sheath (▶ Fig. 6.6). However, in the majority of people, they do not appear to hinder the uniform spread of local anesthetic, so that block of the entire brachial plexus is possible with a single injection in the axillary region.

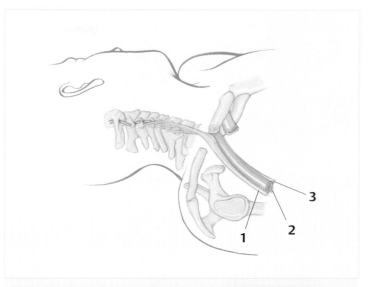

**Fig. 6.1** Brachial plexus in relation to the subclavian (axillary) artery. Note that the cords rotate 90° around the subclavian artery from the infraclavicular region to the axillary region. While the posterior cord is furthest laterally (but deeper) compared with the lateral cord in the infraclavicular region, in the axillary region the names of the cords correspond to their actual positions relative to one another.
1 Lateral cord
2 Posterior cord
3 Medial cord

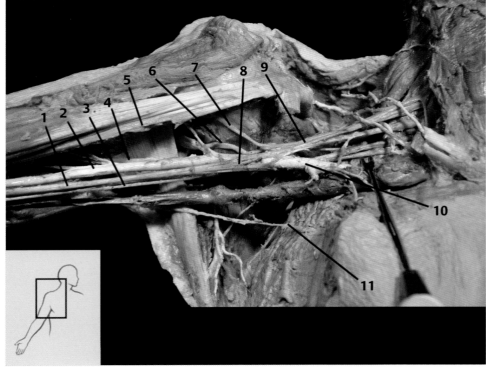

**Fig. 6.2** Brachial plexus in the axillary fossa: anatomical overview.
1 Median nerve
2 Brachial artery
3 Ulnar nerve
4 Radial nerve
5 Coracobrachialis
6 Axillary nerve
7 Musculocutaneous nerve
8 Median nerve with its two roots
9 Lateral cord
10 Subclavian artery
11 Intercostobrachial nerve

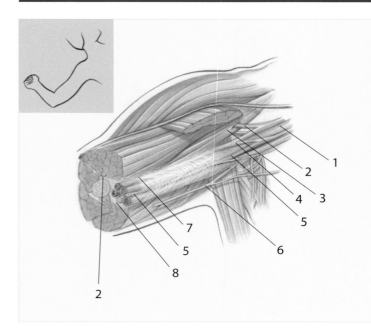

**Fig. 6.3** Axillary plexus: anatomical overview. (Note the neurovascular connective-tissue sheath.)
1 Subclavian artery
2 Musculocutaneous nerve
3 Coracobrachialis muscle
4 Median nerve with its two roots
5 Ulnar nerve
6 Intercostobrachial nerve
7 Median nerve
8 Radial nerve

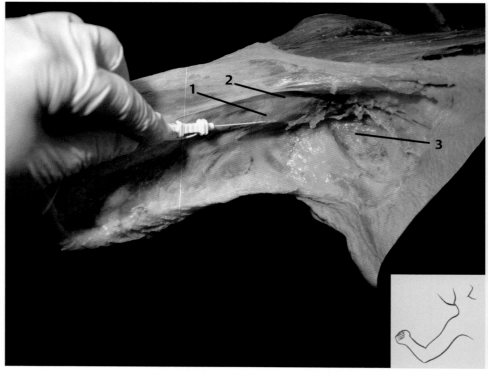

**Fig. 6.4** Brachial plexus in the axillary fossa, deep axillary fascia.
1 Deep axillary fascia with neurovascular bundle below
2 Coracobrachialis
3 Subfascial axillary space

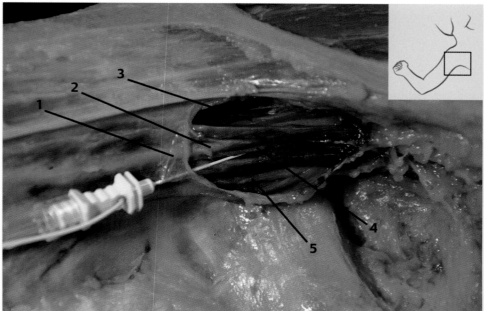

**Fig. 6.5** Brachial plexus in the axillary fossa, deep axillary space opened.
1 Deep axillary fascia
2 Axillary artery
2 Median nerve
4 Radial nerve
5 Ulnar nerve

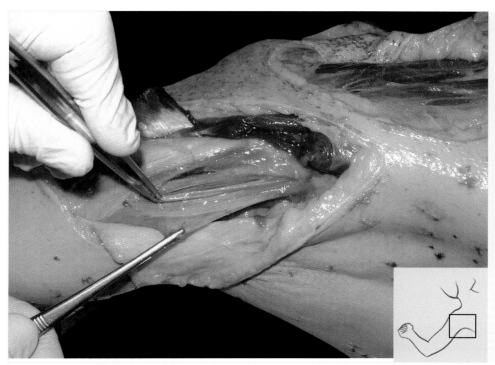

**Fig. 6.6** Axillary plexus with connective-tissue septation.

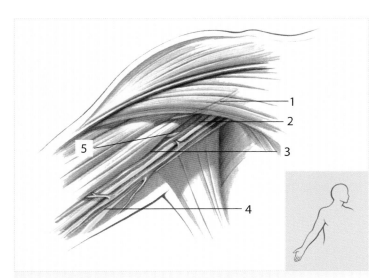

**Fig. 6.7** Axillary plexus anesthesia, anatomical relations.
1 Musculocutaneous nerve
2 Median nerve
3 Axillary artery
4 Ulnar nerve
5 Axillary nerve (situated deeply)

▶ **Localization of the nerves and axillary block.** The musculocutaneous nerve and the axillary nerve leave the neurovascular sheath very far proximally (▶ Fig. 6.7). The axillary nerve is included in the axillary block only in a few cases and the musculocutaneous nerve only if the technique extends very far proximally and a corresponding volume of local anesthetic is used. The radial nerve lies in the axillary region behind the axillary artery and thus, depending on the technique employed, represents the second "problem nerve" in axillary block in addition to the musculocutaneous nerve.

## 6.2 Perivascular Single-Injection Technique ▶

### 6.2.1 Method

The patient lies supine, the arm is abducted about 90°, and the elbow is flexed about 90° and externally rotated. The axillary artery, which can usually be palpated readily, acts as a landmark. The coracobrachialis muscle runs cranial to the axillary artery. The palpating fingers find the gap between the axillary artery and coracobrachialis somewhat distal to the axillary crease. The injection site is located where the lateral edge of pectoralis major crosses the axillary artery (▶ Fig. 6.8).

Following intracutaneous local anesthetic infiltration, a prepuncture is made through the skin for better penetration of the needle used for the block. This needle should have a short bevel (▶ Fig. 6.9) for optimal identification of the neurovascular sheath. The needle is inserted at an angle of about 30 to 45° parallel to the artery in the palpated gap (▶ Fig. 6.8).

After a few millimeters, noticeable resistance is felt, which can be overcome with controlled pressure. Immediately after overcoming this resistance, the needle is lowered and advanced proximally as far as it will go in the neurovascular sheath. A nerve stimulator can now be used to check that the needle is in the correct position. Using small "wobbling movements" different nerves can often be stimulated (median nerve, ulnar nerve, radial nerve) (▶ Fig. 6.10, ▶ Fig. 6.11, ▶ Fig. 6.12, ▶ Fig. 6.13).

The tip of the needle is occasionally behind the median nerve, so it can be helpful to withdraw the needle tip toward the skin (anteriorly) to obtain a response. In contrast to all other blocks, there is no correlation here between the amplitude of the stimulus and the success rate.

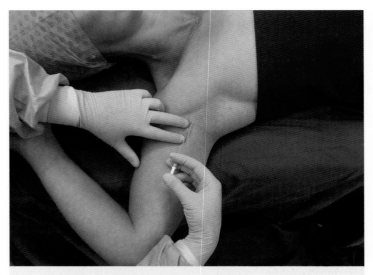

Fig. 6.8 Technique of perivascular axillary plexus anesthesia.

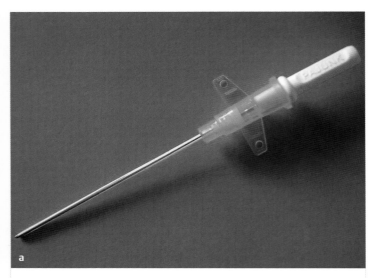

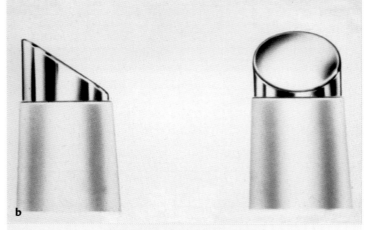

Fig. 6.9 Atraumatic needle for the technique of perivascular axillary block (Source: Pajunk GmbH, Geisingen, with kind permission).
a Needle.
b Needle tip.

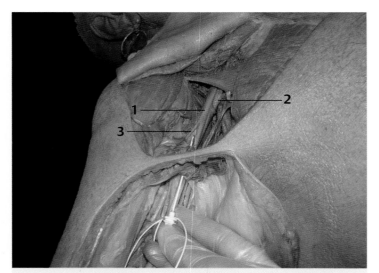

Fig. 6.10 Axillary plexus anesthesia. (Note: the tip of the needle extends almost to the musculocutaneous nerve.)
1 Lateral cord
2 Subclavian artery (axillary)
3 Musculocutaneous nerve

## Material

Single-injection technique: 5 to 7.5 cm long atraumatic needle with a blunt bevel; pencil-point tip is also possible.

Continuous technique: 18G indwelling needle with blunt stylet (e.g., 45° bevel) (▶ Fig. 6.9). After successful placement, remove the stylet, advance a flexible catheter through the indwelling needle (▶ Fig. 6.14), and remove the needle.

For children: 20G indwelling needle with solid steel stylet.

## Practical Note

A response from the musculocutaneous nerve indicates that the needle is in the wrong position (runs in the coracobrachialis muscle after leaving the brachial plexus; see ▶ Fig. 6.3). As an alternative to the use of a nerve stimulator, the correct needle position can also be verified by inducing paresthesia using refrigerated isotonic saline. In terms of effectiveness, this method is similar to the use of a nerve stimulator (Rodriguez et al 1996, Aul 2000), but for patients it is associated with unpleasant paresthesia.

> **Note**
>
> Paresthesia should not be produced deliberately with the needle because of the increased risk of nerve injury.

Axillary plexus anesthesia performed by this method is one of the few techniques that can also be performed without the use of a nerve stimulator and/or ultrasound. For this, an 18G needle with a solid steel stylet, 45° bevel, and rounded edges is helpful to allow the loss of resistance to be felt clearly.

Apart from cold paresthesia and/or a response through the nerve stimulator, the following criteria are regarded as evidence

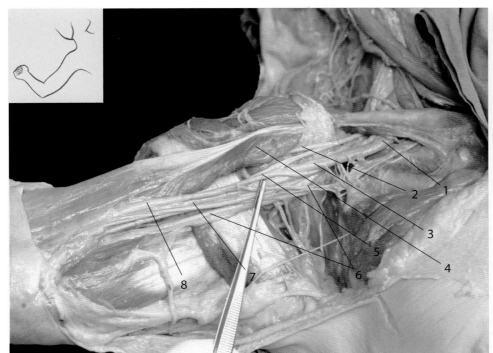

Fig. 6.11 Axillary plexus: anatomical overview.
1 Subclavian artery
2 Musculocutaneous nerve
3 Axillary artery
4 Coracobrachialis
5 Median nerve with two roots
6 Ulnar nerve
7 Axillary artery
8 Median nerve

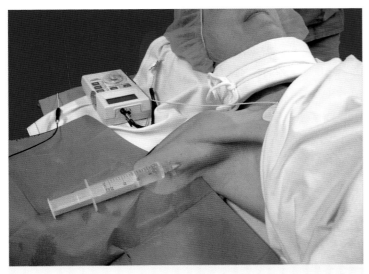

Fig. 6.12 Axillary plexus anesthesia, perivascular technique. Note the tubelike distension due to the injected local anesthetic.

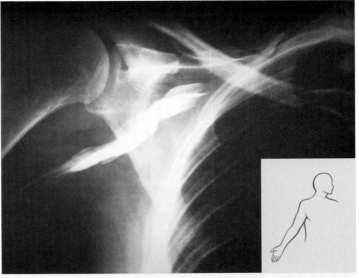

Fig. 6.13 Spread of contrast with perivascular axillary plexus anesthesia technique. Overview: tubelike spread of local anesthetic is clearly visible.

that the needle is in the correct position:
- Clear loss of resistance
- Smooth advancement of the needle

**Note**

The most frequent mistakes in insertion are incorrect orientation (artery not located correctly) and too-deep insertion. The needle must not be advanced deeper (in posterior direction) beyond the point of loss of resistance. (Lower the needle and advance it tangentially according to the procedure in peripheral venipuncture.)

This technique is very well suited to a continuous catheter technique (▶ Fig. 6.14 and ▶ Fig. 6.15).

For a suitable indication, bilateral catheter placement can be combined and performed and used even for severe skin injuries (Neuburger et al 2007) or frostbite.

In order to better reach the radial nerve with perivascular axillary block, use of the same technique, accessing the axillary neurovascular sheath inferior to the axillary artery, has been described (Meier et al 2003). With the patient in the position described above, the incision site in the bicipital medial groove is 3 to 4 cm distal to the intersection of the long head of the triceps brachii muscle with the latissimus dorsi, inferior to the neurovascular sheath. The needle is directed toward the groove between the teres major and the origin of the long head of the triceps brachii muscles. Use of a nerve stimulator and/or ultrasound is recommended.

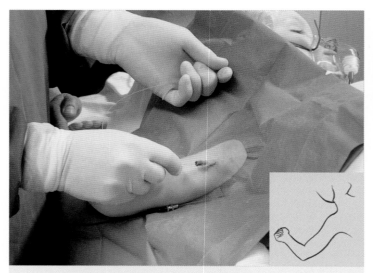

Fig. 6.14 Inserting an indwelling axillary plexus catheter.

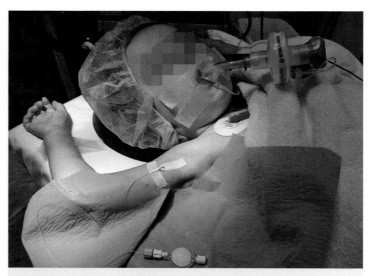

Fig. 6.15 Indwelling axillary plexus catheter.

When using ultrasound, the needle position can be corrected under visual control and the success rate improved (Pfeiffer et al 2008, Geiser et al 2011; Chapter 6.2.2).

## 6.2.2 Perivascular Axillary Block of the Brachial Plexus Using Ultrasound

Linear transducer: 7.5 to 10 MHz
Needle: 5 to 7.5 cm

### Ultrasound Visualization of the Brachial Plexus, Transpectoral in the Short Axis

The transducer is placed transpectorally (after puncture and insertion of the indwelling needle as described in Chapter 6.2) at the site (▶ Fig. 6.16) where the tip of the needle is expected to be (Geiser et al 2011). The axillary artery, positioned in the center of the image (▶ Fig. 6.16) is used for initial orientation. Cranial to the artery is the coracobrachialis muscle, which is shaped like a club in this section, the pectoralis major is anterior, and the subscapularis is posterior. The artery and plexus lie in the angle formed by these three muscles (▶ Fig. 6.16). As in the infraclavicular brachial plexus block, the individual cords/nerves are often difficult to identify in this section before injection of the local anesthetic (▶ Fig. 6.16), so that it is important to place the tip of the needle in relation to the axillary artery (▶ Fig. 6.17). ▶

### Needle Approach and Check of Spread of Local Anesthetic ▶

In a perivascular axillary block of the brachial plexus, the needle is inserted as described in Chapter 6.2 without ultrasound. When using the needle described in Chapter 6.2, the needle shaft is easy to visualize because of its caliber (18G). The position of the tip of the needle is determined by advancing the transducer proximally until the end of the shaft. For this, it is advisable to make continual small movements in the sense of local tissue movements (Chapter 1) for better visualization of the needle. ▶

The optimal needle position is at the caudal lower quadrant immediately adjacent to the axillary artery (▶ Fig. 6.17 and

▶ Fig. 6.18). The needle often reaches this point when it is advanced "blindly." If the needle is not in this position, it is advisable to correct the position. To do so, the needle should be withdrawn perceptibly and then advanced to the desired region under ultrasound guidance. When injecting the local anesthetic, it is important that the local anesthetic spreads below the axillary artery. ▶ The musculocutaneous nerve is in the spread area and, in contrast to "classical" axillary block, does not need to be blocked separately (▶ Fig. 6.19; see Chapter 6.7.1).

### Catheter Placement

The catheter can be placed easily; the spread of the local anesthetic can then be checked by ultrasound further proximally where the tip of the catheter is expected to be.

---

**Tips and Tricks**

- The transducer is placed transpectorally about 5 to 7 cm proximal to the puncture site (depending on the needle used). The area to be disinfected and the drape should be aligned accordingly.
- The puncture site in the axilla should be selected as proximal as possible so that the tip of the needle comes to a stop proximally enough that it is not at the outer border of the pectoralis muscle. Orientation with the transducer is difficult in the "gradient" from the pectoralis muscle down to the axilla.
- The puncture is generally made without using ultrasound. Of course, if the axillary artery is difficult to palpate in the axilla, the entire puncture procedure can be performed using ultrasound. The puncture in the axilla can be made above or below the axillary artery (Chapter 6.2).
- When the local anesthetic is injected, septa are occasionally visualized that prevent spread below the axillary artery, similar to an infraclavicular block. In this case, the needle position should be corrected posteriorly under ultrasound guidance.
- Using ultrasound, excellent success rates (> 90%) and rapid onset times have been described for this technique (Pfeiffer et al 2008, Geiser et al 2011).

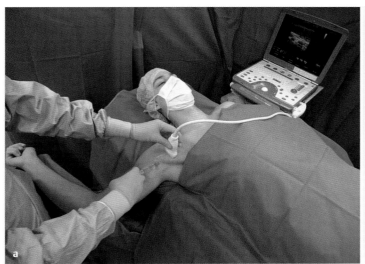

**Fig. 6.16 a–e** Perivascular plexus block, transpectoral section: "sonoanatomy."
**a** Clinical setting.
**b** Anatomical section corresponding to the ultrasound plane at the tip of the needle (unlabeled).
**c** As **b**, but labeled.
**d** Corresponding ultrasound image (unlabeled).
**e** As **d**, but labeled.
1 Pectoralis major
2 Coracobrachialis
3 Musculocutaneous nerve
4 Radial nerve
5 Axillary veins
6 Ulnar nerve
7 Axillary artery
8 Median nerve

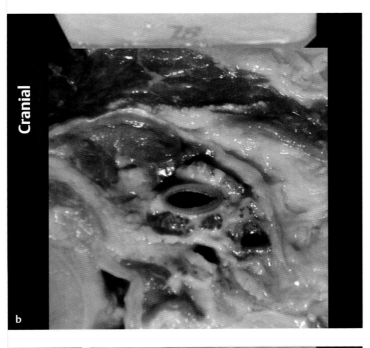

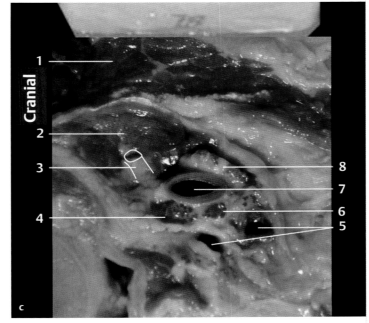

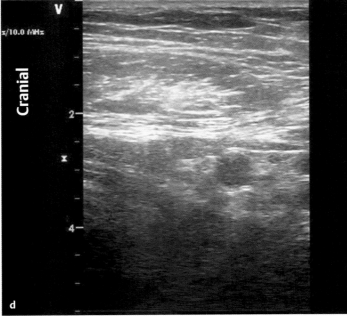

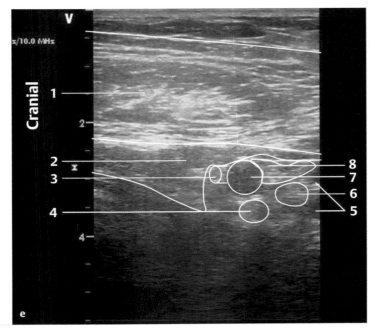

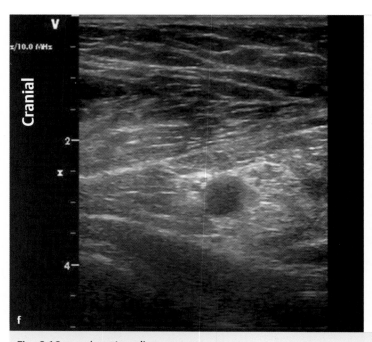
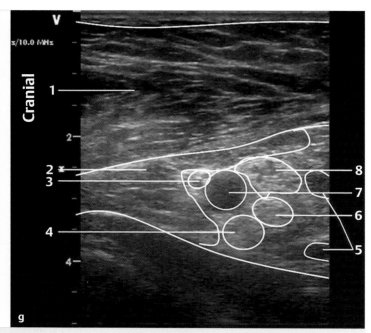

**Fig. 6.16 a–g (continued)**
**f** Same ultrasound plane as **b–e** after injection of a few milliliters of local anesthetic The cords/nerves can be visualized much better.
**g** Partial image **f** with labels.

## 6.3 Sensory and Motor Effects

When this technique is performed correctly, there is reliable sensory and motor block of the median, ulnar, and musculocutaneous nerves (▸ Fig. 6.20; Büttner et al 1987, Büttner and Klose 1991, Aul 2000). There is occasionally incomplete block of the radial nerve.

The incidence of complete block with this technique when ultrasound is not used is 70 to 75% (Büttner et al 1988, Neuburger et al 1998); around 20 to 25% can be supplemented (see below), and around 5% can be classified as complete failures. The results have been improved considerably (Chapter 6.2.2) using a modified technique (Pfeiffer et al 2008, Geiser et al 2011).

| Note |
| --- |
| While the musculocutaneous nerve does not usually pose a problem when an indwelling needle and an adequate volume of local anesthetic are used (see ▸ Fig. 6.10 and ▸ Fig. 6.19; Büttner et al 1987, Büttner and Klose 1991, Aul 2000), the most frequent failures can be attributed to incomplete block of the radial nerve. |

The assumption that placing the arm close to the body while the local anesthetic is being given increases the likelihood of a successful block of the radial nerve (a requirement for this is insertion of an indwelling needle or catheter; Vester-Andersen et al 1986) was not confirmed in a clinical study (Koscielniak-Nielsen et al 1995b).

### 6.3.1 Local Anesthetic, Dosages

Initially: In adults, 30 to 40 mL of a medium-acting (e.g., mepivacaine 1%, prilocaine 1% [10 mg/mL] or a long-acting (ropivacaine 0.5% [5 mg/mL]) local anesthetic is given. An adequate volume is required to sufficiently load the entire neurovascular sheath with the single-shot technique. If the local anesthetic is given through an indwelling catheter, spread as far as the supraclavicular region can be achieved. If the catheter is in the wrong position, the local anesthetic is distributed diffusely in the tissue without effect. Advancing the catheter too far (> 4–5 cm beyond the tip of the needle) or advancing it against resistance should be avoided.

Continuous block: 0.2 to 0.375% (2–3.75 mg/mL) ropivacaine, 6 to 8 mL /h.

## 6.4 Indications and Contraindications

### 6.4.1 Indications

All operative procedures on the elbow, forearm, and hand. In the distal upper arm and elbow region, too, excellent analgesia and anesthesia can be obtained with the axillary block (Schroeder et al 1996). Continuous axillary block is suitable for postoperative pain therapy, physiotherapeutic treatment (e.g., mobilization of stiff joints), prophylaxis and treatment of chronic pain states (CRPS, postamputation pain), sympathetic block (e.g., after replantation of amputated limbs), frostbite, and vasospasm after accidental intra-arterial injection (e.g., of thiopentone).

### 6.4.2 Contraindications

• General contraindications of peripheral blocks
• No special contraindications

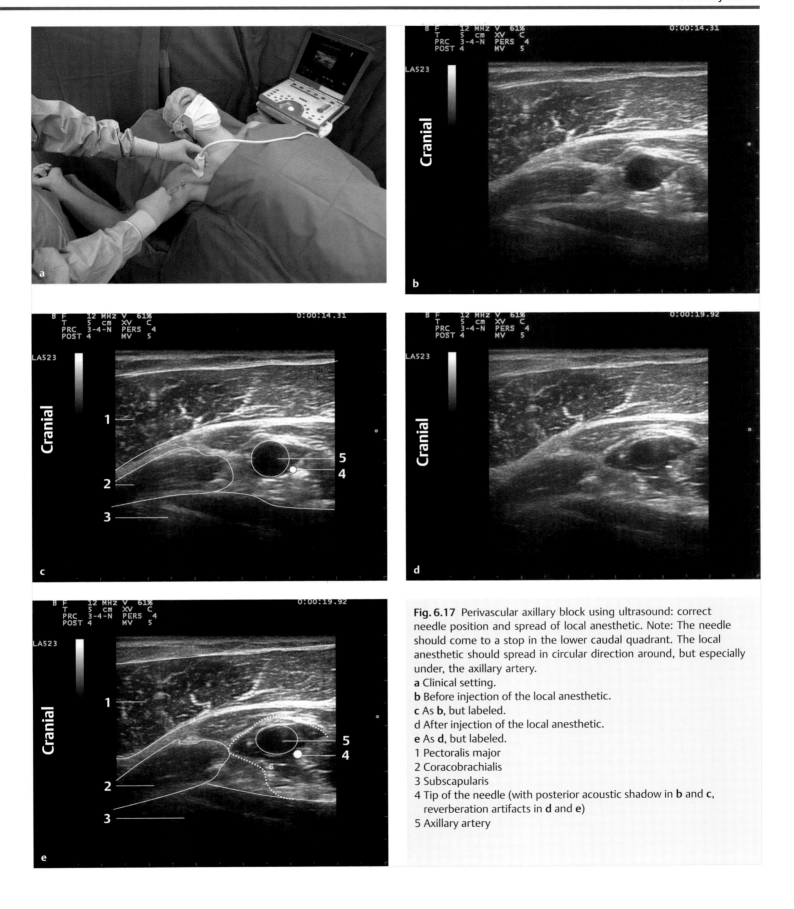

**Fig. 6.17** Perivascular axillary block using ultrasound: correct needle position and spread of local anesthetic. Note: The needle should come to a stop in the lower caudal quadrant. The local anesthetic should spread in circular direction around, but especially under, the axillary artery.

**a** Clinical setting.

**b** Before injection of the local anesthetic.

**c** As **b**, but labeled.

d After injection of the local anesthetic.

**e** As **d**, but labeled.

1 Pectoralis major

2 Coracobrachialis

3 Subscapularis

4 Tip of the needle (with posterior acoustic shadow in **b** and **c**, reverberation artifacts in **d** and **e**)

5 Axillary artery

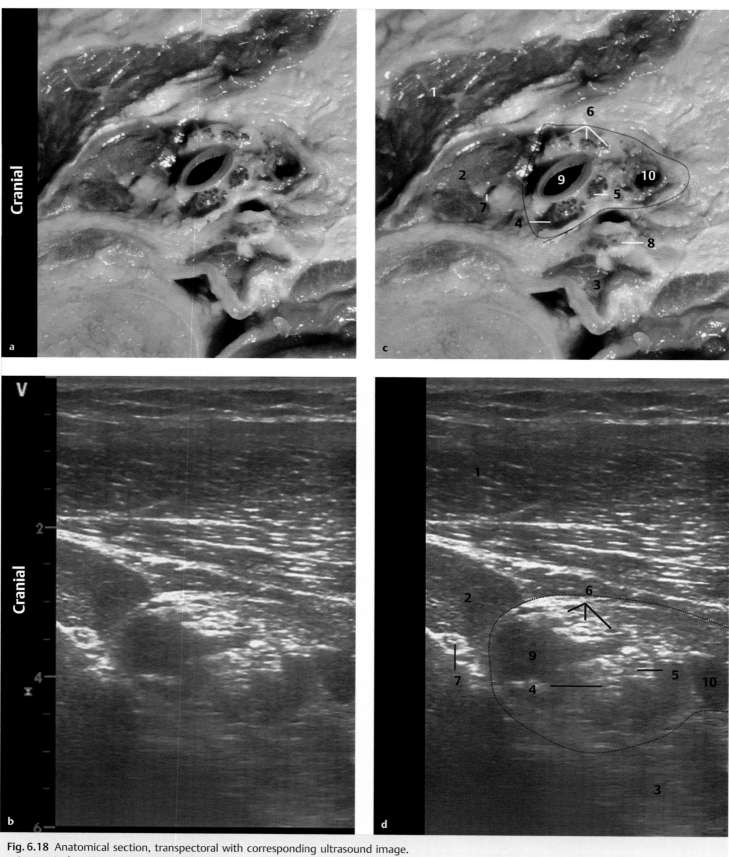

**Fig. 6.18** Anatomical section, transpectoral with corresponding ultrasound image.
**a** Anatomical section, transpectoral.
**b** Ultrasound image corresponding with **a**.
**c** As **a**, but labeled.
**d** As **b**, but labeled.
1 Pectoralis major
2 Coracobrachialis
3 Subscapularis
4 Radial nerve
5 Ulnar nerve
6 Median nerve
7 Musculocutaneous nerve
8 Axillary nerve
9 Axillary artery
10 Axillary vein
Line: deep axillary space
(in the ultrasound image after injection of local anesthetic)

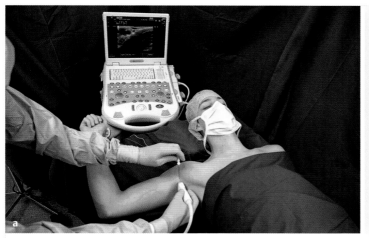

Continued >

Fig. 6.19 a–f Comparison of the position of the musculocutaneous nerve with the rest of the brachial plexus in the axillary (a–c) and transpectoral (d–f) regions. Note: A selective block of the musculocutaneous nerve is always needed in the axilla; the musculocutaneous nerve is included in the perivascular block described here.

a "Classical" technique of axillary block of the brachial plexus (visualization in the axilla) (Chapter 6.7).

b Ultrasound of the axilla.

c As b (labeled).

1 Musculocutaneous nerve

2 Region reached by local anesthetic

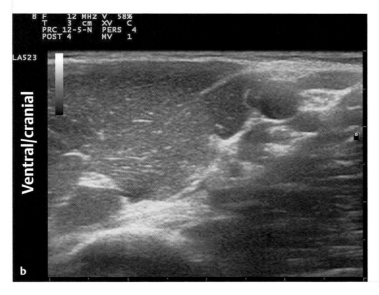

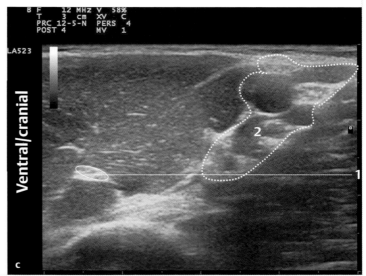

## 6.5 Complications, Side Effects, Method-Specific Problems

- The brachial plexus lies directly subfascially, and the needle is often inserted too deep in the tissue.
- If there are difficulties in identifying the axillary artery, vascular Doppler can be used for assistance.
- An indwelling needle (18G) with a solid stylet has proved to be useful even when a "single-shot" block is performed. If a continuous block is not required, the plastic cannula can at least be left in place until the end of the operation in order to supplement or prolong the block by further injection of local anesthetic.
- The indwelling needle shifts the injection point for the local anesthetic proximally so that the likelihood of successfully blocking the musculocutaneous nerve is high (see ► Fig. 6.10 and ► Fig. 6.19).
- A sufficient volume (30–50 mL in adults) of an adequately concentrated local anesthetic (e.g., mepivacaine 1%) should always be used in order to obtain a successful block.
- When an indwelling needle and an adequate volume are used, there are very few problems with the tourniquet (6.1%) (Büttner et al 1988).
- When a 7.5 cm long 18G needle is used (high axillary plexus anesthesia; Krebs and Hempel 1984), the injection site can be shifted further proximally.

- Vascular puncture with this technique is very rare (1.1%; Büttner et al 1988).
- Nerve injuries are extremely rare with this technique (Krebs and Hempel 1984, Büttner et al 1988).
- An additional block of the superficial cutaneous nerves supplying the inside of the upper arm, particularly the intercostobrachial nerve, is occasionally recommended in the form of subcutaneous infiltration.
- A tourniquet or compression distal to the injection site does not appear to confer any additional advantage (Koscielniak-Nielsen et al 1995a).

## 6.6 Multistimulation Technique, "Midhumeral Approach" According to Dupré

Dupré described the "bloc du plexus brachial au canal huméral" in 1994, which is translated incorrectly in Anglo-American literature as "midhumeral approach." In fact, this technique is performed at the junction of the proximal and middle thirds of the upper arm (► Fig. 6.21).

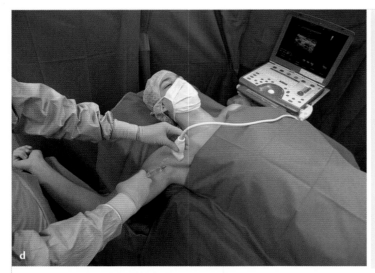

**Fig. 6.19 a–f (continued)**
**d** Perivascular technique (transpectoral image).
**e** Ultrasound image, transpectoral.
**f** As **e** (labeled).

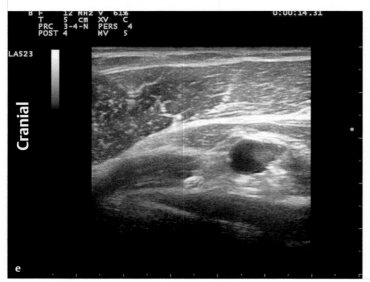

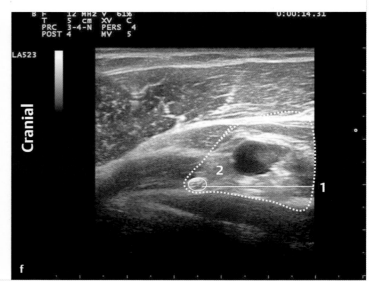

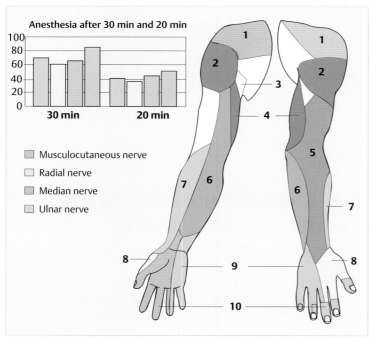

Anesthesia after 30 min and 20 min

- Musculocutaneous nerve
- Radial nerve
- Median nerve
- Ulnar nerve

**Fig. 6.20** Percentages of patients who have reached the stage of anesthesia after 30 and 20 minutes, respectively, following axillary plexus anesthesia with 400 mg mepivacaine (Büttner et al 1987, Büttner and Klose 1991, Aul 2000). Note that the musculocutaneous nerve, which is often described as a problem nerve, is anesthetized with the same frequency as the median nerve, and the radial nerve is not significantly less involved. The ulnar nerve together with the medial cutaneous nerve of the forearm tends to be anesthetized best. Areas 1 and 2 are usually not included in the axillary block, and 3 and 4 can be anesthetized by subcutaneous infiltration on the inside of the upper arm, as they are purely cutaneous nerves.

Sensory innervation of the upper limb:
1 Supraclavicular nerve
2 Axillary nerve (lateral cutaneous of arm)
3 Intercostobrachial nerve
4 Medial cutaneous nerve of the arm
5 Posterior cutaneous nerve of the forearm (radial nerve)
6 Medial cutaneous nerve of the forearm
7 Lateral cutaneous nerve of the forearm (musculocutaneous nerve)
8 Radial nerve
9 Ulnar nerve
10 Median nerve

## 6.6.1 Positioning, Landmarks

The patient lies supine; the arm is abducted 80° and extended on an arm table. The brachial artery is found at the junction of the proximal and middle thirds of the upper arm. The principle is to find and separately block the four main nerves innervating the arm from one injection site by withdrawing the needle under the skin and advancing it in different directions (▶ Fig. 6.21).

## 6.6.2 Method

The **median nerve**, which lies lateral to the brachial artery, is found first. While palpating the brachial artery, the needle is advanced tangentially to the skin proximally and cranially and parallel to the artery under the brachialis fascia; after a typical median nerve motor response is produced, 8 to 10 mL of the local anesthetic is injected (▶ Fig. 6.22, ▶ Fig. 6.23, ▶ Fig. 6.24).

After blocking the median nerve, the needle is drawn back under the skin. By directing the needle anterior–posterior (toward the surface on which the patient is lying) the **ulnar nerve** is now found (▶ Fig. 6.25, ▶ Fig. 6.26, ▶ Fig. 6.27).

After the needle is withdrawn again it is advanced toward the lower edge of the humerus until a motor response is produced in the region of the **radial nerve** (extension of the hand/fingers). A muscle response in the triceps brachii is regarded as unsatisfactory (▶ Fig. 6.28, ▶ Fig. 6.29, ▶ Fig. 6.30).

The **musculocutaneous nerve** is found by advancing the needle horizontally below the belly of the biceps brachii. It is helpful here to elevate the muscle belly a little by pinching it (▶ Fig. 6.31, ▶ Fig. 6.32, ▶ Fig. 6.33).

Per nerve, 8 to 10 mL of local anesthetic is injected. All nerves are found with the aid of the nerve stimulator according to the usual criteria. At the end, the medial cutaneous nerve of the arm is blocked by subcutaneous infiltration.

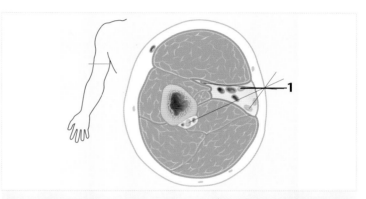

**Fig. 6.21** Anatomy of axillary block, Dupré technique (midhumeral approach).
1 Musculocutaneous nerve
2 Brachial veins
3 Brachial artery
4 Median nerve
5 Radial nerve
6 Medial cutaneous nerve of the forearm
7 Ulnar nerve

**Fig. 6.22** Direction of needle for median nerve block (midhumeral approach).
1 Median nerve block (direction of needle)

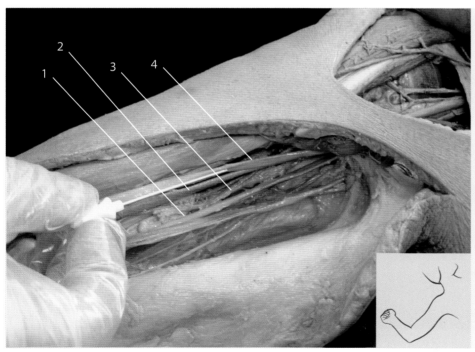

**Fig. 6.23** Direction of needle for median nerve block (midhumeral approach).
1 Ulnar nerve
2 Brachial artery
3 Radial nerve
4 Median nerve

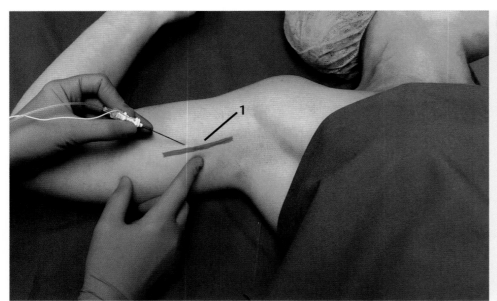

**Fig. 6.24** Direction of needle for median nerve block (midhumeral approach).
1 Course of the brachial artery

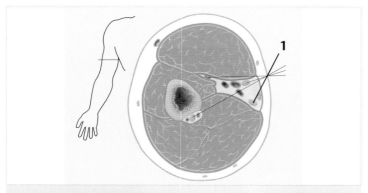

**Fig. 6.25** Direction of needle for ulnar nerve block (midhumeral approach).
1 Ulnar nerve block (direction of needle)

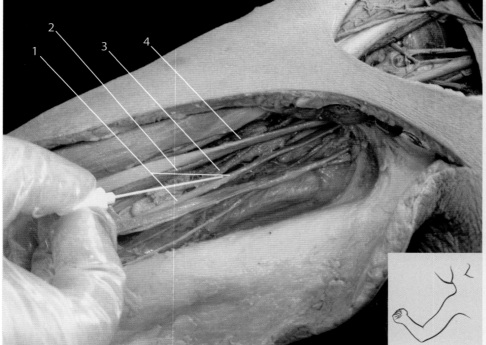

**Fig. 6.26** Direction of needle for ulnar nerve block (midhumeral approach).
1 Ulnar nerve
2 Brachial artery
3 Radial nerve
4 Median nerve

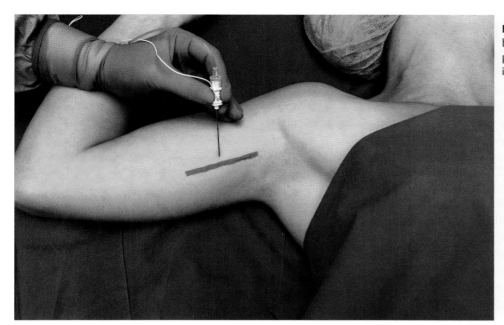

**Fig. 6.27** Direction of needle for ulnar nerve block (midhumeral approach). The needle passes between the skin and the brachial artery in front of the brachial artery.

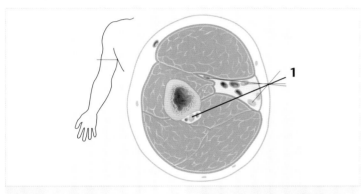

**Fig. 6.28** Direction of needle for radial nerve block (midhumeral approach).
1 Radial nerve block (direction of needle)

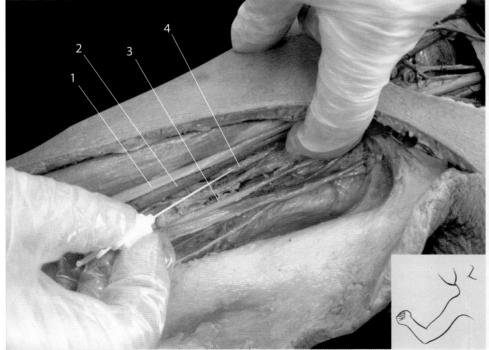

**Fig. 6.29** Direction of needle for radial nerve block (midhumeral approach).
1 Median nerve
2 Brachial artery
3 Ulnar nerve
4 Radial nerve

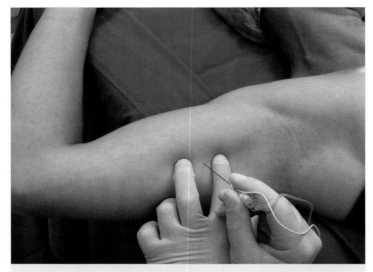

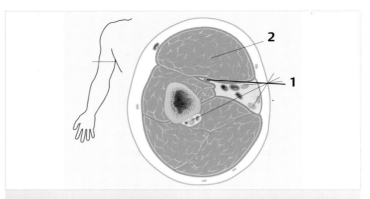

**Fig. 6.31** Direction of needle for musculocutaneous nerve block (midhumeral approach).
1 Musculocutaneous nerve block (direction of needle)
2 Biceps brachii

**Fig. 6.30** Direction of needle for radial nerve block (midhumeral approach). The needle passes between the skin and the brachial artery, that is, below the brachial artery directed toward the humerus.

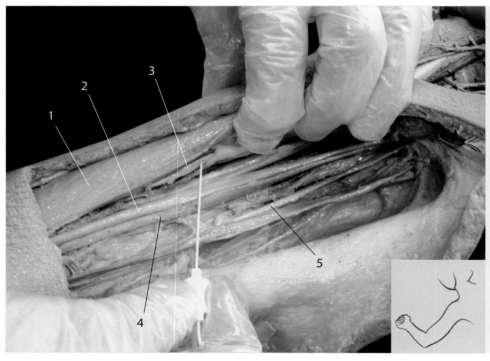

**Fig. 6.32** Direction of needle for musculocutaneous nerve block (midhumeral approach).
1 Biceps brachii
2 Median nerve
3 Musculocutaneous nerve
4 Brachial artery
5 Ulnar nerve

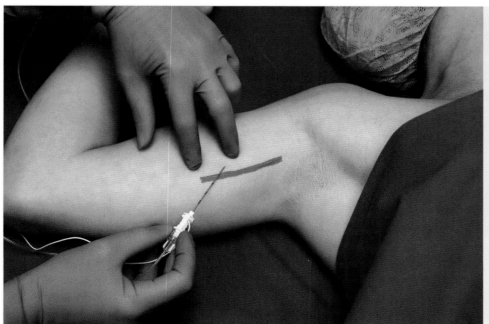

**Fig. 6.33** Direction of needle for musculocutaneous nerve block (midhumeral approach). The biceps muscle is pinched to lift it slightly.

## 6.6.3 Puncture Needle

Needle: 5 to 8 cm, atraumatic, immobile

- This method is not suitable as a continuous technique.
- The success rate is reported as 82.1% (Gaertner et al 1999), 88% (Bouaziz et al 1997), and 95% (Carles et al 2001).
- Completion by selective blocks at the elbow is possible with the aid of the nerve stimulator or ultrasound.
- In addition to the midhumeral approach, a multistimulation technique more proximally in the axilla has been described (Koscielniak-Nielsen et al 1997, 1999a, 1999b). Onset of effect (15 ±7 minutes), success rate (ca. 90%), and the time required to perform the block (5–10 minutes) are similar for the two techniques (Sia et al 2002). One advantage of the distal midhumeral approach compared to a "multistimulation technique" performed directly in the axilla is the fact that the nerves here lie widely separated from each other, so that a nerve injury due to injection into an already anesthetized nerve becomes more unlikely. This method can also be used with a combination of nerve stimulator/ultrasound (▶ Fig. 6.34).
- The success rate in blocking the ulnar nerve is somewhat lower than for the other nerves with this technique (Bouaziz et al 1997).
- The technique allows a differentiated block of the individual nerves. Thus the nerve in whose innervation region the postoperative pain is to be expected can be anesthetized with a long-acting local anesthetic for postoperative pain therapy, while a shorter-acting local anesthetic enables early postoperative restoration of sensation and motor function.

## 6.7 "Classical" Axillary Block of the Brachial Plexus with Ultrasound ▶

Linear transducer: 10 to 12 MHz
Needle: 5 to 7 cm

In what is called the classical technique of axillary block, the local anesthetic is injected directly in the axilla in contrast to the perivascular block described above, in which the puncture is made in the axilla, but the injection site is shifted to the infraclavicular region using an indwelling needle. Without ultrasound, the classical axillary block has a quite variable success rate, sometimes below 70%. The musculocutaneous nerve lies in the axilla outside the neurovascular sheath and must therefore be found and blocked separately. In addition, unlike the perivascular technique described above (Chapter 6.2.2), this technique cannot be used for a continuous block with an indwelling needle. However, with the introduction of ulrasound much better success has been achieved with this technique as well (Soeding et al 2005, Sites et al 2006).

## 6.7.1 Visualization of the Brachial Plexus Using Ultrasound (in the Axilla ▶)

The transducer is placed at the level of the axillary crease in the transverse plane (visualization in the short axis; ▶ Fig. 6.34). The

axillary artery and the nerves lying in the immediate vicinity of the artery are a few centimeters below the skin; the median nerve, which is closest to the surface, is often at a penetration depth of only 1 cm.

To visualize the veins, pressure on the transducer must be reduced.

The position of the veins in relation to the arteries can vary greatly (Retzl et al 2001, Christophe et al 2009). The median nerve is usually located anterior to the artery when the arm is positioned properly (▶ Fig. 6.34). By applying pressure on the transducer, it can be observed that the median nerve glides across the artery from medial to lateral direction.

The ulnar nerve lies somewhat further medially, the radial nerve is deeper, often below the axillary artery and always in close association with the common attachment tendon of the latissimus dorsi and teres major ("conjoined tendon"), which is visualized as a thick white band over the triceps muscle. The musculocutaneous nerve lies between the biceps and the coracobrachialis outside the neurovascular sheath (▶ Fig. 6.35).

Only in very rare cases can all four nerves be visualized simultaneously in one view.

This makes it necessary to change the position of the transducer by shifting and tilting it slightly, so that all four nerves can be clearly identified. If there is any uncertainty, the nerves can be followed further proximally and/or distally and identified based on their typical course. The median nerve runs together with the brachial artery to the cubital fossa, where it lies medial to the artery. The radial nerve runs with the deep brachial artery to the back of the humerus, where it crosses below it at about the middle of the upper arm. The ulnar nerve runs to the ulnar sulcus at the elbow. The course of the musculocutaneous nerve can be followed proximally until it joins the lateral cord or the median nerve. Some nerves in this region are hyperechoic, some are hypoechoic, and some have the typical "honeycomb" structure. For every hypoechoic circular/oval structure, compression and/or color Doppler must be used to differentiate whether it is a vessel or a nerve.

## 6.7.2 Puncture

The needle approach can be "in plane" or "out of plane" (▶ Fig. 6.34).

▶ In-plane technique. ▶ The needle is inserted parallel to the long axis of the transducer in line with the ultrasound beam as seen in ▶ Fig. 6.34b; the distance of the puncture site to the upper edge of the transducer should be selected so the needle enters the beam at a very shallow angle or parallel to the transducer (▶ Fig. 6.34). It is advisable to find first the posterior region in any case because it is impossible to rule out that visibility will be

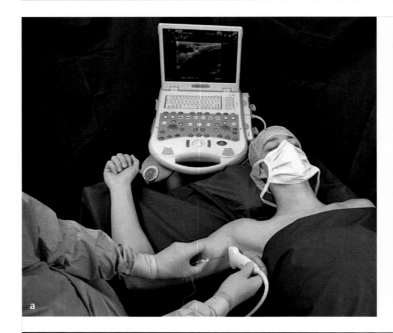

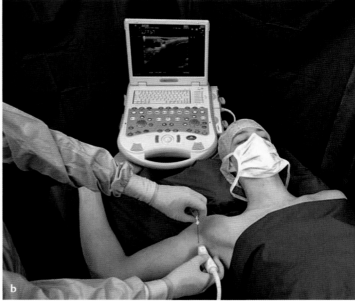

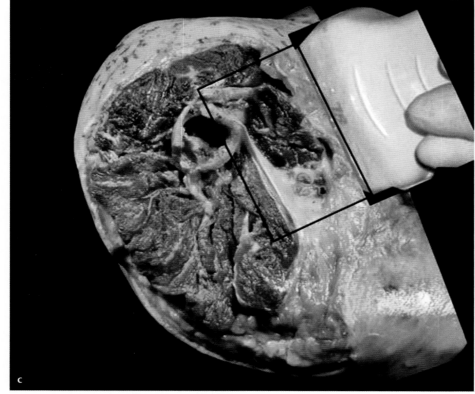

**Fig. 6.34** "Classical" axillary block with ultrasound.
**a** Out-of-plane technique.
**b** In-plane technique.
**c** Anatomical section at the level of the acoustic window (see enlargement in ▶ Fig. 6.35).

impaired by air superimposed on the structures in the background when the local anesthetic is injected.

▶ **Out-of-plane technique.** In an out-of-plane puncture, it is crucial that the local anesthetic also spreads below the axillary artery in order to reach the radial nerve. An attempt should be made to constantly identify the position of the tip of the needle using the hydro-location technique and local tissue movement (Chapter 1).

The question of whether every nerve should be found selectively in an ultrasound-guided block or whether it is sufficient to inject a depot below the axillary artery in the region of the radial nerve is the subject of some controversy (Imasogie et al 2010).

### 6.7.3 Catheter Placement

Continuous technique is not recommended with this technique.

> **Tips and Tricks**
>
> • The "classical" puncture technique is a multistimulation technique with the at least theoretically greater risk of injuring already anesthetized nerves, as neither the nerve stimulator nor the patient can provide information if already anesthetized nerves are accidentally touched. Nerve injuries cannot be completely ruled out even if ultrasound is used.
> • The in-plane technique is generally the preferred method.

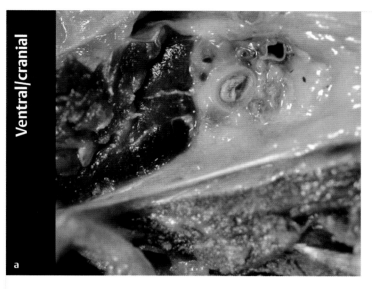
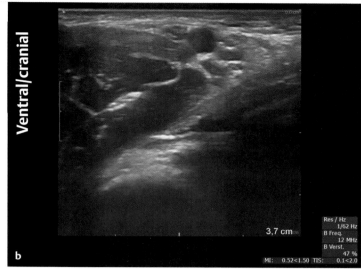
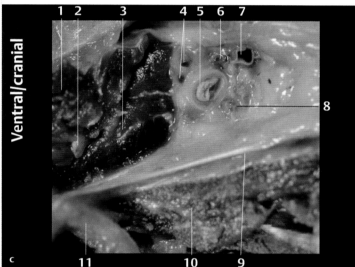
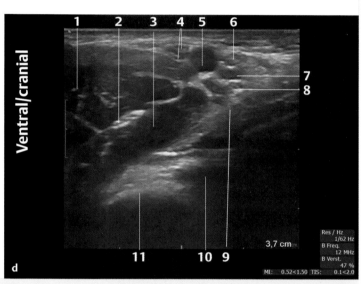

**Fig. 6.35** "Classical": axillary block ("sonoanatomy"), detail from ▶ Fig. 6.34 c.
a Anatomical section (unlabeled).
b Ultrasound image corresponding to a (unlabeled).
c Anatomical section (labeled).
d Ultrasound image corresponding to c (labeled).
1 Biceps muscle
2 Musculocutaneous nerve
3 Coracobrachialis muscle
4 Median nerve

5 Axillary artery
6 Ulnar nerve
7 Vein
8 Radial nerve
9 Common attachment tendon of the latissimus dorsi and teres major ("conjoined tendon")
10 Triceps
11 Humerus

# References

Aul A. Untersuchungen zur Erfolgsrate der axillären Plexus-brachialis-Blockade [Dissertation] Mannheim/Heidelberg: Universität Mannheim/Heidelberg; 2000

Bouaziz H, Narchi P, Mercier FJ et al. Comparison between conventional axillary block and a new approach at the midhumeral level. Anesth Analg 1997; 84: 1058–1062

Büttner J, Kemmer A, Argo A, Klose R, Forst R. Axillary blockade of the brachial plexus. A prospective evaluation of 1133 cases of plexus catheter anesthesia. [Article in German] Reg Anaesth 1988; 11: 7–11

Büttner J, Klose R, Dreesen H. Comparative study of 1% prilocaine and 1% mepivacaine in axillary plexus anesthesia. [Article in German] Reg Anaesth 1987; 10: 70–75

Büttner J, Klose R. Alkalinization of mepivacaine for axillary plexus anesthesia using a catheter. Reg Anaesth 1991; 14: 17–24

Carles M, Pulcini A, Macchi P, Duflos P, Raucoules-Aime M, Grimaud D. An evaluation of the brachial plexus block at the humeral canal using a neurostimulator (1417 patients): the efficacy, safety, and predictive criteria of failure. Anesth Analg 2001; 92: 194–198

Christophe JL, Berthier F, Boillot A et al. Assessment of topographic brachial plexus nerves variations at the axilla using ultrasonography. Br J Anaesth 2009; 103: 606–612

Dupré LJ. Brachial plexus block through humeral approach. [Article in French] Cah Anesthesiol 1994; 42: 767–769

Gaertner E, Kern O, Mahoudeau G, Freys G, Golfetto T, Calon B. Block of the brachial plexus branches by the humeral route. A prospective study in 503 ambulatory patients. Proposal of a nerve-blocking sequence. Acta Anaesthesiol Scand 1999; 43: 609–613

Geiser T, Lang D, Neuburger M, Ott B, Augat P, Büttner J. Perivascular brachial plexus block. Ultrasound versus nerve stimulator. Anaesthesist 2011; 60: 617–624

Imasogie N, Ganapathy S, Singh S, Armstrong K, Armstrong P. A prospective, randomized, double-blind comparison of ultrasound-guided axillary brachial plexus blocks using 2 versus 4 injections. Anesth Analg 2010; 110: 1222–1226

Koscielniak-Nielsen ZJ, Christensen LQ, Pedersen HL, Brushø J. Effect of digital pressure on the neurovascular sheath during perivascular axillary block. Br J Anaesth 1995a; 75: 702–706

Koscielniak-Nielsen ZJ, Horn A, Nielsen PR. Effect of arm position on the effectiveness of perivascular axillary nerve block. Br J Anaesth 1995b; 74: 387–391

Koscielniak-Nielsen ZJ, Stens-Pedersen HL, Lippert FK. Readiness for surgery after axillary block: single or multiple injection techniques. Eur J Anaesthesiol 1997; 14: 164–171

Koscielniak-Nielsen ZJ, Nielsen PR, Nielsen SL, Gardi T, Hermann C. Comparison of transarterial and multiple nerve stimulation techniques for axillary block using a high dose of mepivacaine with adrenaline. Acta Anaesthesiol Scand 1999a; 43: 398–404

Koscielniak-Nielsen ZJ, Rotbøll Nielsen P, Sørensen T, Stenør M. Low dose axillary block by targeted injections of the terminal nerves. Can J Anaesth 1999b; 46: 658–664

Krebs P, Hempel V. Eine neue Kombinationsnadel für die hohe axilläre Plexus brachialis-Anästhesie. Anästh Intensivmed 1984; 25: 219

Meier G, Maurer H, Bauereis C. Axillary brachial plexus block. Anatomical investigations to improve radial nerve block. [Article in German] Anaesthesist 2003; 52: 535–539

Neuburger M, Kaiser H, Rembold-Schuster I. Vertical infraclavicular brachial-plexus blockade. A clinical study of reliability of a new method for plexus anesthesia of the upper extremity. [Article in German] Anaesthesist 1998; 47: 595–599

Neuburger M, Büttner J, Lang D. Case report: bilateral block of the brachial plexus—approaches, dosage and effectiveness. [Article in German] Anasthesiol Intensivmed Notfallmed Schmerzther 2007; 11–12: 770–773

Pfeiffer K, Weiss O, Krodel U, Hurtienne N, Kloss J, Heuser D. Ultrasound-guided perivascular axillary brachial plexus block. A simple, effective and efficient procedure. [Article in German] Anaesthesist 2008; 57: 670–676

Retzl G, Kapral S, Greher M, Mauritz W. Ultrasonographic findings of the axillary part of the brachial plexus. Anesth Analg 2001; 92: 1271–1275

Rodríguez J, Bárcena M, Alvarez J. Axillary brachial plexus anesthesia: electrical versus cold saline stimulation. Anesth Analg 1996; 83: 752–754

Schroeder LE, Horlocker TT, Schroeder DR. The efficacy of axillary block for surgical procedures about the elbow. Anesth Analg 1996; 83: 747–751

Sia S, Lepri A, Campolo MC, Fiaschi R. Four-injection brachial plexus block using peripheral nerve stimulator: a comparison between axillary and humeral approaches. Anesth Analg 2002; 95: 1075–1079

Sites BD, Beach ML, Spence BC et al. Ultrasound guidance improves the success rate of a perivascular axillary plexus block. Acta Anaesthesiol Scand 2006; 50: 678–684

Soeding E, Sha S, Royse CE, Marks P, Hoy G, Royse AG. A randomized trial of ultrasound-guided brachial plexus anaesthesia in upper limb surgery. Anaesth Intensive Care 2005; 33: 719–725

Vester-Andersen T, Broby-Johansen U, Bro-Rasmussen F. Perivascular axillary block VI: The distribution of gelatine solution injected into the axillary neurovascular sheath of cadavers. Acta Anaesthesiol Scand 1986; 30: 18–22

# 7 Selective Blocks of Individual Nerves in the Upper Arm, at the Elbow, and Wrist

## 7.1 Radial Nerve Block (Middle of Upper Arm) ▶

### 7.1.1 Anatomy

The radial nerve passes under the middle of the humerus in the radial groove to reach the outside of the upper arm and then enters the elbow on the radial side of the flexor aspect (▶ Fig. 7.1, ▶ Fig. 7.2, ▶ Fig. 7.3).

### 7.1.2 Method

The arm is positioned as for perivascular axillary plexus anesthesia. In the middle of the upper arm, the gap between the flexors and extensors is found. The posterior border of the humerus is palpated. Coming from below (below the brachial artery), the posterior border of the humerus is found with a 4 to 8 cm long needle (▶ Fig. 7.2). On bone contact, an attempt is made to

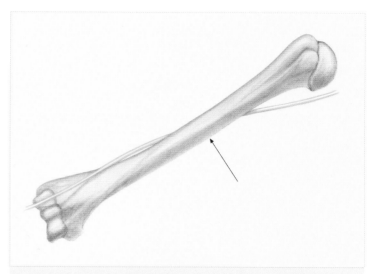

**Fig. 7.1** Selective radial nerve block in the mid-upper arm. The posterior border of the humerus is sought.

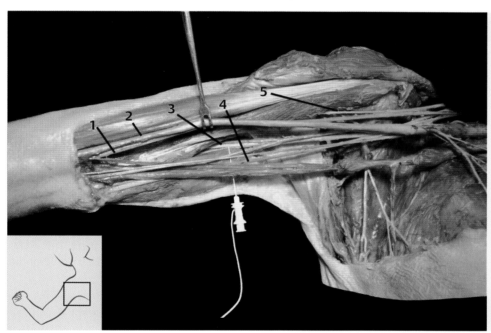

**Fig. 7.2** Selective radial nerve block.
1 Median nerve
2 Brachial artery
3 Radial nerve
4 Ulnar nerve
5 Musculocutaneous nerve

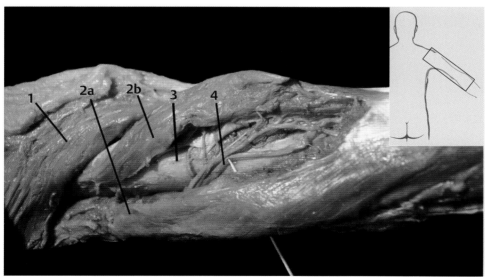

**Fig. 7.3** Selective radial nerve block in the middle of the right upper arm, view from dorsal, dissection in prone position.
1 Deltoid muscle
2a Long head of the triceps brachii muscle
2b Lateral head of the triceps brachii muscle
3 Humerus
4 Radial nerve with deep brachial artery

113

advance the needle a little further under the humerus. The technique should generally be performed with the nerve stimulator and an immobile needle or using ultrasound, particularly if an axillary block has already been performed. When there is a clear response to a corresponding stimulus and pulse duration, 8 to 10 mL of the local anesthetic is injected with repeated aspiration.

## Material

Needle: 4 to 8 cm

> **Tips and Tricks**
>
> The motor response should be in the hand (extension of the wrist or fingers).

## Sensory and Motor Effects

Sensory and motor loss in the region of the radial nerve distal to the injection site.

## Indications

▶ **Supplement to brachial plexus anesthesia.** It has proved useful to perform this block in combination with (supplementing) a perivascular block (▶ Fig. 7.4) if the radial nerve was not specifically stimulated when the axillary block was performed. Unlike the "multistimulation technique," this method is associated with directly finding only one nerve and is presumably preferable from the aspects of time required and patient acceptance, and is comparable with the multistimulation technique with respect to effectiveness. Using ultrasound is helpful (Chapter 7.13).

## 7.1.3 Radial Nerve Block of the Upper Arm Using Ultrasound

Linear transducer: 10 to 12 MHz
Needle: 6 cm

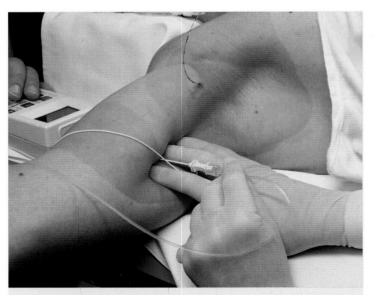

**Fig. 7.4** Selective radial nerve block of the mid-upper arm. Note the indwelling plexus catheter. This block can be used to supplement a brachial plexus block.

## Ultrasound Orientation

The arm is abducted as for a perivascular axillary plexus block or as described in Chapter 7.1. The transducer is placed in the short axis in the middle of the upper arm so the radial nerve is visible as a strongly hyperechoic structure in the region of the radial groove at the posterior edge of the humerus (▶ Fig. 7.5). From here, the nerve can be followed proximally for a certain distance, but can no longer be found at half the distance between the anterior segment of the acromion and the lateral epicondyle in 99% of patients (Foxall et al 2007). In the region of the radial groove, the radial nerve is accompanied by the deep brachial artery, whose position with respect to the radial nerve is variable (Foxall et al 2007).

## Needle Insertion

The needle is inserted using the in-plane or out-of-plane technique.

## Catheter Placement

Placement of a catheter is not described.

# 7.2 Blocks at the Elbow ▶

## 7.2.1 Anatomy

After passing under the humerus, the radial nerve appears at the elbow on the radial side between the brachioradialis and the brachialis muscles lateral to the biceps tendon (▶ Fig. 7.6). Here it divides into a sensory superficial branch and a thicker, mainly motor deep branch (▶ Fig. 7.7).

The lateral cutaneous nerve of the forearm is the sensory terminal branch of the musculocutaneous nerve and provides the sensory innervation of the radial side of the forearm. It lies on the radial side; since it is already epifascial lateral to the biceps tendon it is very superficial (▶ Fig. 7.7).

The median nerve, which crossed the brachial artery from lateral direction at the upper arm, passes through the elbow medial (on the ulnar side) to the brachial artery (mnemonic: median nerve—medial; ▶ Fig. 7.6 and ▶ Fig. 7.7).

The ulnar nerve passes through the ulnar groove and lies subfascially dorsal to the medial epicondyle and then disappears between the two heads of the flexor carpi ulnaris muscle (▶ Fig. 7.8 and ▶ Fig. 7.9).

## 7.2.2 Radial Nerve Block (Elbow)

The extended arm is abducted and externally rotated and the forearm is supinated. The biceps tendon can be palpated easily. The puncture site is 1 to 2 cm lateral (radial) to the biceps tendon at the level of the intercondylar line. The (stimulation) needle is advanced slightly proximally and laterally in the direction of the lateral epicondyle of the humerus (▶ Fig. 7.10). After producing a response, 5 mL of local anesthetic is injected.

The block can also be performed using a nerve stimulator or ultrasound guidance.

> **Practical Note**
>
> A catheter can also be inserted here.

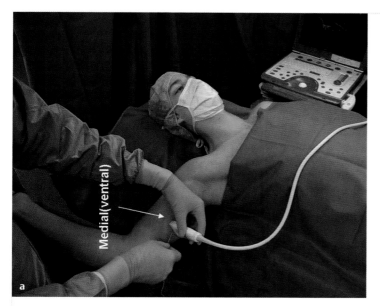
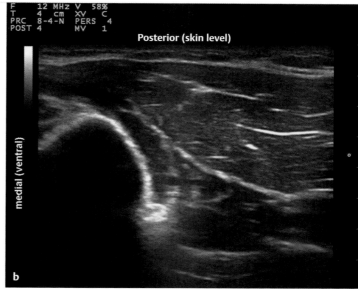
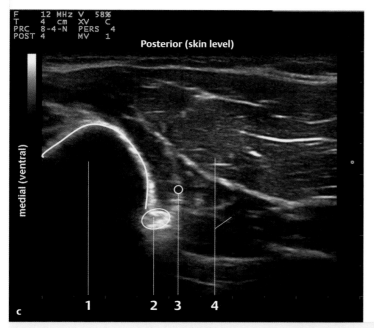
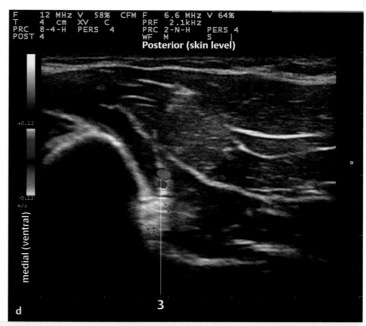

**Fig. 7.5** Visualization of the radial nerve in the region of the radial groove (mid-upper arm).
a Clinical setting in the out-of-plane technique.
b In ultrasound.
c As **b**, but labeled.
d As **b**, but with Doppler (CFM).

1 Humerus with osseous acoustic shadow
2 Radial nerve
3 Deep brachial artery
4 Triceps

## 7.2.3 Musculocutaneous Nerve Block (Elbow)

The lateral cutaneous nerve of the forearm, a sensory terminal branch of the musculocutaneous nerve, is already very superficial in the elbow region. It is blocked by subcutaneous infiltration lateral to the biceps tendon in the direction of the lateral epicondyle of the humerus with a 24G or 25G needle about 5 cm long (▶ Fig. 7.11 and ▶ Fig. 7.12).

The technique can be readily combined with the technique of radial nerve block at the elbow.

**Practical Note**

The creation of a Cimino shunt in conduction anesthesia is an indication for a combined radial nerve and musculocutaneous nerve block.

## 7.2.4 Median Nerve Block (Elbow)

The extended arm is abducted and externally rotated and the forearm is supinated. The pulse of the brachial artery is palpated on the intercondylar line. Medial to the artery, a 24G needle is

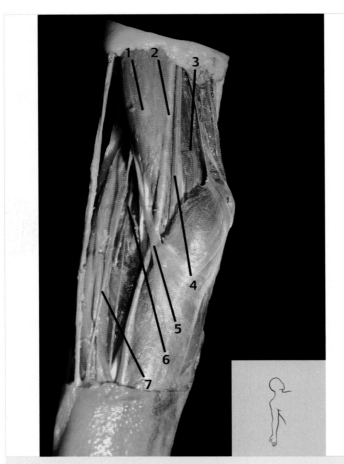

**Fig. 7.6** Anatomy of a right cubital fossa.
1 Biceps brachii
2 Brachial artery
3 Brachialis
4 Median nerve
5 Bicipital aponeurosis
6 Radial nerve
7 Lateral cutaneous nerve of the forearm

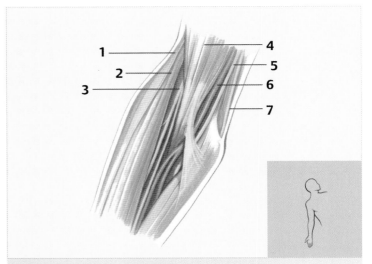

**Fig. 7.7** Cubital fossa, right arm.
1 Posterior cutaneous nerve of the forearm
2 Brachioradialis muscle
3 Radial nerve
4 Biceps brachii muscle
5 Median nerve
6 Brachial artery
7 Ulnar nerve

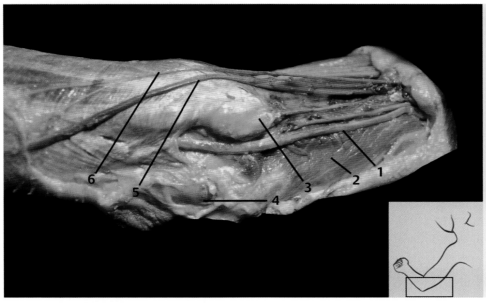

**Fig. 7.8** Ulnar nerve in the ulnar groove, right arm, view from medial.
1 Ulnar nerve
2 Triceps brachii muscle
3 Medial epicondyle
4 Olecranon
5 Basilic vein of the forearm
6 Anterior branch of the medial cutaneous nerve of the forearm

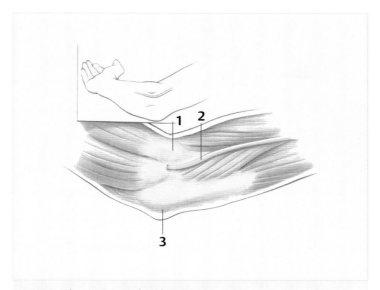

Fig. 7.9 Ulnar nerve in the ulnar groove.
1 Medial epicondyle of the humerus
2 Ulnar nerve
3 Olecranon

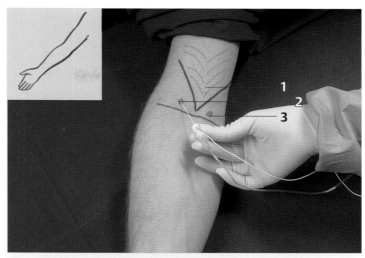

Fig. 7.10 Radial nerve block, right elbow.
1 Biceps brachii muscle
2 Puncture site in the radial nerve
3 Brachial artery

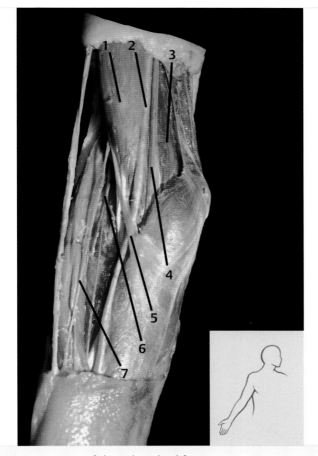

Fig. 7.11 Anatomy of the right cubital fossa.
1 Biceps brachii muscle
2 Brachial artery
3 Brachialis muscle
4 Median nerve
5 Bicipital aponeurosis
6 Radial nerve
7 Lateral cutaneous nerve of the forearm

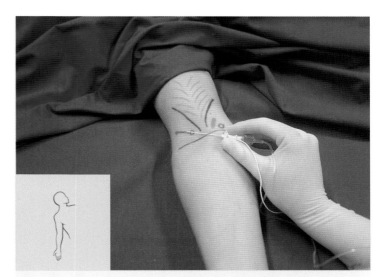

Fig. 7.12 Lateral cutaneous nerve of the forearm block (terminal branch of the musculocutaneous nerve), right arm, here subcutaneous!

advanced parallel to the artery in proximal direction at an angle of about 45° to the skin with stimulation (▶ Fig. 7.13 and ▶ Fig. 7.14). When there is a corresponding response after 1 to 2 cm, approximately 5 mL of the local anesthetic is injected.

### Practical Notes

The median nerve is always medial to the artery (mnemonic: median—medial).
A catheter can also be inserted here (▶ Fig. 7.15).

## 7.2.5 Ulnar Nerve Block (Elbow)

The extended arm is abducted and externally rotated and the elbow is flexed by 90°. The ulnar groove is located between the medial epicondyle of the humerus and the olecranon. The ulnar nerve is often palpated easily here. The ulnar nerve is in the ulnar

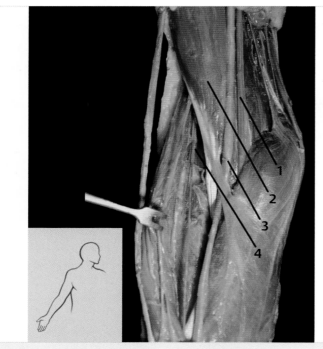

Fig. 7.13 Anatomy of the right cubital fossa, median nerve.
1 Median nerve
2 Biceps brachii muscle
3 Brachial artery
4 Radial nerve

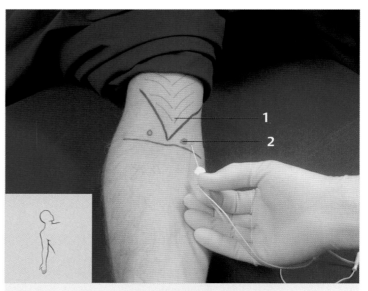

Fig. 7.14 Median nerve block in the cubital fossa medial to the brachial artery.
1 Biceps brachii muscle
2 Brachial artery

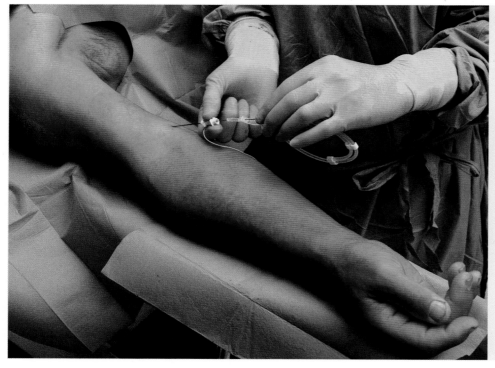

Fig. 7.15 Median nerve catheter.

groove only when the elbow is flexed (▶ Fig. 7.16 and ▶ Fig. 7.17). Because of the risk of pressure injury, the needle should not be inserted directly into the ulnar groove but about 1 to 2 cm proximal to it (▶ Fig. 7.18). The needle should be introduced tangentially to the nerve. Using a 3.5 to 5 cm immobile needle and a nerve stimulator, approximately 5 mL of the local anesthetic is injected when there is a corresponding motor response.

### Practical Notes

The ulnar nerve is in the ulnar groove only when the elbow is flexed. The volume should be kept low, because the ulnar nerve is very sensitive to pressure or tension.

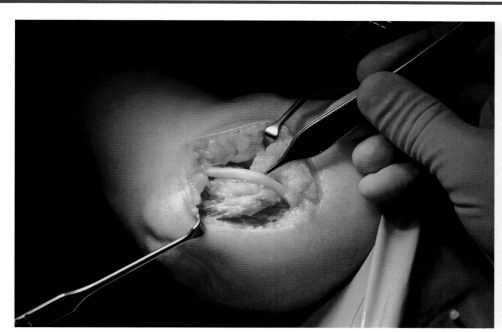

**Fig. 7.16** Ulnar nerve, operative findings in an ulnar sulcus syndrome, right arm.

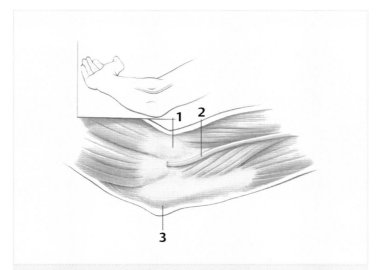

**Fig. 7.17** Ulnar nerve in the ulnar fossa.
1 Medial epicondyle of the humerus
2 Radial nerve
3 Olecranon

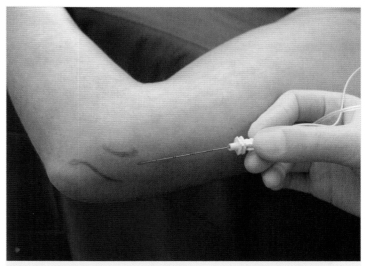

**Fig. 7.18** Ulnar nerve block, right arm.

Remarks on block techniques in the elbow and further distal:
- A continuous technique (catheter placement) for the three nerves (radial, ulnar, median) is possible (Lurf and Leixnering 2008, 2009, 2010; Büttner and Meier 2011; see ▶ Fig. 7.15).
- ▶ Fig. 7.19 shows an ulnar nerve catheter at the forearm for pain therapy. It was placed under ultrasound guidance.

## 7.2.6 Individual Nerve Blocks with Ultrasound (Elbow)

Linear transducer: 10 to 12 MHz
Needle: 6 cm

### Ultrasound Orientation

Three of the four nerves supplying the arm can be found and punctured in the elbow region using ultrasound (▶ Fig. 7.20). The musculocutaneous nerve can no longer be clearly visualized here.

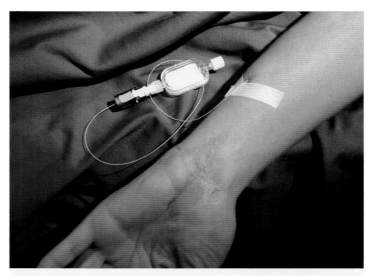

**Fig. 7.19** Ulnar nerve catheter at the forearm. Placed under ultrasound guidance.

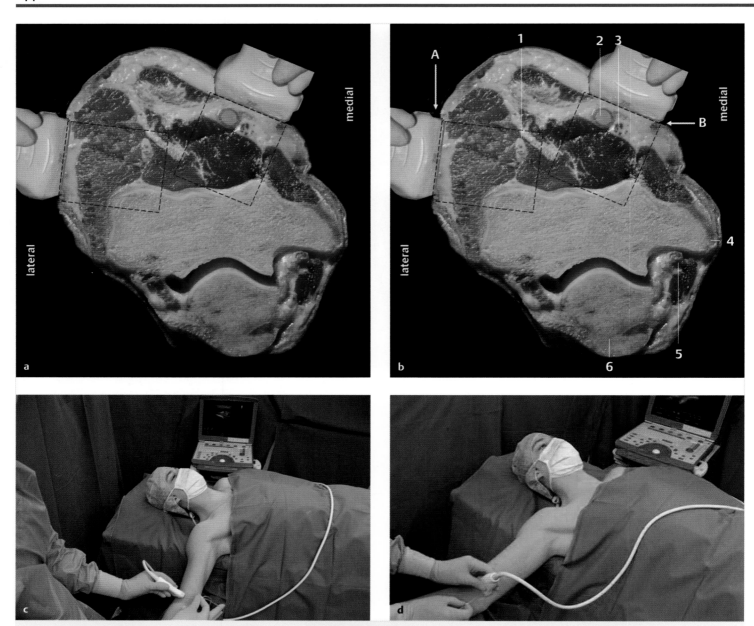

**Fig. 7.20** Ultrasound-guided visualization of the peripheral nerves at the elbow: anatomical section in the region of the epicondyles.

**a** Anatomical section in the region of the epicondyles.

**b** As **a**, but labeled.

**c** Blockage of the radial nerve in the sectional plane.

**d** Blockage of the median nerve in the sectional plane.

1 Radial nerve

2 Brachial artery

3 Median nerve

4 Humerus (medial epicondyle)

5 Ulnar nerve (in the ulnar groove)

6 Olecranon

**A** Transducer position and acoustic window for a radial nerve block (see also ► Fig. 7.21 and ► Fig. 7.24)

**B** Transducer position and acoustic window for a medial nerve block (see also ► Fig. 7.22)

The ulnar nerve should be blocked further proximal or distal to the ulnar groove.

► **Radial nerve.** The radial nerve can be best found about 4 to 5 cm proximal to the elbow in the short axis (► Fig. 7.21). It is embedded between the brachial muscle (medial) and the brachioradialis and extensor carpi radialis muscles and is readily visualized as a hyperechoic structure with the typical "honeycomb" pattern. The transducer is placed lateral (at the edge) proximal to the lateral epicondyle. The nerve is located at the anterior lateral border of the humerus at a depth of 1 to 2 cm (McCartney et al 2007).

► **Median nerve.** The median nerve is located in the elbow region medial (on the ulnar side) to the brachial artery at a depth of generally less than 1 cm (McCartney et al 2007). Here and in the further distal course, it has the "honeycomb" structure typical for peripheral nerves. The nerve is visualized in the short axis at the elbow; its course can be easily followed by sliding the transducer distally down to the wrist (► Fig. 7.22).

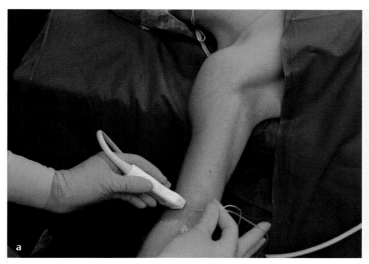

**Fig. 7.21** Visualization of the radial nerve proximal to the elbow (short axis) with ultrasound, in-plane needle approach.
**a** Clinical setting.
**b** Ultrasound image (unlabeled).
**c** Ultrasound image (labeled).
1 Humerus
2 Radial nerve

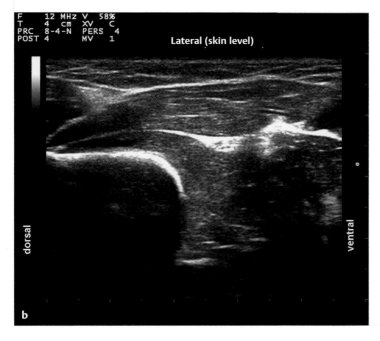

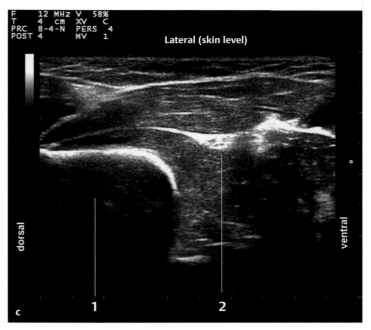

▶ **Ulnar nerve.** The ulnar nerve should not be looked for directly in the ulnar groove. It can be found distal to or 4 to 5 cm proximal to the medial epicondyle in the short axis. Proximal to the medial epicondyle, it is usually at a depth of less than 1 cm (▶ Fig. 7.23).

## Needle Approach

The *radial nerve* block is best performed in plane proximal to the elbow (▶ Fig. 7.24). When the needle is withdrawn, the lateral cutaneous nerve of the forearm can be anesthetized due to infiltration of the musculocutaneous nerve and/or its sensory terminal branch. The *median nerve* and the *ulnar nerve* can each be found and blocked in plane or out of plane.

## Catheter Placement

A catheter can be placed in the region of all three nerves.

| Practical Note |
| --- |
| The median nerve and ulnar nerve can be found and blocked in the entire forearm using ultrasound. |

# 7.3 Blocks at the Forearm ("Wrist Block")

## 7.3.1 Anatomy

The median nerve at the wrist is on the palmar side between the tendon of flexor carpi radialis (radial side) and the palmaris longus tendon. It passes through the carpal tunnel into the palm of the hand (▶ Fig. 7.25 and ▶ Fig. 7.26).

The ulnar nerve runs on the palmar side beside the tendon of flexor carpi ulnaris and passes here into the palm of the hand. Lying immediately adjacent to each other in order from medial (ulnar) to lateral are:
• the tendon of flexor carpi ulnaris,
• the ulnar nerve, and
• the ulnar artery (▶ Fig. 7.25 and ▶ Fig. 7.26).

The *superficial branch* of the radial nerve has only sensory fibers at the wrist. About 7 to 8 cm proximal to the wrist, the nerve, which has been on the flexor surface until then, passes under the brachioradialis tendon and now crosses the outer border of the wrist to reach the extensor side of the forearm (▶ Fig. 7.27). It is

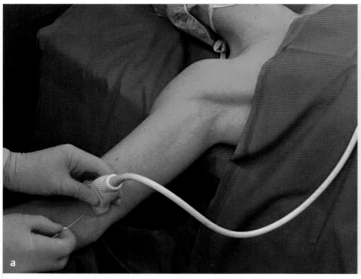

**Fig. 7.22** Visualization of the median nerve at the elbow (see also ▶ Fig. 7.20).
**a** Clinical setting, out-of-plane approach.
**b** Ultrasound image (unlabeled).
**c** Ultrasound image (labeled).
**d** Corresponding anatomical section (unlabeled).
**e** Corresponding anatomical section (labeled).
1 Brachial artery
2 Median nerve
3 Humerus

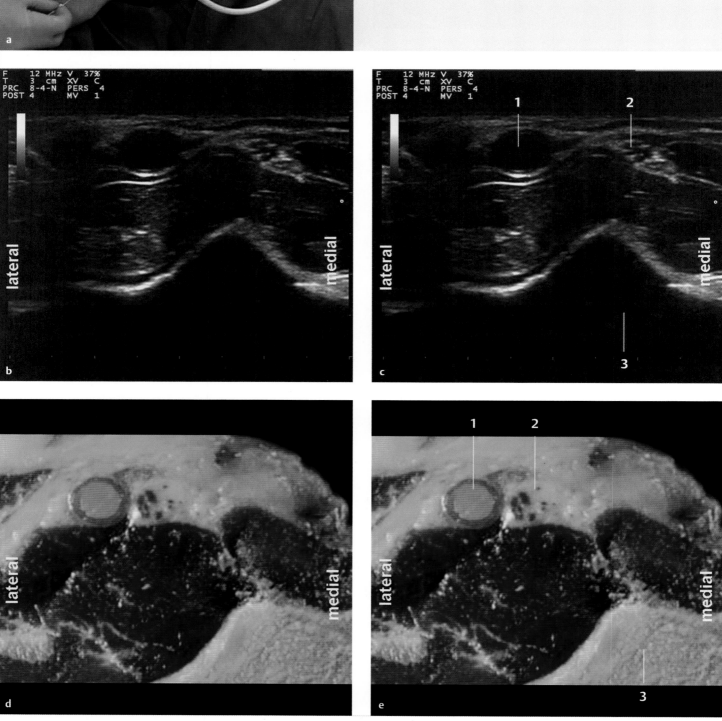

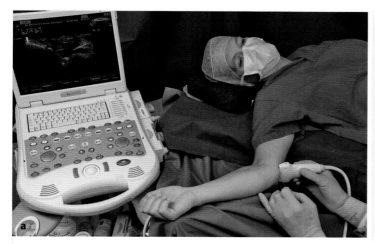

**Fig. 7.23** Visualization of the ulnar nerve proximal to the elbow (short axis) using ultrasound, out-of-plane approach.
**a** Clinical setting, out-of-plane approach.
**b** Ultrasound image (unlabeled).
**c** Ultrasound image (labeled).
1 Medial epicondyle
2 Ulnar nerve

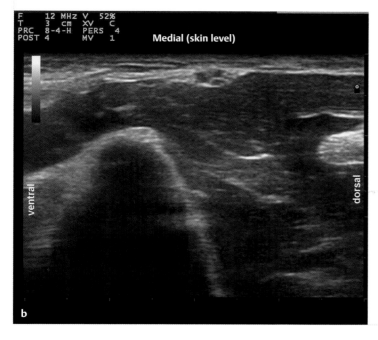

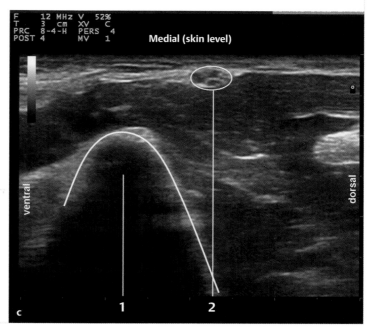

mainly epifascial here and can accordingly be blocked by subcutaneous infiltration.

## 7.3.2 Median Nerve Block (Wrist)

Abducted extended arm, forearm supinated. When the patient's fist is clenched tightly, the tendons of flexor carpi radialis and palmaris longus are readily shown. Directing the needle tangentially toward the nerve, a short 24G or 25G needle is introduced between the two tendons in the region of the wrist crease (▶ Fig. 7.28 and ▶ Fig. 7.29). When paresthesia is produced, the needle is withdrawn minimally and about 3 mL of the local anesthetic is injected. Often the palmaris longus muscle has not developed. In these cases the needle must be inserted on the ulnar side of the flexor carpi radialis tendon. Subsequent subcutaneous infiltration in the radial and ulnar direction ensures a pain-free block of the ulnar and radial nerves.

## 7.3.3 Ulnar Nerve (Wrist)

The needle is inserted three to four finger widths proximal to the wrist directly radial to the tendon of flexor carpi ulnaris; a 25G needle is advanced slowly tangentially toward the nerve (▶ Fig. 7.30 and ▶ Fig. 7.31); when paresthesia is produced, the needle is withdrawn minimally and about 3 mL of the local anesthetic is injected. If no paresthesia is produced, a depot is injected under the tendon of flexor carpi ulnaris. In every case, the block should be supplemented with a subcutaneous injection medial to the tendon of flexor carpi ulnaris in the direction of the ulnar styloid process in order to block the dorsal branch as well.

## 7.3.4 Radial Nerve (Wrist)

Starting from the "anatomical snuff box," subcutaneous infiltration is performed with 5 mL of local anesthetic along the extensor pollicis longus muscle in the direction of the dorsum of the wrist. After withdrawing the needle, further subcutaneous infiltration is performed at a right angle to the previous needle direction toward the palm. A further 5 mL of local anesthetic is given.

Alternatively, a subcutaneous ring infiltration can be injected with local anesthetic on the radial side (▶ Fig. 7.32 and ▶ Fig. 7.33).

## 7.3.5 Block of Individual Nerves with Ultrasound

Linear transducer: 12 MHz
Needle: 5 cm

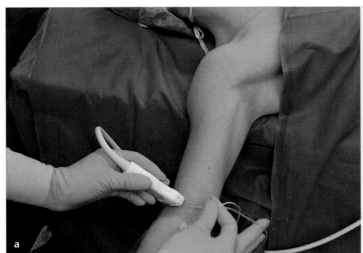

**Fig. 7.24** Radial nerve block in the elbow.
**a** Clinical setting.
**b** Ultrasound image before injection of local anesthetic.
**c** As **b**, but labeled.
**d** Ultrasound image after injection of local anesthetic.
**e** As **d**, but labeled.
1 Radial nerve
Dashed line: space filled with local anesthetic.

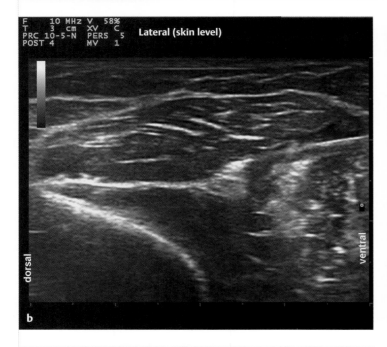

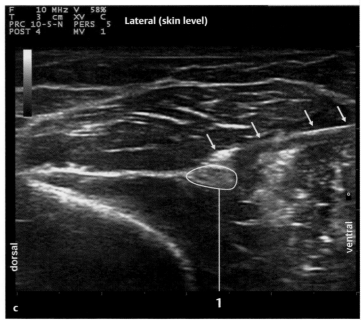

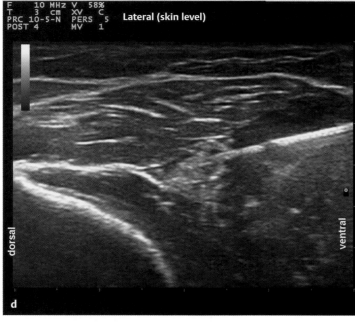

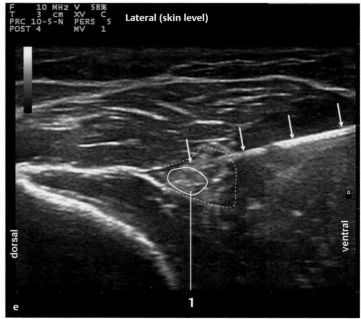

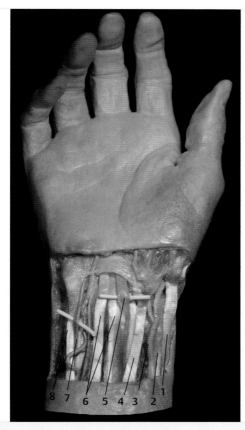

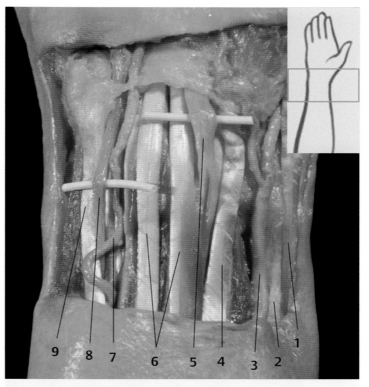

**Fig. 7.25** Anatomy of a right palmar distal forearm region. The palmaris longus muscle is not developed. Block of the median nerve and the ulnar nerve (dissection by Miriam Petrac).
1 Abductor pollicis longus muscle
2 Brachioradialis muscle
3 Radial artery
4 Flexor carpi radialis muscle
5 Median nerve (marked with a yellow band)
6 Tendons of the flexor digitorum superficialis
7 Ulnar nerve marked with a yellow band with ulnar artery
8 Flexor carpi ulnaris

**Fig. 7.26** Anatomy of a right palmar distal forearm region. The palmaris longus muscle is not developed. Block of the median nerve and the ulnar nerve (dissection by Miriam Petrac).
1 Abductor pollicis longus muscle (tendon)
2 Brachioradialis muscle (tendon)
3 Radial artery
4 Flexor carpi radialis
5 Median nerve marked with a yellow band
6 Flexor digitorum superficialis (tendons)
7 A. ulnaris
8 Ulnar nerve marked with a yellow band
9 Flexor carpi ulnaris (tendon)

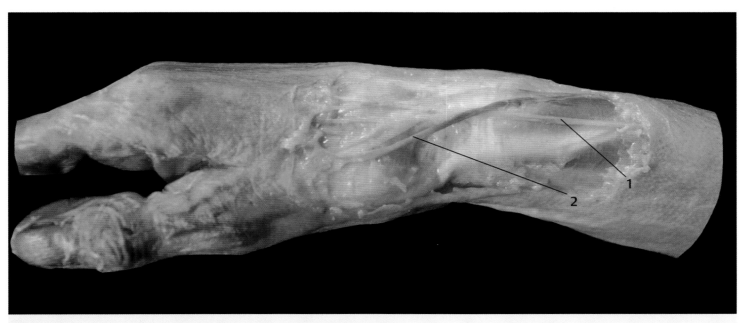

**Fig. 7.27** Terminal branches of the superficial branch of the radial nerve.
1 Superficial branch of the radial nerve
2 Cephalic vein of the forearm

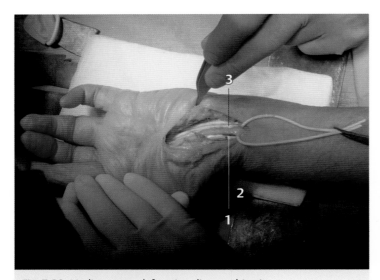

**Fig. 7.28** Median nerve, left wrist, dissected in situ.
1 Tendon of the flexor carpi radialis
2 Median nerve
3 Tendon of the palmaris longus

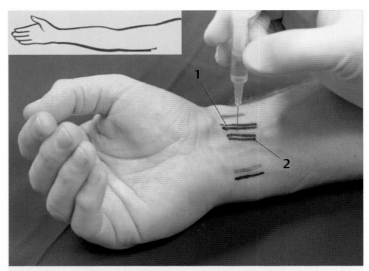

**Fig. 7.29** Median nerve block at the wrist.
1 Tendon of the flexor carpi radialis
2 Tendon of the palmaris longus

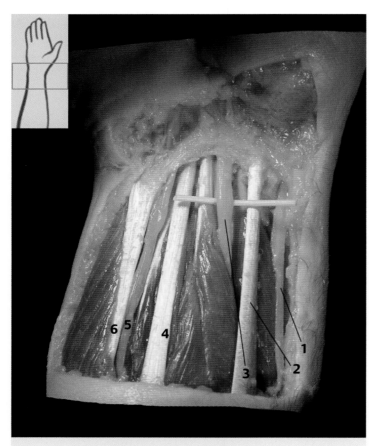

**Fig. 7.30** Right distal forearm at the wrist.
1 Radial artery
2 Flexor carpi radialis
3 Median nerve marked with a yellow band
4 Flexor digitorum superficialis
5 Ulnar artery
6 Flexor carpi ulnaris (hidden by the ulnar nerve)
Caution: The palmaris longus is not developed.

## Ultrasound Orientation

Proximal to the wrist, the median nerve and ulnar nerve can be readily visualized using ultrasound. The terminal branches of the radial nerve can no longer be visualized here; they are blocked by subcutaneous infiltration (Chapter 7.3).

▶ **Median nerve.** The median nerve can be visualized along its entire course from the elbow to the wrist; it is marked by a "honeycomb" structure. In the distal forearm, it lies about 0.6 to 1.0 cm below the skin (McCartney et al 2007; ▶ Fig. 7.34). A puncture directly in the wrist crease is unfavorable for a distal block because the nerve is difficult to distinguish from the surrounding tendons here (▶ Fig. 7.35). The different anisotropic behavior of tendons and nerve can be used for differentiation (Chapter 1). It is better to find the median nerve some 8 to 10 cm proximal to the wrist in the short axis (▶ Fig. 7.36).

▶ **Ulnar nerve.** The ulnar nerve lies in the distal forearm medial (ulnar) to the ulnar artery. It has the typical "honeycomb" structure of peripheral nerves. It is found in the short axis about 5 to 8 cm proximal to the wrist crease (▶ Fig. 7.37), where its branches (dorsal branch and palmar branch of the ulnar nerve) can also be found.

## Needle Approach

All needle insertions can be made out of plane or in plane.

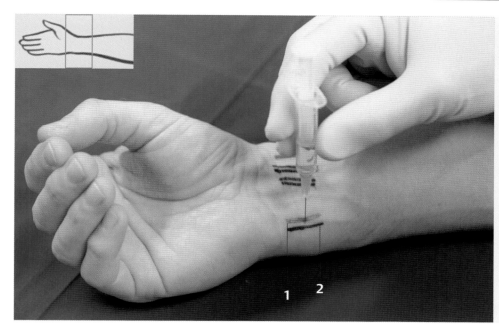

**Fig. 7.31** Ulnar nerve block at the wrist.
1 Ulnar artery
2 Flexor carpi ulnaris

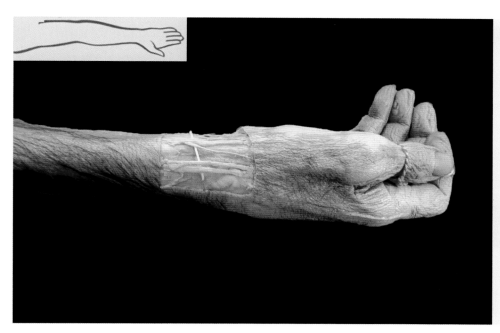

**Fig. 7.32** Terminal branches of the superficial branch of the radial nerve, right wrist.

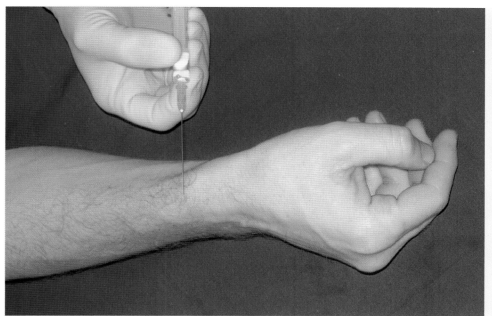

**Fig. 7.33** Radial nerve block at the wrist: subcutaneous infiltration from the radial side.

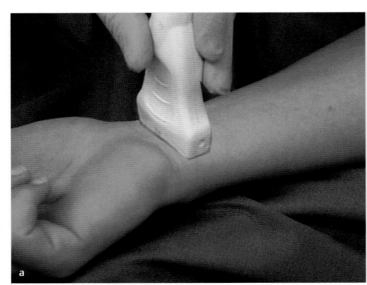

**Fig. 7.34** Anatomical section at the wrist crease.
**a** Transducer position for visualizing the median nerve.
**b** Anatomical section.
**c** With labeling and acoustic window, as visualized in ▶ Fig. 7.35.
* Flexor tendons (for close-up, see ▶ Fig. 7.35)
1 Median nerve
2 Ulnar artery
3 Ulnar nerve
4 Ulna
5 Radius

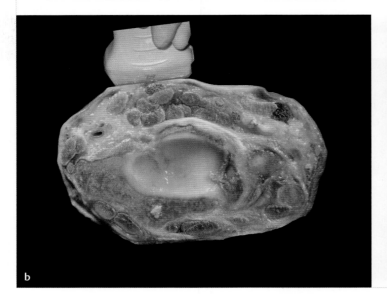

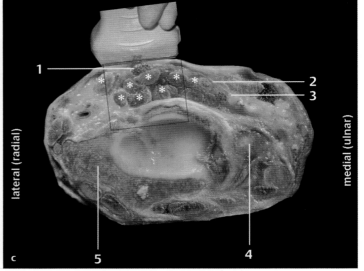

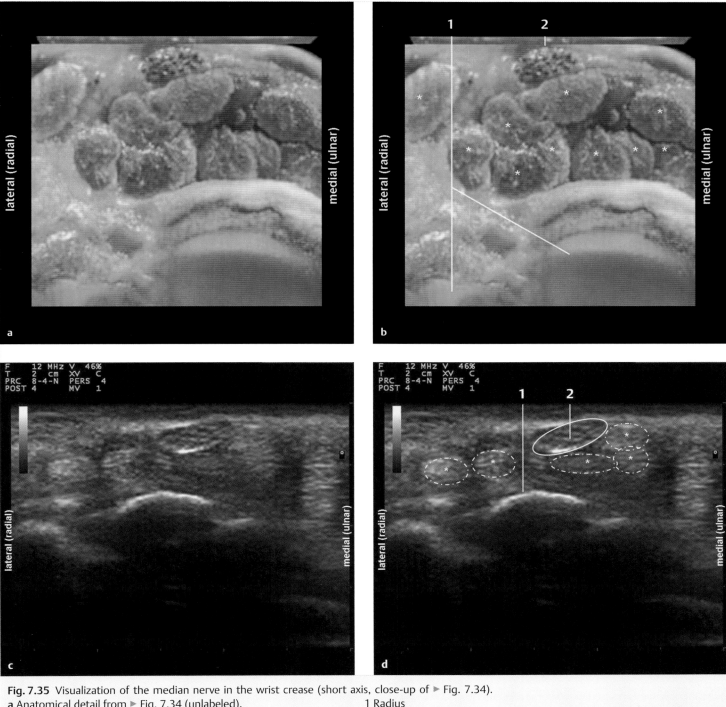

**Fig. 7.35** Visualization of the median nerve in the wrist crease (short axis, close-up of ▸ Fig. 7.34).
**a** Anatomical detail from ▸ Fig. 7.34 (unlabeled).
**b** As **a**, but labeled.
**c** Corresponding ultrasound image (unlabeled).
**d** As **c**, but labeled.

1 Radius
2 Median nerve
* Flexor tendons

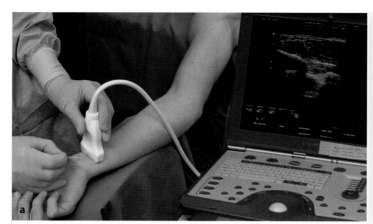

**Fig. 7.36** Visualization of the median nerve about 8 cm proximal to the wrist crease using ultrasound (short axis, out-of-plane approach).
**a** Clinical setting.
**b** Ultrasound image (unlabeled).
**c** Ultrasound image (labeled).
1 Radius
2 Median nerve
3 Ulna

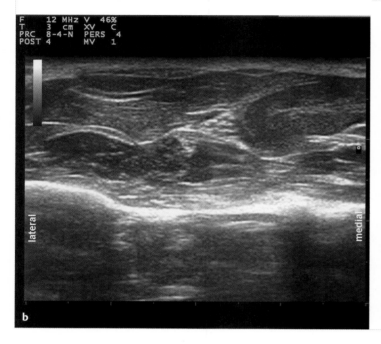

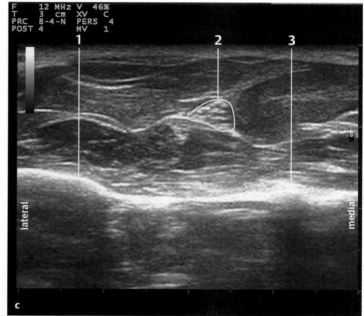

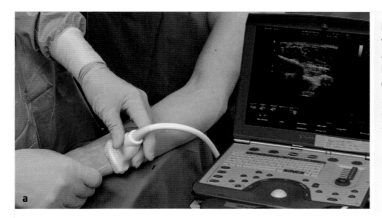

**Fig. 7.37** Visualization of the ulnar nerve about 8 cm proximal to the wrist crease using ultrasound (short axis, out-of-plane approach).
a Clinical setting.
b Ultrasound image (unlabeled).
c Like **b**, but labeled.
1 Ulnar artery
2 Ulnar nerve
3 Ulna

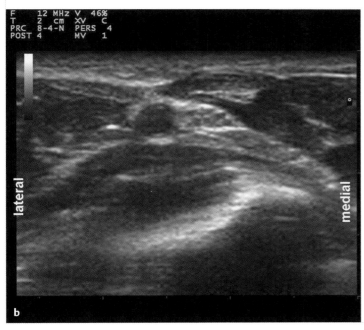

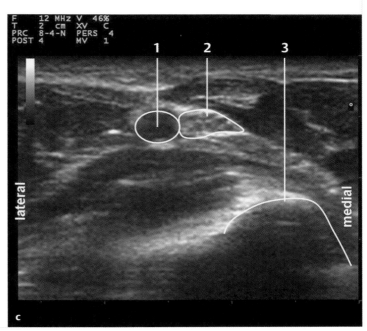

# References

Büttner J, Meier G. Memorix Periphere Regionalanästhesie. Stuttgart: Thieme; 2011

Foxall GL, Skinner D, Hardman JG, Bedforth NM. Ultrasound anatomy of the radial nerve in the distal upper arm. Reg Anesth Pain Med 2007; 32: 217–220

Lurf M, Leixnering M. Ultrasound-guided placement of a median nerve catheter in the forearm. Pain-free mobilisation following arthrolysis and tenolysis. [Article in German] Anaesthesist 2008; 57: 686–688

Lurf M, Leixnering M. Ultrasound-guided ulnar nerve catheter placement in the forearm for postoperative pain relief and physiotherapy. Acta Anaesthesiol Scand 2009; 53: 261–263

Lurf M, Leixnering M. Sensory block without a motor block: ultrasound-guided placement of pain catheters in the forearm. Acta Anaesthesiol Scand 2010; 54: 257–258

McCartney CJL, Xu D, Constantinescu C, Abbas S, Chan VW. Ultrasound examination of peripheral nerves in the forearm. Reg Anesth Pain Med 2007; 32: 434–439

# Part 3

## Lower Limb

# 8 General Overview

## 8.1 Lumbosacral Plexus

The anterior rami of the lumbar, sacral, and coccygeal spinal nerves together form the lumbosacral plexus (▶ Fig. 8.1 and ▶ Fig. 8.2). The lumbar plexus and the sacral plexus are connected by the fourth lumbar nerve to the lumbosacral plexus. This nerve is bifurcated (nervus furcalis) and belongs to both the lumbar plexus (femoral nerve and obturator nerve) and the sacral plexus (L4 segment for the lumbosacral trunk, see ▶ Fig. 8.3).

▶ **Parts relevant for anesthesia.** In contrast to the upper limb, there is no peripheral technique that allows the entire lumbosacral plexus to be anesthetized with one injection, so that for complete "one-legged anesthesia" the lumbar plexus and the sacral plexus (or the parts of them relevant for the leg) must be anesthetized separately.

The parts of the lumbar plexus relevant for anesthesia of the leg are (▶ Fig. 8.4):
- Femoral nerve
- Lateral cutaneous nerve of the thigh
- Obturator nerve

The parts of the *sacral plexus* relevant for innervation of the leg are (▶ Fig. 8.5 and ▶ Fig. 8.6):
- Sciatic nerve with its terminal branches
- Posterior cutaneous nerve of the thigh

### Note

Two injections must generally be made, as complete anesthesia cannot be reliably achieved with a single injection (Gligorijevic 2000).

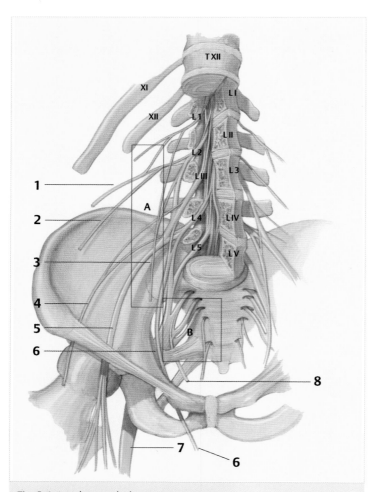

**Fig. 8.1** Lumbosacral plexus, anterior view.
A Lumbar plexus
1 Iliohypogastric nerve
2 Ilioinguinal nerve
3 Genitofemoral nerve
4 Lateral cutaneous nerve of the thigh
5 Femoral nerve
6 Obturator nerve
B Sacral plexus
7 Sciatic nerve
8 Pudendal nerve

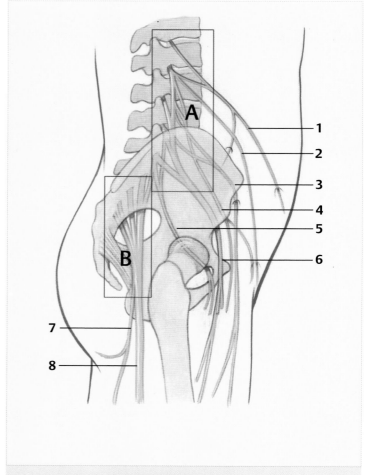

**Fig. 8.2** Lumbosacral plexus, lateral view.
A Lumbar plexus
1 Iliohypogastric nerve
2 Ilioinguinal nerve
3 Lateral cutaneous nerve of the thigh
4 Genitofemoral nerve
5 Obturator nerve
6 Femoral nerve
B Sacral plexus
7 Posterior cutaneous nerve of the thigh
8 Sciatic nerve

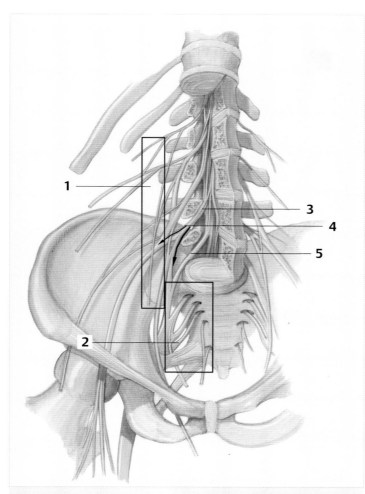

Fig. 8.3 The nervus furcalis arises from the root of L4 and gives off branches to the lumbar plexus and the sacral plexus.
1 Lumbar plexus
2 Sacral plexus
3 Root from L4
4 Nervus furcalis (note division into a branch to the lumbar plexus and a branch to the sacral plexus)
5 Root of L5

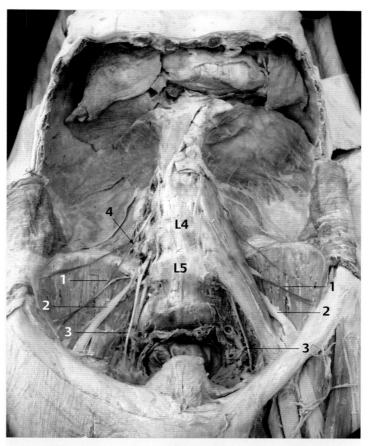

Fig. 8.4 Lumbar plexus, anterior view via the abdominal cavity: the psoas major muscle has been removed on the right.
1 Lateral cutaneous nerve of the thigh
2 Femoral nerve
3 Obturator nerve
4 Destination of needle tip in psoas compartment block

## 8.1.1 Lumbar Plexus

The lumbar plexus is formed by fibers from the 12th thoracic segment and the anterior rami of the 1st to 4th lumbar nerves. Segments L1–L4 are usually involved in the formation of the femoral nerve, the obturator nerve, and the lateral cutaneous nerve of the thigh. The plexus passes peripherally after its exit from the intervertebral foramina, usually covered by the psoas major muscle (▸ Fig. 8.4).

The genitofemoral nerve and the lateral cutaneous nerve of the thigh leave the plexus soon after the iliohypogastric and ilioinguinal nerves have split off.

▸ **Nerves relevant for anesthesia.** The individual nerves of the lumbar plexus relevant for anesthesia are as follows:
- The lateral cutaneous nerve of the thigh (L2/3) passes over the iliacus muscle medial to the anterior superior iliac spine under the inguinal ligament; it is a purely sensory nerve innervating the skin on the lateral side of the thigh.
- The obturator nerve (L2–L4) leaves the plexus medial to the psoas major muscle and passes through the obturator canal together with the obturator vein and artery to the inside of the

thigh. An accessory obturator nerve, which innervates the capsule of the hip joint, is found in 9% of people. The obturator nerve has a very variable sensory area of innervation in the medial thigh and provides motor innervation to the adductors.
- The femoral nerve (L1–L4) is the largest nerve of the lumbar plexus and provides the sensory innervation of the front of the thigh, while its sensory terminal branch, the saphenous nerve, innervates the inside of the lower leg as far as the ankle. The femoral nerve passes anterior to the psoas major muscle under the inguinal ligament through the muscular lacuna and is the motor nerve for the quadriceps femoris, sartorius, and pectineus muscles.

## 8.1.2 Sacral Plexus

The sacral plexus constitutes the lower part of the lumbosacral plexus and is the biggest nerve plexus in the human body. The plexus is formed by the junction of the anterior rami of the five sacral nerves and the coccygeal nerve. It also receives a substantial trunk, the lumbosacral trunk, from the lumbar nerves, which is composed of the entire anterior ramus of the fifth lumbar nerve and fibers from the fourth lumbar nerve (▸ Fig. 8.5). The

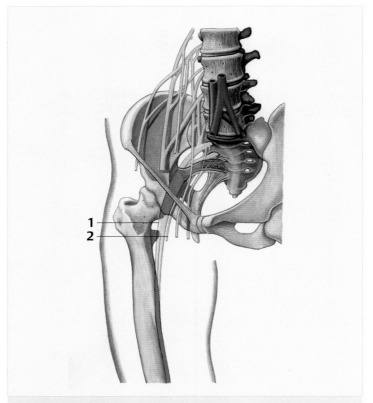

**Fig. 8.5** Course of the sciatic nerve, the main nerve from the sacral plexus.
1 Sciatic nerve
2 Posterior cutaneous nerve of the thigh

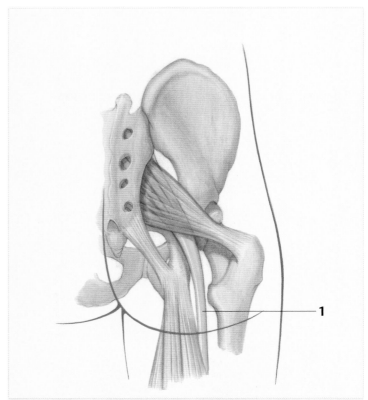

**Fig. 8.6** Sciatic nerve, posterior view.
1 Sciatic nerve

sacral plexus provides the nerves for the parts of the lower limb that are not supplied by the lumbar plexus, that is, for some of the hip muscles, for the flexor side of the thigh, and for all the muscles of the lower leg and foot. It also innervates the skin in part of the buttock area, the posterior side of the thigh, and the posterior, fibular, and anterior side of the lower leg and foot.

▶ **Sciatic plexus.** For anesthesia of the leg, only the so-called sciatic plexus is of importance. It derives its roots from part of the anterior ramus of the 4th lumbar nerve and from the entire anterior ramus of the 5th lumbar nerve, which together form the lumbosacral trunk, and from the anterior rami of the 1st and 2nd and part of the 3rd sacral nerve. The anterior ramus of the 1st sacral nerve is not only the biggest branch of the lumbosacral plexus, but also the biggest anterior ramus overall.

All roots of the plexus converge from their exit sites toward the greater sciatic foramen, so that the plexus forms a triangular sheet, the tip of which points toward the infrapiriform foramen where the sciatic nerve emerges. The nerve plexus lies largely on the piriformis muscle and is covered in pelvic direction by the parietal peritoneum or the tissue beneath it, the parietal fascia of the pelvis, and branches of the iliac artery. Both the superior and inferior gluteal arteries are related to the plexus in that the former passes between the lumbosacral trunk and the root of the 1st sacral nerve, the latter between the 2nd and 3rd sacral nerves.

The articular rami, which supply parts of the hip capsule, and the periosteal branches, which innervate the periosteum of the ischial tuberosity, the greater trochanter, and the lesser trochanter, are derived from the sciatic plexus.

▶ **Nerves relevant for anesthesia.** The following are the nerves relevant for anesthesia of the lower limb (Meier 2003):
• The posterior cutaneous nerve of the thigh (S1–S3), a purely sensory nerve, leaves the pelvis minor through the infrapiriform foramen and passes a long distance subfascially, but close to the fascia lata downward on the back of the thigh toward the back of the knee.
• The sciatic nerve (L4–S3) is the biggest nerve in the body. It derives its fibers from all the roots of the sacral plexus and innervates the entire lower leg and foot, the ischiocrural muscles of the thigh, and the small external rotators of the hip. It leaves the pelvis through the infrapiriform foramen and then passes downward in the middle third between the ischial tuberosity and the greater trochanter. The proximal part of the popliteal fossa is the furthest point at which it will divide into its two terminal branches: the tibial nerve for the flexor muscles of the ankle and sole of the foot and the common fibular nerve (also known as the common peroneal nerve) for the extensor side of the ankle and the dorsum of the foot.
• The *tibial nerve* supplies the motor innervation to the flexor muscles of the ankle and is responsible for the flexors of the toes and foot. It provides sensory innervation to the skin of the lateral lower leg and the sole of the foot, and after joining the communicating branch of the fibular nerve it innervates the lateral margin of the heel and foot as the *sural nerve* and its terminal branch the *lateral dorsal cutaneous nerve*. Complete anesthesia of the tibial nerve makes plantar flexion of the foot nearly impossible while spreading and closing of the toes are rendered completely impossible.

• The *common fibular nerve* (L4–S2) runs in the popliteal fossa lateral to the tibial nerve and medial to the biceps femoris muscle as far as its attachment to the head of the fibula. Distally from this point it winds around the neck of the fibula to pass posteriorly through the intermuscular septum of the leg to reach the peroneal compartment. Here it enters the gap between the origins of the fibularis longus muscle (also known as the peroneus longus) and immediately divides into its two branches. One of them is predominantly sensory (superficial fibular nerve) and the other is mainly motor (deep fibular nerve). The superficial fibular nerve supplies "little muscle and a lot of skin," namely motor supply only to the fibular muscles but sensory innervation to the skin of the lower leg and with its medial and intermediate dorsal cutaneous nerves to the skin of the dorsum of the foot and the toes. The deep fibular nerve in contrast supplies "a lot of muscles and little skin," namely motor supply to extensor muscles of the lower leg and sensory supply only to the sides of the first and second toes facing each other (also called the first interdigital space).

# 8.2 Historical Overview—Lower Limb

In 1784, the English surgeon James Moore (1762–1860) published a small book with the title "A Method of Preventing or Diminishing Pain in Several Operations of Surgery." Among other things, it described the isolated anesthesia of the sciatic nerve. At that time, Moore suggested to surgeon John Hunter at St. George's Hospital in London that he compress the sciatic nerve with a metal clamp to perform a foot amputation with as little pain as possible. The attempt was successful, but the method did not become established because the pain caused by the strong compression was almost as severe as the pain caused by the surgical procedure.

▶ **Development of a hollow needle.** In 1853, a hollow needle was developed by Alexander Wood from Edinburgh that allowed drugs to be injected under the skin. In the same year, Charles Gabriel Pravaz from France introduced a glass syringe that could be used in combination with Wood's hollow needle to inject drugs.

▶ **Cocaine.** In 1860, chemists Albert Niemann and Wilhelm Lossen from Göttingen succeeded for the first time in isolating the main alkaloid of the coca plant, which Niemann named "cocaine." Thomas Moreno y Maiz from Peru reported in 1868 that injecting a cocaine solution into the thigh of bullfrogs led to complete anesthesia. Moreno y Maiz concluded his article with the question: "Could cocaine be used as a local anesthetic? The future will tell."

▶ **Development of new local anesthetics.** The conditions for performing regional anesthesia were thus already present in the 19th century. But it was not until the first half of the 20th century that the development of new local anesthetics (novocaine, procaine, lidocaine) gave new impetus leading to progress in performing peripheral nerve blocks.

▶ **Block of the lower limb with multiple injections.** Nyström described the block of the lateral cutaneous nerve of the thigh as far back as 1904. Läwen then combined this with a femoral nerve block. In 1911—the same year that Hirschel from Heidelberg and Kulenkampff from Zwickau also reported on their techniques for an upper limb block—an article was published by A. Läwen, who was a senior physician in the department of surgery in Leipzig at the time, titled: "On Conduction Anesthesia of the Lower Limb, with Remarks on the Technique of Injections of the Sciatic Nerve for Treatment of Sciatica." Läwen succeeded in anesthetizing the entire lower limb with multiple separate injections in the vicinity of the sciatic and femoral nerves. However, he himself considered the method to be of only limited use for clinical routine because of the multiple injections.

▶ **Transgluteal technique.** In 1923, some 12 years later, the founder of the American Society of Regional Anesthesia, Gaston Labat, described the transgluteal technique of sciatic nerve block in his book "Regional Anesthesia." Paralumbar anesthesia techniques were also described at the start of the last century, and as early as 1929, Braun described a series of techniques for lumbar plexus block.

▶ **Psoas compartment block.** In the hopes of having found a method with a paravertebral approach that would allow a block of the entire lumbosacral plexus with one injection, the term "combined lumbosacral plexus anesthesia" was coined by Winnie in 1974 (Winnie et al 1974). Two years later Chayen et al (1976) described a comparable technique and called it "psoas compartment block" (PCB).

Brands and Callahan (1978) described a continuous technique of the psoas compartment block that was performed based on the technique introduced by Chayen. However, they entered between the costal process of L3 and L4 and then advanced an epidural catheter over an 18G needle into the psoas compartment.

▶ **Inguinal paravascular technique: 3-in-1 block.** The work of Alan Winnie, who described the inguinal paravascular technique of the lumbar plexus block ("3-in-1 block"; Winnie et al 1973) was immensely important for the development of continuous regional anesthesia. Winnie had developed the concept of a common fascia space between the psoas major and the iliac muscles for the femoral nerve, obturator nerve, and lateral cutaneous nerve of the thigh and postulated that the nerves of the lumbar plexus could be anesthetized by the spread of local anesthetic via the iliopsoas fascia (iliac fascia).

In the following years, continuous methods were also described, both for the psoas compartment block and in 1980 for the first time, the continuous "3-in-1" block by Rosen. The "3-in-1" block was widely used, especially in combination with a sciatic nerve block.

▶ **Posterior transgluteal sciatic nerve block.** The sacral plexus block in the form of a sciatic nerve block can be performed as a posterior, anterior, lateral, or popliteal technique. The Labat posterior transgluteal technique is often cited and is now considered the standard technique. In 1998, Sutherland described a posterior but very complicated approach that makes a continuous technique possible (Sutherland 1998). Other modifications have been described over the years. It is conspicuous that they are mostly case reports and there are no studies with larger numbers of cases.

▶ **Parasacral sciatic nerve block.** Mansour (1993) reported on a parasacral block of the sciatic nerve. Morris added the possibility of continuous anesthesia by catheter placement (Morris and Lang 1997) to widen the range of posterior parasacral block techniques.

▶ **Anterior sciatic nerve block.** In 1963, Beck described the anterior sciatic nerve block (Beck 1963). The landmarks used in Beck's anterior technique are difficult to find in obese patients or patients with a hip replacement on the side to be anesthetized. In 1999, Chelly published an article with new guidelines for the anterior sciatic nerve block technique that simplify anatomical orientation.

▶ **Continuous anterior sciatic nerve block.** Meier et al investigated the optimal conditions for the continuous technique of the anterior sciatic nerve block during intensive anatomical studies. As the result of these studies, Meier described a continuous anterior sciatic nerve block which is reliable and easy to perform (Meier and Heinrich 1995, Meier et al 1999). A continuous technique is used especially postoperatively to treat pain in the popliteal fossa and for pain syndromes of the lower leg and foot.

▶ **Knee block.** A method of sciatic nerve block that has been in use for many years is the so-called "knee block," a block of the tibial and fibular nerves in the popliteal fossa. This method has been proven for decades as a single dose "popliteal nerve block" in the popliteal fossa. In recent years, continuous popliteal sciatic nerve blocks have been described that can be used not only for pain therapy, but also to improve circulation in the foot.

▶ **Distal sciatic nerve block.** Several groups have been working on the possibilities of a distal sciatic nerve block. Vloka et al worked very intensively on the anatomical situation in the popliteal fossa and published their impressive anatomical studies in 1996. In the same year, Singelyn et al (1997) and Meier et al (1999) described a method for continuous distal sciatic nerve block. Singelyn selects an approach 10 cm cranial to the popliteal fossa in the midline, Meier lateral to the proximal border of the popliteal fossa.

▶ **Foot block.** Nerve blocks at the lower leg, ankle, and foot were already performed and described by many authors at the start of the 20th century, but only very little research into this has been published. In 1967, Nolte and Dam published a method that makes complete anesthesia of the foot possible through a combination of individual peripheral blocks and they called this technique "foot block." This method originated in Iceland. The foot block was used there very successfully and with no appreciable side effects for surgical treatment of foot injuries that are very common in fishermen. These techniques are still significant for outpatient care and to supplement regional anesthesia (Meier 2010).

## 8.3 Sensory Innervation of the Leg

The sensory innervation of the leg (▶ Fig. 8.7) can be variable. There are regions where two nerves can overlap to provide the sensory innervation. In particular, the division of the sensory

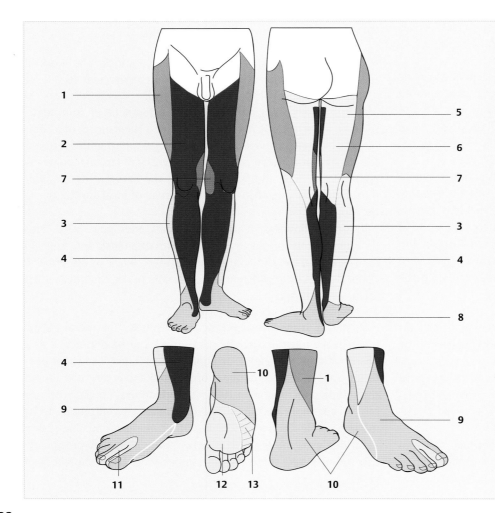

**Fig. 8.7** Sensory innervation of the lower limb. Blue: area of the femoral nerve and its branches. Yellow: area of the sciatic nerve and its branches. Light blue: area of the lateral cutaneous nerve of the thigh. Green: area of the obturator nerve.
1 Lateral cutaneous nerve of the thigh
2 Femoral nerve
3 Fibular nerve
4 Saphenous nerve
5 Sciatic nerve
6 Posterior cutaneous nerve of the thigh
7 Obturator nerve
8 Posterior tibial nerve
9 Superficial fibular nerve
10 Sural nerve
11 Deep fibular nerve
12 Medial plantar nerve
13 Lateral plantar nerve (tibial nerve)

innervation of the anterior and medial parts of the thigh is very variable.

In most cases, a femoral nerve block in conjunction with a sciatic nerve block is adequate for complete anesthesia of the leg. The obturator nerve does not appear to be consistently involved in the sensory innervation of the knee. However, for complex knee operations (e.g., total knee replacement), an additional block of the obturator nerve or a psoas compartment block as an alternative to femoral nerve block should be performed.

The question of which area of skin receives its sensory innervation from the obturator nerve cannot be answered clearly, and occasionally the obturator nerve does not appear to have any "area" of its own.

▶ **Bony innervation.** In individual cases, clinical experience also contradicts the periostal innervation of the lower limb generally accepted today (▶ Fig. 8.7). The head of the tibia is considered to be innervated mainly by parts of the sciatic nerve; however, in clear contradiction to this, a selective femoral nerve block is extremely effective for postoperative pain management of a fracture of the head of the tibia, which is often very painful after surgery.

The bony innervation of the femur close to the hip is also inconsistent with the usually successful pain therapy by means of femoral nerve block after hip fractures. One explanation might be that the soft tissue (innervated by the femoral nerve) is primarily responsible for the pain.

▶ **Motor response.** ▶

## 8.3.1 Innervation of the Bones (Innervation of Periosteum)

Relevant anatomical relations (periosteal innervation) for anesthesia and pain therapy:

- The periosteum of the femur is innervated posteriorly and anteriorly by the sciatic nerve in the upper third, by the obturator nerve in the middle third, and in the distal third laterally by the sciatic nerve and medially by the femoral and obturator nerves.
- The knee joint is innervated by branches of the femoral and sciatic nerves anteriorly, and posteriorly by branches of the sciatic, obturator, and saphenous nerves.
- With the exception of the lateral head of the tibia and the head of the fibula (supplied by the common fibular nerve), the periosteum of the tibia and fibula is supplied by the tibial nerve (important for lower leg amputations, fractures).
- The ankle receives its sensory supply from the tibial and sural nerves.
- The periosteum of the tarsal bones is innervated by the sural nerve and parts of the tibial nerve, and the metatarsals and the phalanges are innervated by the deep fibular nerve and terminal branches of the tibial nerve (Wagner 1994).

The motor responses are detailed in the videos on the MediaCenter. ▶

## References

Beck GP. Anterior approach to sciatic nerve block. Anesthesiology 1963; 24: 222–224

Brands E, Callahan V. Continuous lumbar plexus block. Anaesth Intens Care 1978; 256–258

Chayen D, Nathan H, Chayen M. The psoas compartment block. Anesthesiology 1976; 45: 95–99

Chelly JE, Delaunay L. A new anterior approach to the sciatic nerve. Anesthesiology 1999; 91: 1655-1660

Dam W, Nolte H. Anästhesie unter primitiven Bedingungen und während Massenkatastrophen. Wehrdienst und Gesundheit 1967; Bd. 15, Wehr und Wissen, Darmstadt: 225-231

Gligorijevic S. Lower extremity blocks for day surgery. Tech Reg Anesth Pain Manage 2000; 4: 30–37

Mansour NY. Reevaluating the sciatic nerve block: another landmark for consideration. Reg Anesth 1993; 18: 322–323

Meier G, Heinrich Ch. Sciatic nerve block: A comparison of three different techniques. 24th Central European Congress on Anesthesiology. Bologna: Monduzzi; 1995: 509–512

Meier G. Der kontinuierliche Ischiadikusblock zur Anästhesie und postoperativen Schmerztherapie. Anaesthesist 1996; 45 S2: 100

Meier G. Der kontinuierliche anteriore Ischiadicuskatheter (KAI). In: Mehrkens HH, Büttner J, ed Kontinuierliche periphere Leitungsblockaden. Munich: Arcis; 1999: 47–48

Meier G, Bauereis Ch, Meier Th. Kontinuierliche distale Ischiadicusblockaden zur Schmerztherapie. Schmerz 1999; S1: 74–75

Meier G. Nervenblockaden an den unteren Extremitäten. In: Niesel HC, Van Aken H, ed Lokalanästhesie, Regionalanästhesie, Regionale Schmerztherapie. 2nd ed Stuttgart: Thieme; 2003: 306–393

Meier G. Nervenblockaden an den unteren Extremitäten. In: Van Aken H, Wulf H, eds. Lokalanästhesie, Regionalanästhesie, Regionale Schmerztherapie. 3rd ed. Stuttgart: Thieme; 2010

Morris GF, Lang SA. Continuous parasacral sciatic nerve block: two case reports. Reg Anesth 1997; 22: 469–472

Platzer W. Color Atlas of Human Anatomy Vol 1. Locomotor System. 7th edition. Stuttgart: Thieme; 2014

Rosenblatt RM. Continuous femoral anesthesia for lower extremity surgery. Anesth Analg 1980; 59: 631–632

Singelyn FJ, Aye F, Gouverneur JM. Continuous popliteal sciatic nerve block: an original technique to provide postoperative analgesia after foot surgery. Anesth Analg 1997; 84: 383–386

Sutherland IDB. Continuous sciatic nerve infusion: expanded case report describing a new approach. Reg Anesth Pain Med 1998; 23: 496–501

Vloka JD, Hadzić A, Kitain E et al. Anatomic considerations for sciatic nerve block in the popliteal fossa through the lateral approach. Reg Anesth 1996a; 21: 414–418

Vloka J, Hadzić A, Lesser J et al. Presence and anatomical characteristics of a common perineural sheath in the popliteal fossa. Reg Anesth 1996b; 21: 13

Wagner F. Beinnervenblockaden. In: Niesel HC, ed. Regionalanästhesie, Lokalanästhesie, Regionale Schmerztherapie. Stuttgart: Thieme; 1994: 417–521

Winnie AP, Ramamurthy S, Durrani Z. The inguinal paravascular technic of lumbar plexus anesthesia: the "3-in-1 block". Anesth Analg 1973; 52: 989–996

Winnie AP, Ramamuethy S, Durrani Z, Radojinic R. Plexus blocks for lower extremity surgery. New answers to old problems. Anesthesiol Rev 1974; 1: 11–16

# 9 Psoas Block

## 9.1 Anatomical Overview

The anterior rami of the first four lumbar nerves lie between the deep and the superficial origins of the psoas major muscle and form the lumbar plexus. The ramus of the fourth lumbar nerve divides into cranial, medial, and caudal branches:

- The cranial part supplies the femoral nerve.
- The medial part supplies the obturator nerve.
- The caudal branch combines with the anterior ramus of the fifth lumbar nerve to form the lumbosacral trunk, which is involved in forming the sacral plexus (▶ Fig. 9.1 and ▶ Fig. 9.2).

▶ **Iliohypogastric nerve and ilioinguinal nerve.** The first branch from the lumbar plexus, the iliohypogastric nerve, lies at the lateral border of the psoas major muscle. It is usually followed by the ilioinguinal nerve, passing through the psoas muscle and running almost parallel.

▶ **Genitofemoral nerve.** The next nerve passing through psoas major is the genitofemoral nerve, which divides at a variable level into the genital branch and the femoral branch.

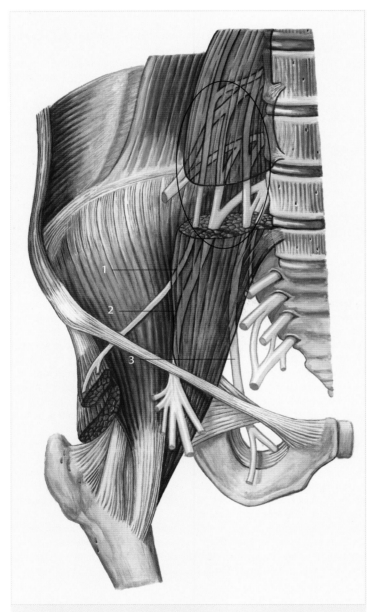

**Fig. 9.1** The lumbar plexus penetrates the psoas major muscle. The area of the psoas major and the lumbar plexus has to be found so that the local anesthetic can be injected here.
1 Lateral cutaneous nerve of the thigh
2 Femoral nerve
3 Obturator nerve
Oval region included by the block.

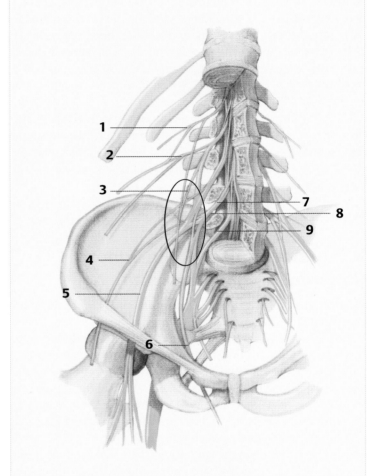

**Fig. 9.2** Anatomy of the lumbar plexus. The lumbar plexus is formed from the anterior rami of the nerve roots of T12 and L1–L4. It gives branches to the sacral plexus (nervus furcalis). With the psoas block a block of the obturator nerve can be expected, contrary to the femoral nerve block.
1 Iliohypogastric nerve
2 Ilioinguinal nerve
3 Genitofemoral nerve
4 Lateral cutaneous nerve of the thigh
5 Femoral nerve
6 Obturator nerve
7 Root of L4
8 Nervus furcalis (connecting L4/L5)
9 Root of L5, going to the sacral plexus
Oval region included in psoas block.

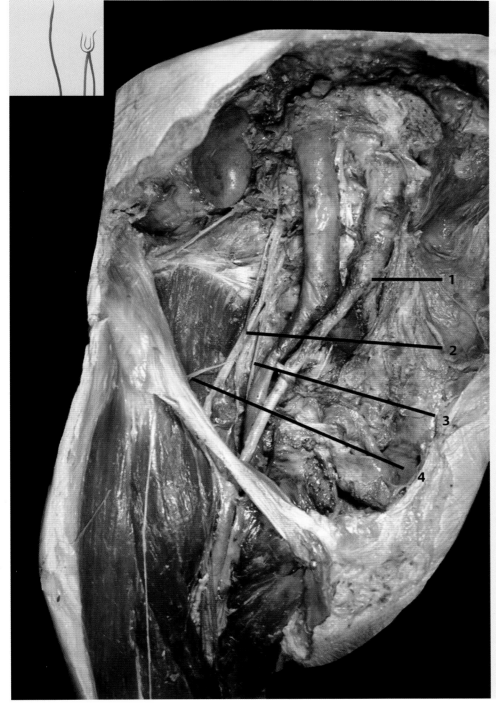

**Fig. 9.3** Lumbar plexus.
1 Bifurcation of the abdominal aorta corresponding to L4
2 Femoral nerve
3 Obturator nerve
4 Lateral cutaneous nerve of the thigh

▶ **Lateral cutaneous nerve of the thigh.** A further branch of the lumbar plexus lying at the lateral border of the psoas major muscle is the lateral cutaneous nerve of the thigh, which reaches the muscular lacuna far laterally close to the anterior superior iliac spine.

▶ **Femoral nerve.** The biggest branch, the femoral nerve, runs in the groove between the iliacus and psoas major muscles and passes through the muscular lacuna to the thigh.

▶ **Obturator nerve.** The last branch, the obturator nerve, is the only one that runs medial to the psoas major muscle and reaches the obturator canal after passing beneath the external iliac artery and vein and crossing the linea terminalis of the lesser pelvis. It passes through and perforates the parietal pelvic fascia to reach the obturator canal (▶ Fig. 9.2 and ▶ Fig. 9.3).

**Note**

There is no evidence of a compartment in the anatomical sense. The lumbar plexus permeates the psoas muscle. The term "psoas compartment block" should be replaced by "psoas block."

## 9.2 Technique of Psoas Block ▶

### 9.2.1 Classical Technique (according to Chayen)

The technique, originally called "psoas compartment block", was described in 1976 by Chayen (Chayen et al 1976). In the following years, other versions of the technique were published, including continuous anesthesia (e.g., Geiger 1999).

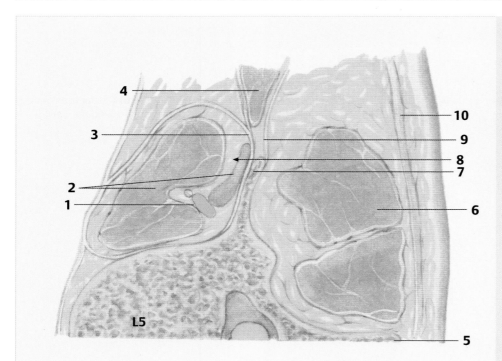

Fig. 9.4 Anatomy at the level of the puncture site for psoas block (transverse section).
1 Lumbar plexus, nerve roots
2 Psoas major muscle
3 Psoas fascia
4 Quadratus lumborum muscle
5 Spinous process
6 Erector spinae muscle
7 Transverse process
8 Direction of needle
9 Transversalis fascia
10 Thoracolumbar fascia

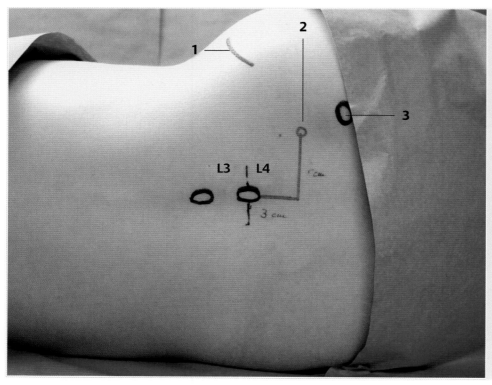

Fig. 9.5 Psoas block can be performed in the lateral decubitus or sitting position. The injection site is 3 cm below the spinous process of L4 and 5 cm lateral to the interspinal line. Occasionally, 5 cm is too far laterally, so a distance of 4 to 4.5 cm should be selected in slim patients.
1 Iliac crest
2 Injection site
3 Posterior superior iliac spine

The position of the lumbar plexus between the fasciae of the psoas major muscle, quadratus lumborum, and the vertebral bodies allows a cranial block of the lumbar plexus (Platzer 2014; ▸ Fig. 9.4).

## Landmarks

A dorsal line between the iliac crests marks the spinous process of the 4th lumbar vertebra. A 3-cm interspinal line is drawn caudally from the spinous process of L4. From the caudal end of this line, a 5-cm line is drawn laterally at a right angle toward the side to be blocked. This second line ends a little before the medial border of the iliac crest, cranial to the posterior superior iliac spine, and corresponds to the insertion site (▸ Fig. 9.5).

## Position of the Patient

The patient is positioned on his or her side with the legs drawn up and the spine flexed with the side to be anesthetized uppermost (▸ Fig. 9.6). Alternatively, the patient may assume a sitting position, similar to that used for neuraxial anesthesia (▸ Fig. 9.7).

## Method

Using continuous stimulation with a current of 0.5 to 1.0 mA, a needle 10 to 12 cm long is advanced at a right angle to the skin in strictly sagittal direction (▸ Fig. 9.6, ▸ Fig. 9.7, ▸ Fig. 9.8). Contact between the needle tip and the transverse process of the 5th lumbar vertebra is first sought at a depth of 5 cm to a maximum

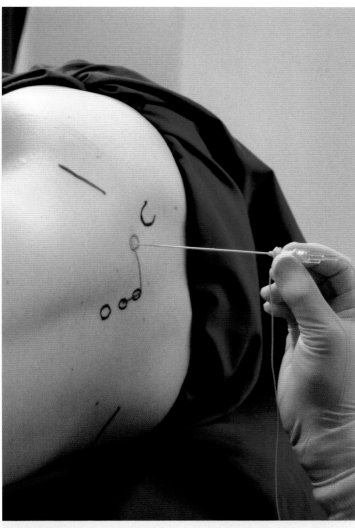

**Fig. 9.6** The needle must be directed strictly sagittally in psoas block, that is, perpendicular to all planes.

**Fig. 9.7 a, b** Psoas block can be performed in the lateral decubitus or sitting position. The injection site is 3 cm below the spinous process of L4 and 5 cm lateral to the interspinal line. The 5 cm distance occasionally proves to be too far laterally, so a distance of 4 to 4.5 cm should be selected in slim patients. The needle must be directed strictly sagittally in psoas block. After about 5 to 8 cm the costal (transverse) process of L5 is usually encountered. After withdrawing the needle slightly, it is advanced further cranial to the process. A further 2 cm (up to 2.5 cm) deeper than the transverse process, a loss of resistance is felt when the transversalis fascia or quadratus lumborum is penetrated if an appropriate needle and technique are used. The nerve stimulator shows a response in the quadriceps muscle when the lumbar plexus is reached. A response in the region of the foot can occasionally be observed; in this case parts of the L4 root passing to the sacral plexus have been stimulated, and this indicates that the needle direction is too medial.

1 Spinous process of L4
2 Iliac crest
3 Posterior superior iliac spine
4 Transverse process of L5

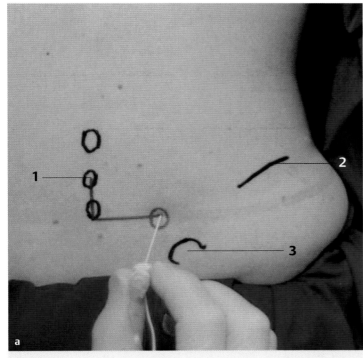

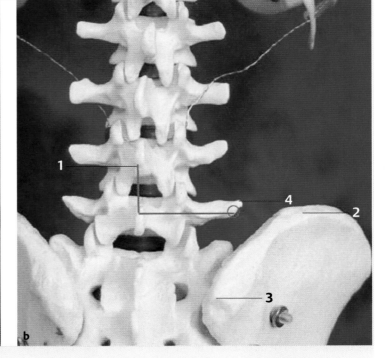

**Fig. 9.7**

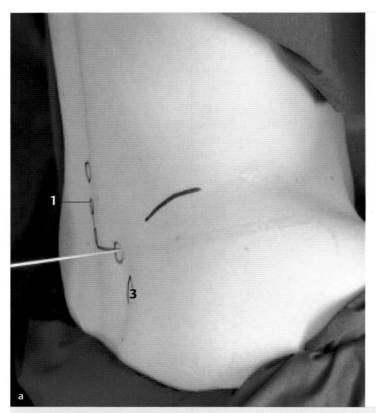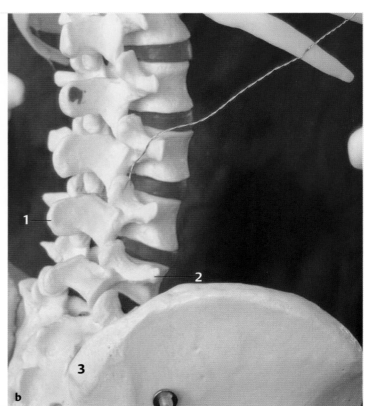

**Fig. 9.8 a, b** The needle must be directed strictly sagittally in psoas block, that is, perpendicular to all planes. The transverse process of L5 is usually encountered after about 5 to 8 cm. After withdrawing the needle slightly, it is advanced cranial to the process. Contact with the transverse process is helpful for depth orientation and the needle should not be advanced more than 2 to 2.5 cm after bone contact, in general never deeper than 11 cm.
1 Spinous process of L4
2 Transverse process of L5
3 Posterior superior iliac spine

of 8 cm (▶ Fig. 9.7 and ▶ Fig. 9.8). After making bone contact and withdrawing the needle about 4 cm, the needle is changed to a more cranial direction and advanced again.

> **Note**
>
> The needle should never be advanced more than 2.5 cm beyond the first bone contact, and never more than 11 cm overall (▶ Fig. 9.8).

When the needle has passed the transverse process of the 5th lumbar vertebra, the loss of resistance after passing through the quadratus lumborum muscle and transversalis and psoas fascia indicates that the psoas compartment has been reached (▶ Fig. 9.9, ▶ Fig. 9.10, ▶ Fig. 9.11, ▶ Fig. 9.12, ▶ Fig. 9.13).

Muscle contractions of the quadriceps (anterior thigh) indicate that the tip of the needle is in the correct position close to the femoral nerve (▶ Fig. 9.14). The desired response corresponds to the motor block obtained by femoral nerve blockade.

After careful aspiration, a test dose of 3 mL of local anesthetic is injected to exclude an incorrect intrathecal position. This is followed by injection of 40 mL of a medium-acting or long-acting local anesthetic. After each 10 mL, aspiration should be repeated to exclude an accidental intravascular position. Initially, 40 mL of prilocaine 1% or mepivacaine 1% (10 mg/mL) or 30 mL of prilocaine 1% (10 mg/mL) and 10 mL of ropivacaine 0.75% (7.5 mg/mL) can be injected (Büttner and Meier 1999, Geiger 1999, Meier and Büttner 2001).

## Continuous Psoas Block

The anatomical orientation corresponds to the landmarks given by Chayen (see above). The puncture is made with a 12-cm stimulation needle, which allows a catheter to be introduced. When advancing the needle, the transverse process of the 5th lumbar vertebra does not absolutely have to be contacted. Contractions of the quadriceps indicate the immediate vicinity of the femoral nerve.

After correct stimulation, negative aspiration, and a test dose of a local anesthetic (3 mL of a medium-acting local anesthetic to exclude an intrathecal position), 30 mL of local anesthetic is injected. The catheter is advanced caudally (▶ Fig. 9.15). Slight resistance at the end of the needle during advancement is normal and is caused by the transition of the needle tip to the tissue. This slight resistance is usually easily overcome (Geiger 1999).

A trial aspiration is performed to exclude an intravascular position and another test dose is given through the catheter to exclude an intrathecal position.

Initially, 20 mL of prilocaine 1% (10 mg/mL) and 10 mL of ropivacaine 0.5% (5 mg/mL) can be injected; for continuous administration, 5 to 15 mL/h of ropivacaine 0.2% (2 mg/mL) can be injected or bolus injections of 20 mL of ropivacaine 0.2 to 0.375% (2–3.75 mg/mL) can be given. The maximum recommended dose of ropivacaine is 37.5 mg/h (Büttner and Meier 1999, Meier 2001, Meier and Büttner 2001; ▶ Fig. 9.16 and ▶ Fig. 9.17).

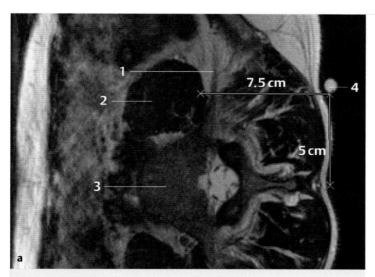

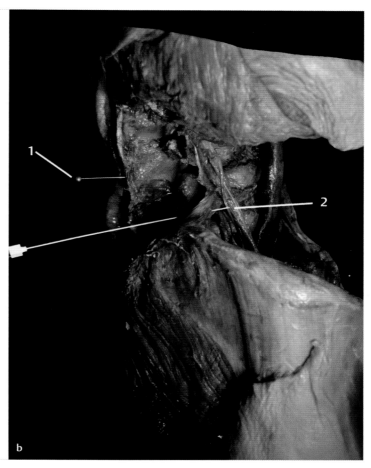

**Fig. 9.9 a, b** MRI scan of the injection site for psoas block.
**a** NMR scan at the level of the injection site. Note the depth of
7.5 cm at which the psoas major muscle is
reached (average male, 75 kg, 185 cm).
1 Transverse process of L5
2 Psoas major muscle
3 L5
4 Injection site, marked
**b** Lumbar plexus.
1 Needle in the spinous process of L4
2 Femoral nerve

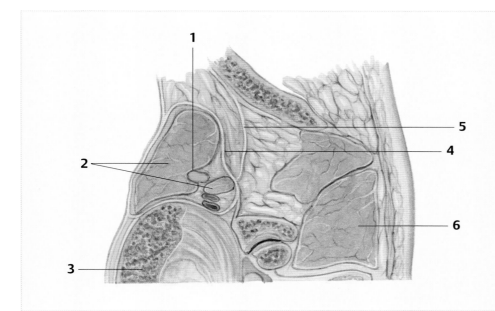

**Fig. 9.10** Diagram of anatomy corresponding to
the plane of the MR image in ▶ Fig. 9.9.
1 Lumbar plexus
2 Psoas major muscle
3 L5
4 Psoas fascia
5 Transversalis fascia
6 Erector spinae muscle

## 9.2.2 Psoas Blockade with Ultrasound

Curved array: 2 to 5 MHz
Penetration depth: 10 to 15 cm
Needle: 10 to 12 cm

### Ultrasound Orientation

An overview of the position of the kidneys is possible in the *frontal plane* (▶ Fig. 9.19). The neural structures in the psoas muscle can usually not be visualized in adults by ultrasound due to the large skin-to-nerve distance. The nerves run in the posterior third of the psoas major muscle.

In the next step, the distance from the skin to the costal processes (transverse processes) can be determined in the *parasagittal plane (long axis)* using ultrasound (▶ Fig. 9.19). In the long axis, the transducer is moved laterally from the sagittal plane starting from the level of L4/5 toward the side to be anesthetized. First the articular process becomes visible, appearing as a more or less continuous, wavy hyperechoic line with interrupted acoustic shadows below it caused by the bony structures of the articular process (▶ Fig. 9.20). When the transducer is moved

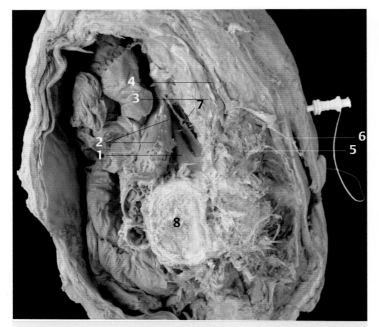

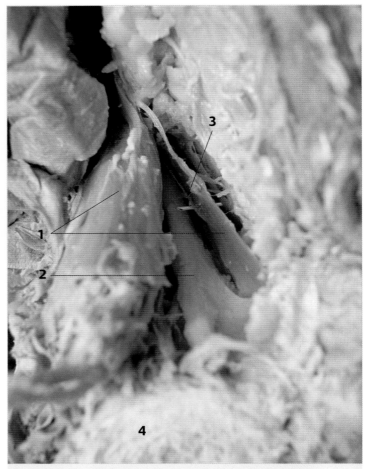

**Fig. 9.11** Cross-section through a torso at the level of L5, view from above. The lumbar plexus lies embedded with its nerve roots in the psoas major muscle. On passing through the quadratus lumborum muscle with the transversalis fascia, a "loss of resistance" is felt. However, the block should generally be performed with the nerve stimulator.
1 Lumbar plexus
2 Psoas major muscle (muscle layers divided to show the lumbar plexus)
3 Quadratus lumborum muscle
4 Transversalis fascia
5 Erector spinae muscle
6 Thoracolumbar fascia
7 Needle tip
8 Vertebral body

**Fig. 9.13** Enlarged detail of ▶ Fig. 9.11.
1 Psoas major muscle (muscle layers divided to show the lumbar plexus)
2 Nerve roots of the lumbar plexus
3 Needle tip
4 Vertebral body

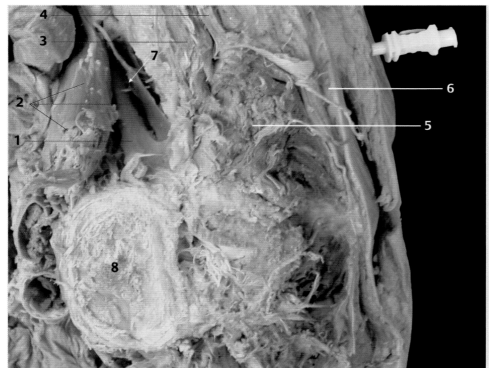

**Fig. 9.12** Cross-section through a torso at the level of L5, view from above. Enlarged detail of ▶ Fig. 9.11.
1 Lumbar plexus
2 Psoas major muscle (muscle layers divided to show the lumbar plexus)
3 Quadratus lumborum muscle
4 Transversalis fascia
5 Erector spinae muscle
6 Thoracolumbar fascia
7 Needle tip
8 Vertebral body

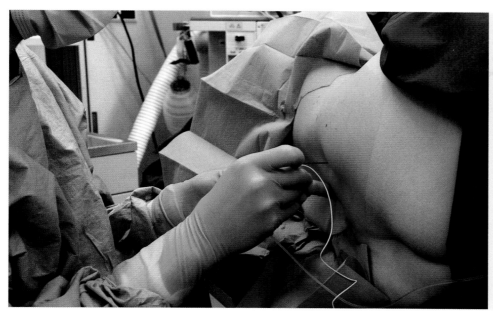

**Fig. 9.14** The response to the nerve stimulator is expected in the quadriceps muscle. Aspiration is always undertaken before injection of the local anesthetic. Both before injecting through the needle and before injecting through the indwelling catheter, a test dose (3 mL of a medium-acting local anesthetic) must be given to exclude an
intrathecal position as in epidural anesthesia.

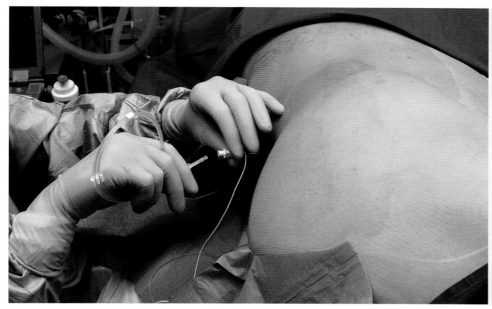

**Fig. 9.15** The psoas block can also be performed as a continuous technique. The catheter is advanced about 5 cm beyond the tip of the needle.

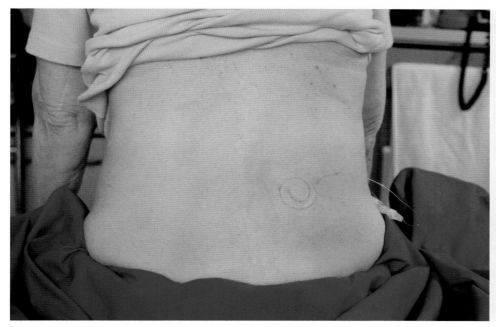

**Fig. 9.16** Psoas catheter.

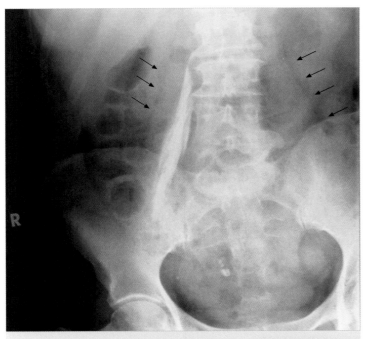

**Fig. 9.17** Spread of contrast with correct psoas block. Note the shadow of the psoas edge.
→, Psoas edge shadow

further laterally, the costal processes (transverse processes) come into view, visualized as intermittent bony acoustic shadows interspersed with soft tissue (psoas major; ▶ Fig. 9.20). When the transducer is moved further laterally, the lateral border of the transverse processes can be visualized as the loss of the acoustic shadows. The kidney may appear in the image here.

This method gives greater certainty with respect to the estimated penetration depth of the needle (Ilfeld et al 2010).

The median depth of the costal process was determined to be 5.0 cm (interquartile 4.5–5.5 cm; range 3.5–7.5 cm). To produce a response using the nerve stimulator, the needle must be advanced another 2.5 cm (interquartile 2.0–3.0 cm; range 0.2–4.0 cm). The lumbar plexus thus lies at a depth of 7.5 cm (interquartile 7.0–8.0; range 5.0–9.5 cm) (Ilfeld et al 2010).

This study (Ilfeld et al 2010) showed that the injection site described by Capdevilla et al (2002) at the junction from the middle to the lateral third on a transverse line from L4 to a line running parallel to the spine through the posterior superior iliac spine was too lateral by 0.75 cm in 50% of the patients examined. This is largely consistent with the results of a study by Heller et al (2009).

**Fig. 9.18** Visualization of the structures at risk in a psoas block in the frontal plane.
**a** Clinical setting.
**b** Ultrasound scan.
1 Kidney (cranial)
2 Psoas major muscle

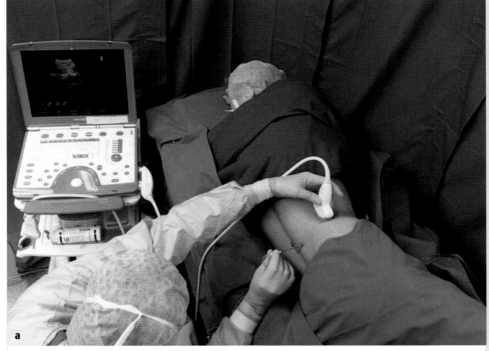

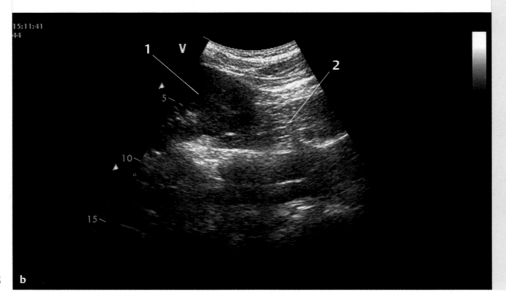

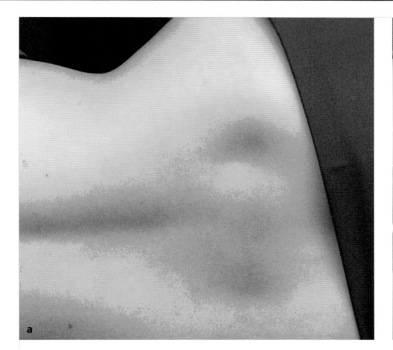

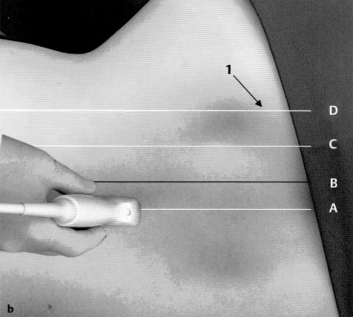

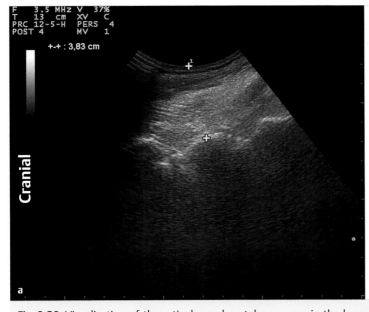

**Fig. 9.19** Psoas block: visualization of the articular process and costal processes (transverse processes) in the long axis for orientation regarding the estimated depth at which the lumber plexus can be expected.
**a** Clinical setting.
**b** Clinical setting, labeled.
**c** Projection of lines A to D onto the skeleton.
A Sagittal plane at the level of the spinous process
B Parasagittal plane at the level of the articular process
C Parasagittal plane at the level of the costal processes (transverse processes)
D Parallel to the long axis through the posterior superior iliac spine
1 Posterior superior iliac spine

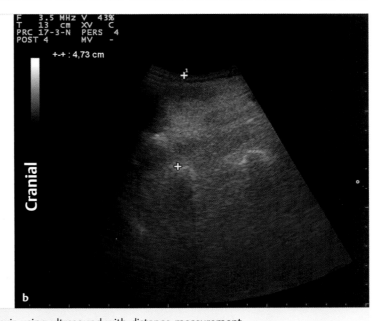

**Fig. 9.20** Visualization of the articular and costal processes in the long axis using ultrasound with distance measurement.
**a** Articular process (corresponds to line B in ► Fig. 9.19c), measured distance to skin: 3.83 cm. **b** Costal processes (transverse processes) (corresponds to line C in ► Fig. 9.19c), measured distance to skin: 4.73 cm.

In the plane between the transverse processes of L4/5, the transducer is then rotated in the *transversal plane.* Immediately lateral to the spinous process, the typical structure of the articular process can be visualized in cross-section with the bony acoustic shadow. The psoas major can often be visualized further laterally and somewhat deeper. At an even greater penetration depth behind the psoas major, a hyperechoic line can be seen that marks the junction from the psoas major to the peritoneal cavity. Intestinal movement can often be seen beneath it. The sagittal diameter of the psoas major at the level of L4/5 is reported to be 4.7 ± 0.4 cm (Takai et al 2011); at L3/4 the sagittal diameter is somewhat smaller (about 4 cm).

### Needle Approach

The transducer is rotated at the level of L3/4 from the sagittal plane to the transverse plane and adjusted so the space between the costal process allows a view of the deeper level (▶ Fig. 9.21). The target is the posterior third of the psoas major, as this is where the lumbar plexus runs. This technique should be performed only with the simultaneous use of the nerve stimulator. The puncture is made in plane from medial to lateral or from lateral to medial (▶ Fig. 9.21). There is a greater risk in a lateral to medial puncture that an accidental subarachnoidal puncture can lead to high spinal anesthesia.

For another promising technique ("Shamrock Method": Sauter et al 2013) the transducer is placed transversally in the flank (like ▶ Fig. 9.18 a, but turned 90° in the transverse plane). By moving it dorsally and tilting it caudally, the transverse process and vertebral body of L4 are visualized on the medial side of the quadratus lumborum muscle. With the psoas muscle anteriorly, the erector spinae muscle posteriorly and the quadratus lumborum muscle situated at the apex of the transverse process, a well recognizable pattern of a shamrock with three leaves can be seen. By tilting the transducer more caudally until the transverse process of L4 disappears, this probe position permits an in-plane postero-anterior needle approach.

### Catheter Placement

A catheter can be placed.

---

**Tips and Tricks**

- Orientation of the anticipated depth of the costal processes is helpful in any case to obtain information on the maximum penetration depth of the needle.
- Visualization is difficult in obese patients.
- Ultrasound-guided blocks should be performed only by persons very experienced in performing ultrasound-guided regional anesthesia.
- The technique should be conducted with the simultaneous use of a nerve stimulator.

---

## 9.3 Sensory and Motor Effects

There is a complete block of the lumbar plexus. While the iliohypogastric, ilioinguinal, and genitofemoral nerves are not important for leg innervation, the following nerves are usually fully anesthetized by psoas block:

- The lateral cutaneous nerve of the thigh (L2/3) passes over the iliacus muscle medial to the anterior superior iliac spine under the inguinal ligament and is a purely sensory nerve innervating the skin of the lateral side of the thigh.
- The obturator nerve (L2–L4) leaves the plexus medial to the psoas muscle and passes together with the obturator artery and nerve through the obturator canal to the inside of the thigh. In 9% of people an accessory obturator nerve is found that innervates the capsule of the hip joint. The obturator nerve has a very variable sensory area of innervation on the medial thigh and provides motor innervation to the adductors.
- The femoral nerve (L1–L4) is the biggest nerve of the lumbar plexus and provides the sensory innervation of the front of the thigh and the inside of the lower leg as far as the ankle. It passes anterior to the psoas major muscle below the inguinal ligament through the muscular lacuna and is responsible for the motor innervation of the quadriceps femoris, sartorius, and pectineus muscles.

## 9.4 Indications and Contraindications

### 9.4.1 Indications

- All operations on the lower limb (including hip, knee, and ankle joint replacement) can be performed under lumbar plexus block in combination with a sciatic nerve block (sacral plexus).
- Pain therapy after operations on the knee or hip (e.g., after cruciate ligament surgery, synovectomy, total joint replacement).
- Wound management, skin grafting in the anterior and lateral thigh.
- Mobilization (early mobilization after surgery, painless physiotherapy).

### 9.4.2 Contraindications

- General contraindications (see Chapter 20.2).
- Coagulation disorders: in contrast to all other peripheral blocks, the same rules apply with regard to coagulation as for neuraxial blocks (Gogarten et al 2007).
- Peritoneal infection.
- Relative: major alterations of the spine (e.g., kyphoscoliosis).

## 9.5 Complications, Side Effects, Method-Specific Problems

- Bilateral anesthesia (epidural-like spread)
- Total spinal anesthesia (Morisot 1979, Auroy et al 2002) or epidural anesthesia (▶ Fig. 9.22, ▶ Fig. 9.23, ▶ Fig. 9.24)

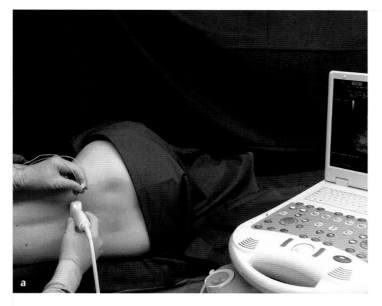

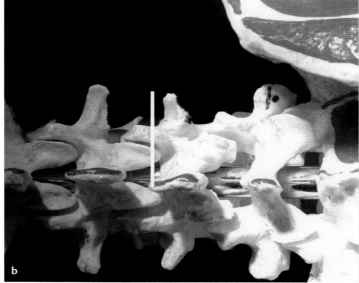

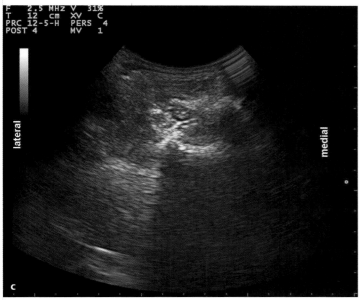

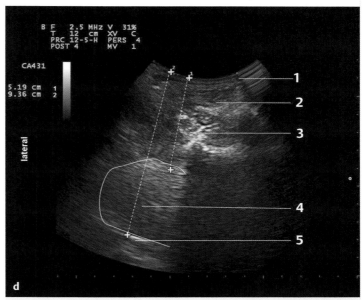

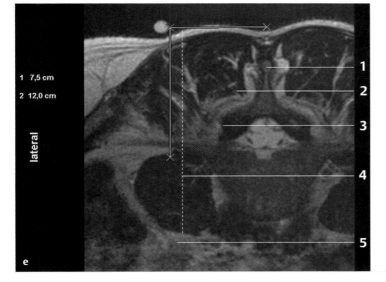

**Fig. 9.21** Visualization of the psoas major muscle and in-plane puncture of the lumbar plexus at the level of L3/4 using ultrasound.
**a** Clinical setting.
**b** Acoustic window indicated on the skeleton (white line).
**c** Ultrasound image in the transverse plane between the costal processes L3/L4.
**d** Corresponds to **c** with labeling and distance measurement.
**e** Analogue MRI image.
1 Spinous process
2 Erector spinae muscle
3 Articular process
4 Psoas major muscle
5 Junction from the psoas major muscle to the peritoneal cavity

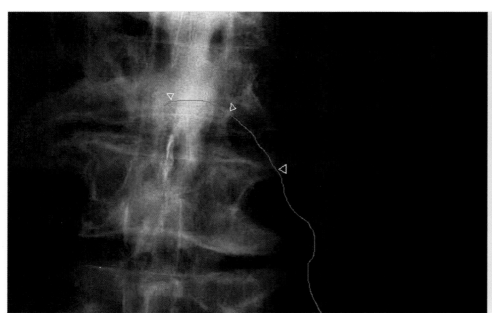

Fig. 9.22 Advancing the catheter too far can lead to an epidural position with corresponding spread and effect of the local anesthetic (see contrast medium). For this reason the patient requires adequate monitoring after injection of the local anesthetic, as a test dose does not exclude an epidural position. By withdrawing the catheter 7.5 cm, a correct catheter position was obtained in this case. (Source: H. Kaiser, Rechbergklinik Bretten, with kind permission.)

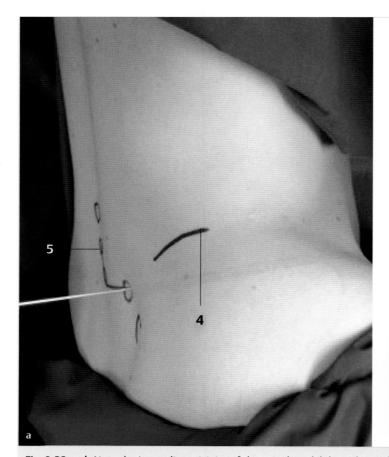

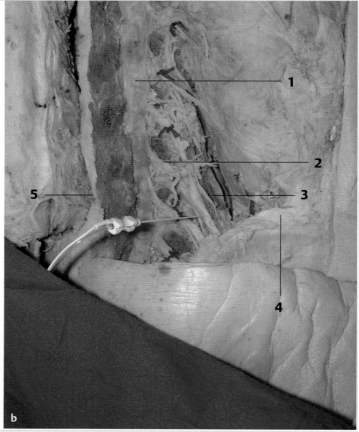

Fig. 9.23 a, b Note the immediate vicinity of the spinal cord: bilateral anesthesia, disorders of bladder function, and even high spinal anesthesia with cardiocirculatory arrest have been described. The good vascularization may lead to hematoma with temporary neurological impairment. With regard to coagulation, the rules applying to neuraxial blocks should be followed in psoas block. By comparison, these rules can be followed more liberally with other peripheral blocks.

1 Dura mater
2 Nerve roots
3 Lumbar plexus in psoas major muscle
4 Iliac crest
5 Spinous process of L4

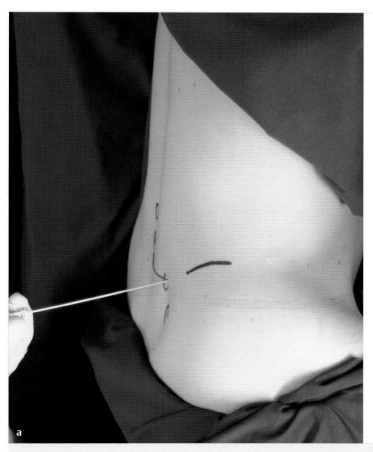
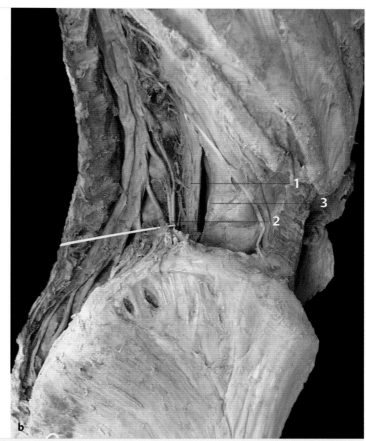

**Fig. 9.24 a, b** Psoas block, lateral view. Because of the risk of penetrating the peritoneal cavity, the depth of needle penetration should not exceed 11 cm.
1 Psoas major muscle
2 Lumbar plexus
3 Peritoneum

- Peritoneal injection (Farny et al 1994a, 1994b; ▶ Fig. 9.24)
- Retroperitoneal hematoma (Klein et al 1997, Weller et al 2003). Note the contraindications!
- Subcapsular hematoma of the kidney (rare; Aida et al 1996; ▶ Fig. 9.25)
- Infection (psoas abscess with continuous technique, Neuburger et al 2005; ▶ Fig. 9.26)
- Systemic toxicity from the local anesthetic due to accidental intravascular injection (Auroy et al 2002)
- Nerve damage (e.g., femoral nerve damage, Al-Nasser and Palacios 2004)

## 9.6 Remarks on the Technique

▶ **Anatomy.** In anatomical investigations, Farny et al (1994a, 1994b) found that the average distance between the skin and the femoral nerve is 9.0 cm (± 1.4 cm) in women and 9.9 cm (± 2.1 cm) in men. Farny therefore considered peritoneal injection to be possible with a needle length of 11 cm or more. For this reason, the needle should not be longer than 10 to 12 cm or should at least not be advanced further.

The landmarks described by Chayen do not necessarily correspond with the anatomical circumstances. Heller et al (2009) demonstrated great variability in an anatomical study. Nerve stimulation is thus indispensable and ultrasound is very helpful even with the possibilities and limitations described in Chapter 9.2.2.

**Practical Notes**

- Because of the risk of renal puncture, the orientation lines should start from L4, not from L3.
- Contact with the transverse process of L5 is helpful for orientation. The needle should be advanced a maximum of 2 (–2.5) cm beyond this distance (Gray et al 2004, Awad and Duggan 2005).
- Nerve stimulation should be used. Combination with a loss of resistance technique can simplify the procedure.
- Ultrasound-guided needle insertion is becoming more and more common today (Gray et al 2004, Sauter et al 2013; see also Chapter 9.2.2).
- It is relatively easy to identify the transverse costal process of L4/L5, thus allowing depth measurement (no more than 2 cm beyond the first bony contact of the needle).
- Excessively deep injection (over 11 cm) should be avoided (see below).
- A test dose is indispensable (exclusion of an intrathecal position).
- A volume of 30 mL of the local anesthetic is required for sufficient anesthesia.
- If the lateral cutaneous nerve of the thigh has a very high origin from the plexus, incomplete anesthesia of the outside of the thigh is possible (rare compared to inguinal lumbar plexus block; Bruelle et al 1998).
- An intrathecal or epidural position can be excluded by a radiological check of the catheter's position.

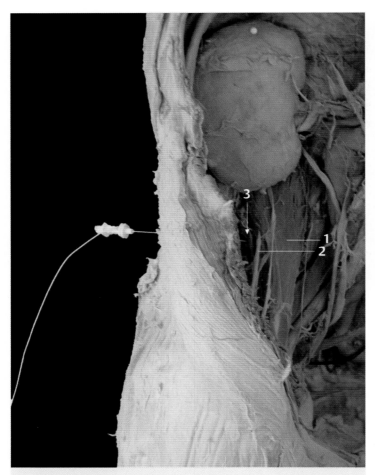

Fig. 9.25 Psoas block, anterior view. Note the safe distance from the lower pole of the kidney when L4 is the reference level for determining the puncture site.
1 Psoas major muscle
2 Lumbar plexus
3 Needle tip

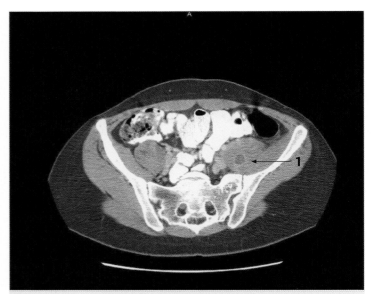

Fig. 9.26 In rare cases a psoas catheter can cause a psoas abscess. In this case the abscess healed without surgical intervention and without sequelae.
1 Psoas abscess on the left after psoas catheter

▶ **Peripheral nerve stimulation.** Peripheral nerve stimulation (PNS) facilitates performance and improves the success rate (Mehrkens et al 1987, Parkinson et al 1989, Vaghadia et al 1992, Ayers and Kayser 1999). The nerve stimulator should therefore not be dispensed with in this technique (Kaiser et al 1990). The combination of PNS and loss of resistance technique is recommended.

Needles with a short-bevel or pencil-point tip have therefore also proved to be suitable for this technique. Contraction of the vastus muscles or the adductors should be produced. Contact of the needle with the transverse process of the 5th lumbar vertebra is helpful for anatomical orientation (Chayen et al 1976, Parkinson and Mueller 1989, Parkinson et al 1989).

> **Note**
>
> If the direction of the needle is corrected, this should only be in cranial direction over the transverse process and not in medial direction.

The transverse process of the 5th lumbar vertebra is very short, so if the needle is directed medially there can be a response from parts of the sacral plexus (sciatic nerve) (▶ Fig. 9.7), as the lumbosacral trunk lies furthest medially and paravertebrally while the femoral nerve lies in the middle of the lumbosacral plexus. This

often leads to an unwanted paravertebral, epidural-like spread of anesthesia with the corresponding side effects, but without achieving complete lumbosacral plexus anesthesia (Ayers and Kayser 1999, Gligorijevic 2000).

▶ **Bilateral effects.** However, even when performed correctly, bilateral spread of the block must be anticipated. The incidence is between 8% and 88% (Parkinson et al 1989, Geiger 1999, Vaghadia et al 1992, Rogers and Ramamurthy 1996). The bilateral effects can probably be attributed to diffusion of the local anesthetic into the epidural space (Geiger 1999, Farny et al 1994a, 1994b, Hahn et al 1996).

▶ **Distance to the interspinal line.** Occasionally the 5 cm distance from the interspinal line proves to be too great and a distance of 4 to 4.5 cm can be selected in slim patients, although directing the needle medially must be strictly avoided here as well. A variant using a distance of 3 cm from the interspinal line has also been described with good results (3 cm caudally and 3 cm on the side to be blocked from L4; Pandin et al 2002). A further variation uses the transverse costal process of L4 as a landmark (Awad and Duggan 2005). The costal process of L4 is located about 4 cm lateral to the spinous process; the needle must be directed in a strictly sagittal direction. With the aid of a nerve simulator, the needle is advanced to a maximum of 2 cm below the spinous process under nerve stimulation until the desired response is obtained.

▶ **Monitoring the patient.** The monitoring of patients must be similar to that in neuraxial anesthesia, as an incorrect intrathecal or epidural position cannot be absolutely ruled out. Accidental spinal anesthesia and high epidural anesthesia have been described (Gentili et al 1998). In a review article involving a total of 394 psoas blocks, Auroy reported one cardiocirculatory arrest with fatal outcome, two cases of acute respiratory insufficiency (complete respiratory paralysis) as a result of accidental intrathecal injection of the local anesthetic, and one seizure due to intravascular injection of the local anesthetic (Auroy et al 2002). This represents a major complication rate of 0.8% associated with this technique!

▶ **Check of position.** An intrathecal or epidural catheter position can also be excluded by a *subsequent radiograph* (Douglas and Bush 1999). Initial studies suggest that the use of *ultrasound* may improve and facilitate orientation and checking of the catheter position in psoas block as in other areas (brachial plexus, femoral nerve) in the future (Kirchmair et al 2000a, 2000b).

The lateral cutaneous nerve of the thigh often leaves the lumbar plexus very far cranially, so incomplete anesthesia in the area supplied by this nerve is possible even when the psoas block is performed correctly (Bruelle et al 1998). Inserting the needle using L3 for orientation instead of L4 confers no advantages (Bartmann et al 1993), and the risk of a subcapsular hematoma of the kidney is increased (Aida et al 1996).

▶ **Coagulation disorders.** In discussions of the side effects or complications of the technique, there are few reports on its use in patients with coagulation disorders. Theoretically, psoas block has a better risk/benefit ratio in patients under anticoagulant therapy compared to epidural anesthesia. Psoas blocks have been described under anticoagulation with no complications (Ayers and Kayser 1999).

> **Note**
>
> Psoas block should only be performed in patients with coagulation disorders in justified, exceptional cases, as complications must be taken into account.

Case descriptions report extensive retroperitoneal hematomas after psoas blocks with impairment of the psoas muscle (Klein et al 1997, Weller et al 2003). In one case, the block was performed under prophylactic administration of enoxaparin; reversible plexus injury occurred (Klein et al 1997). In another case, the anticoagulation was given after performing the continuous psoas block but before withdrawing the indwelling catheter. There were no neurological deficits but there was a drop in hemoglobin necessitating a transfusion and causing renal failure and ileus. In a third case with normal coagulation status, a hematoma requiring transfusion involving considerable impairment of the patient but no neurological deficits occurred despite perioperative discontinuation of continuous administration of unfractionated heparin (Weller et al 2003).

> **Note**
>
> With respect to coagulation, unlike all other peripheral blocks, the rules that apply to neuraxial blocks also apply to the psoas block (Gogarten et al 2007).

In comparison with general anesthesia or neuraxial anesthesia, patients have better circulatory stability under a psoas block.

▶ **Psoas–sciatic nerve block.** For most operations on the leg, particularly when they are performed with a tournique at the

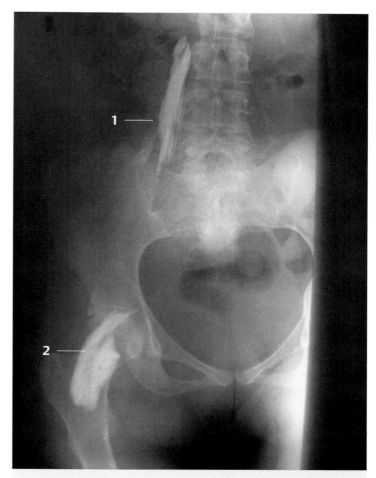

**Fig. 9.27** Spread of contrast in combined psoas and sciatic nerve block. Initially, about 30 mL of a 1% (10 mg/mL) medium-acting local anesthetic (prilocaine/mepivacaine) in combination with 15 (–20) mL of 0.375% (3.75 mg/mL) ropivacaine or 10 mL of ropivacaine 0.75% (7.5 mg/mL) can be given in each catheter.
1 Spread of contrast in psoas block
2 Spread of contrast in sciatic nerve block

thigh, the combination of psoas and sciatic nerve block is necessary for anesthesia. For this combination, relatively large volumes of local anesthetic are required. The sciatic nerve is adequately blocked with 20 to 25 mL of local anesthetic, while volumes of 30 mL are required for block of the lumbar plexus in the psoas region (▶ Fig. 9.27). The systemic toxicity of the local anesthetic has to be considered.

> **Note**
>
> A combination of 30 mL of a medium-acting local anesthetic with 20 mL of ropivacaine 0.75% (7.5 mg/mL) or 40 mL of ropivacaine 0.375% (3.75 mg/mL) is possible for combined psoas and sciatic nerve block.

▶ **Advantages.** The advantage of a psoas–sciatic nerve block compared to an inguinal femoral nerve–sciatic nerve block in knee operations is based on the more complete lumbar plexus anesthesia, which also includes the option of obturator nerve block (Uckunkaya et al 2000, Luber et al 2001). The hip is innervated by branches of the lumbar plexus and the sacral plexus (Birnbaum et al 1997). Cranial anesthesia of the lumbar plexus can also be used successfully in combination with a sciatic nerve

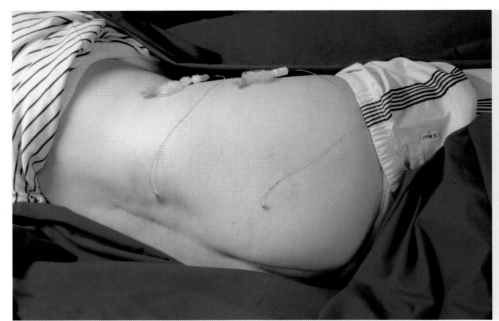

**Fig. 9.28** Psoas block can be used in conjunction with posterior proximal sciatic nerve block for complete anesthesia of the entire leg (also as a continuous technique). In the continuous technique both catheters can, for example, each be infused with 6 mL of 0.33% (3.3 mg/mL) ropivacaine per hour.

block and sedation of the patient for anesthesia for operations on the hip (total hip replacement; Geiger et al 1994, Chudinov et al 1999, Mitchell 1999, Türker et al 2000, de Visme et al 2000, Bruckenmeier et al 2001).

Further studies have indicated a beneficial effect with regard to diminished blood loss in hip operations (Twyman et al 1990, Stevens et al 2000). In addition to the positive results with regard to good intraoperative anesthesia with comparatively less impairment of the hemodynamic parameters, the continuous technique also offers the possibility of postoperative pain therapy (► Fig. 9.28).

## 9.7 Summary

Psoas block can be performed in sitting position or with the patient lying on his or her side. It consists of a cranial approach to the lumbar plexus with a high success rate. The procedure requires sterile conditions, comparable with epidural anesthesia. Full supervision and monitoring of the patient must be ensured. During this monitoring, the possibility of the development of epidural-like spread or spinal anesthesia must be borne in mind. Peritoneal infections, coagulation disorders, and major abnormalities of the spine must be regarded as contraindications. In combination with sacral plexus block, the technique leads to sufficient anesthesia in operations on the leg and is well suited for pain therapy and mobilization with operations on the hip and knee.

## References

Aida S, Takahashi H, Shimoji K. Renal subcapsular hematoma after lumbar plexus block. Anesthesiology 1996; 84: 452–455

Al-Nasser B, Palacios JL. Femoral nerve injury complicating continuous psoas compartment block. Reg Anesth Pain Med 2004; 29: 361–363

Auroy Y, Benhamou D, Bargues L et al. Major complications of regional anesthesia in France: The SOS Regional Anesthesia Hotline Service. Anesthesiology 2002; 97: 1274–1280

Awad IT, Duggan EM. Posterior lumbar plexus block: anatomy, approaches, and techniques. Reg Anesth Pain Med 2005; 30: 143–149

Ayers J, Kayser EF. Continuous lower extremity techniques. Tech Reg Anesth Pain Manage 1999; 3: 47–57

Bartmann E, Mehrkens HH, Geiger P, Herrmann M. Anatomic examinations to optimize the paravertebral approach to the psoas compartment. Surgical and radiologic anatomy. J Clin Anat 1993; 15: 3

Birnbaum K, Prescher A, Hessler S, Heller KD. The sensory innervation of the hip joint—an anatomical study. Surg Radiol Anat 1 997; 19: 371–375

Bruckenmeier CC, III, Xenos JS, Nilsen SM. Lumbar plexus block with perineural catheter and sciatic nerve block for total hip arthroplasty. J Arthroplasty 2002; 17: 499–502

Bruelle P, Cuvillon P, Ripart J, Eledjam JJ. Sciatic nerve block: parasacral approach. Reg Anesth 1998; 23: 78

Büttner J, Meier G. Kontinuierliche periphere Techniken zur Regionalanästhesie und Schmerztherapie—Obere und untere Extremität. Bremen: Uni-Med; 1999

Capdevila X, Macaire P, Dadure C et al. Continuous psoas compartment block for postoperative analgesia after total hip arthroplasty: new landmarks, technical guidelines, and clinical evaluation. Anesth Analg 2002; 94: 1606–1613

Chayen D, Nathan H, Chayen M. The psoas compartment block. Anesthesiology 1976; 45: 95–99

Chudinov A, Berkenstadt H, Salai M, Cahana A, Perel A. Continuous psoas compartment block for anesthesia and perioperative analgesia in patients with hip fractures. Reg Anesth Pain Med 1999; 24: 563–568

de Visme V, Picart F, Le Jouan R, Legrand A, Savry C, Morin V. Combined lumbar and sacral plexus block compared with plain bupivacaine spinal anesthesia for hip fractures in the elderly. Reg Anesth Pain Med 2000; 25: 158–162

Douglas I, Bush D. The use of patient-controlled boluses of local anaesthetic via a psoas sheath catheter in the management of malignant pain. Pain 1999; 82: 105–107

Farny J, Drolet P, Girard M. Anatomy of the posterior approach to the lumbar plexus block. Can J Anaesth 1994a; 41: 480–485

Farny J, Girard M, Drolet P. Posterior approach to the lumbar plexus combined with a sciatic nerve block using lidocaine. Can J Anaesth 1994b; 41: 486–491

Geiger P, Bartmann E, Gelowicz-Maurer M, Mehrkens HH. Combined sciatic nerve plus continuous paravertebral lumbar plexus block in orthopaedic knee surgery. XIII Annual ASRA-Congress, Barcelona (special abstract issue); 1994: 57

Geiger P. Der Psoas-Kompartment-Block. In: Mehrkens HH, Büttner J, eds. Kontinuierliche periphere Leitungsblockaden zur postoperativen Analgesie. Munich: Arcis; 1999: 29–42

Gentili M, Aveline C, Bonnet F. [Total spinal anesthesia after posterior lumbar plexus block] [Article in French] Ann Fr Anesth Reanim 1998; 17: 740–742

Gligorijevic P. Lower extremity blocks for day surgery. Tech Reg Anesth Pain Manage 2000; 4: 30–37

Gogarten W, Van Aken H, Büttner J et al. Rückenmarksnahe Regionalanästhesien und Thromboembolieprophylaxe/antithrombotische Medikation. Anästh Intensivmed 2007; 48: 109–124

Gray A, Collins AB, Schafhalter-Zoppoth I. An introduction to femoral nerve and associated lumbar plexus nerve blocks under ultrasonic nerve guidance. Tech Reg Anesth Pain Manage 2004; 8: 155–163

Hahn MB, McQuillan PM, Sheplock GJ. Regional Anesthesia: an Atlas of Anatomy and Techniques. St. Louis: Mosby; 1996

Heller AR, Fuchs A, Rössel T et al. Precision of traditional approaches for lumbar plexus block: impact and management of interindividual anatomic variability. Anesthesiology 2009; 111: 525–532

Ilfeld BM, Loland VJ, Mariano ER. Prepuncture ultrasound imaging to predict transverse process and lumbar plexus depth for psoas compartment block and perineural catheter insertion: a prospective, observational study. Anesth Analg 2010; 110: 1725–1728

Kaiser H, Niesel HC, Hans V. Fundamentals and requirements of peripheral electric nerve stimulation. A contribution to the improvement of safety standards in regional anesthesia. [Article in German] Reg Anaesth 1990; 13: 143–147

Kirchmair L, Entner T, Burger R et al. Ultrasound (US) guided psoas compartment block (PCB): Anatomical fundamentals. Int Monitor Reg Anesth 2000; 12: 197

Kirchmair L, Entner T, Burger R et al. Ultrasound (US) guided psoas compartment block (PCB): Verification of a new technique with CT. Int Monitor Reg Anesth 2000; 12: 199

Klein SM, D'Ercole F, Greengrass RA, Warner DS. Enoxaparin associated with psoas hematoma and lumbar plexopathy after lumbar plexus block. Anesthesiology 1997; 87: 1576–1579

Luber MJ, Greengrass R, Vail TP. Patient satisfaction and effectiveness of lumbar plexus and sciatic nerve block for total knee arthroplasty. J Arthroplasty 2001; 16: 17–21

Mehrkens HH, Schleinzer W, Geiger P. Successful peripheral regional anaesthesia by aid of an improved nerve stimulator. Abstract 6. Annual Meeting, ESRA. Paris; 1987

Meier G. Peripheral nerve block of the lower extremities. [Article in German] Anaesthesist 2001; 50: 536–557, quiz 557, 559

Meier G, Büttner J. Regionalanästhesie—Kompendium der peripheren Blockaden. Munich: Arcis; 2001

Mitchell ME. Regional anesthesia for hip surgery. Tech Reg Anesth Pain Manage 1999; 3: 94–106

Morisot P. Les blocs du membre inférieur. Encyclop Med-chir Anesthesie 1979; 363: 23

Neuburger M, Lang D, Büttner J. Abscess of the psoas muscle caused by a psoas compartment catheter. Case report of a rare complication of peripheral catheter regional anaesthesia. [Article in German] Anaesthesist 2005; 54: 341–345

Pandin PC, Vandesteene A, d'Hollander AA. Lumbar plexus posterior approach: a catheter placement description using electrical nerve stimulation. Anesth Analg 2002; 95: 1428–1431

Parkinson S, Mueller JB. A simple technique for continuous lumbar sympathetic blockade. Anesth Analg 1989; 68: 218

Parkinson SK, Mueller JB, Little WL, Bailey SL. Extent of blockade with various approaches to the lumbar plexus. Anesth Analg 1989; 68: 243–248

Platzer W. Color Atlas of Human Anatomy Vol 1. Locomotor System. 7th edition. Stuttgart: Thieme; 2014

Rogers NR, Ramamurthy P. Lower extremity blocks. In: Brown DL, ed. Regional Anesthesia and Analgesia. 1st ed. Philadelphia: Saunders; 1996: 284–285

Sauter AR, Ullensvang K, Bendtsen TF, Børglum J. The "Shamrock Method" a new and promising technique for ultrasound guided lumbar plexus block. Br J Anaesth. 2013: e-letter (http://bja. oxfordjournals.org/forum/topic/brjana_el%3B9814)

Stevens RD, Van Gessel E, Flory N, Fournier R, Gamulin Z. Lumbar plexus block reduces pain and blood loss associated with total hip arthroplasty. Anesthesiology 2000; 93: 115–121

Takai Y, Katsumata Y, Kawakami Y, Kanehisa H, Fukunaga T. Ultrasound method for estimating the cross-sectional area of the psoas major muscle. Med Sci Sports Exerc 2011; 43: 2000–2004

Türker G, Uckunkaya N, Yilmazlar A. Postoperative analgesia with psoas compartment block after prosthetic hip surgery. Int Monitor Reg Anesth 2000; A12: 246

Twyman R, Kirwan T, Fennelly M. Blood loss reduced during hip arthroplasty by lumbar plexus block. J Bone Joint Surg Br 1990; 72: 770–771

Uckunkaya N, Türker G, Yilmazlar A et al. Combined psoas compartment and sciatic nerve blocks for lower limb surgery. Int Monitor Reg Anesth 2000; A12: 196

Vaghadia H, Kapnoudhis P, Jenkins LC, Taylor D. Continuous lumbosacral block using a Tuohy needle and catheter technique. Can J Anaesth 1992; 39: 75–78

Weller RS, Gerancher JC, Crews JC, Wade KL. Extensive retroperitoneal hematoma without neurologic deficit in two patients who underwent lumbar plexus block and were later anticoagulated. Anesthesiology 2003; 98: 581–585

# 10 Inguinal Paravascular Lumbar Plexus Anesthesia (Femoral Nerve Block)

## 10.1 Anatomical Overview

The femoral nerve arises within the psoas muscle, usually from the anterior divisions of the four large roots L1–L4 but sometimes only from L2–L4, and is the largest nerve of the lumbar plexus (► Fig. 10.1). It passes in the fascial space between psoas major and iliacus through the muscular lacuna to the thigh (► Fig. 10.2). The iliopectineal fascia separates the muscular lacuna and thus the femoral nerve from the vascular lacuna through which the lymphatic vessels and the femoral artery and vein run. After giving off a few superficial cutaneous branches (anterior cutaneous branches), it lies under the fascia lata and the iliac fascia in the femoral trigone (Woodburne 1983, Hahn et al 1996, Platzer 2014; ► Fig. 10.3 and ► Fig. 10.4).

In the region of the inguinal ligament, the femoral nerve is about 1 cm lateral to the artery, where it usually soon fans out (► Fig. 10.5 and ► Fig. 10.6).

The femoral nerve provides the sensory innervation of the anterior thigh and is involved in the innervation of the hip and knee joints and of the femur. It provides the motor supply to the knee extensors and hip flexors.

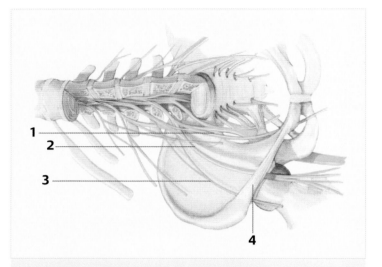

**Fig. 10.1** Anatomical overview of the lumbar plexus and the femoral nerve.
1 Obturator nerve
2 Femoral nerve
3 Lateral cutaneous nerve of the thigh
4 Inguinal ligament

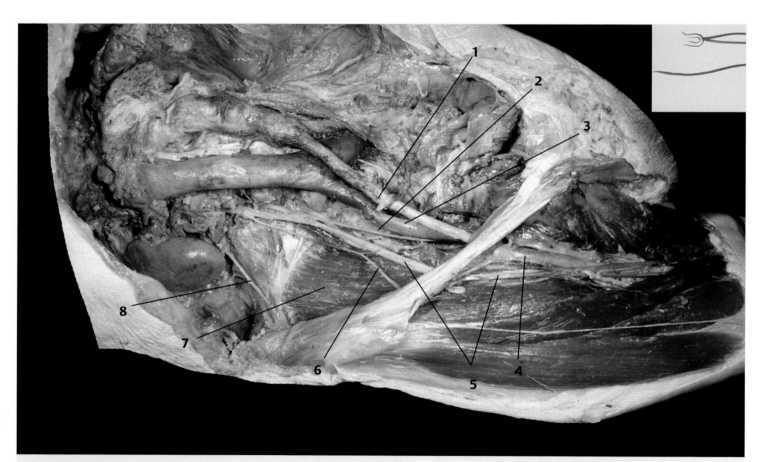

**Fig. 10.2** Lumbar plexus.
1 Common iliac artery
2 Obturator nerve
3 External iliac vein
4 Femoral artery
5 Femoral nerve
6 Lateral cutaneous nerve of the thigh
7 Iliacus muscle
8 Ilioinguinal nerve

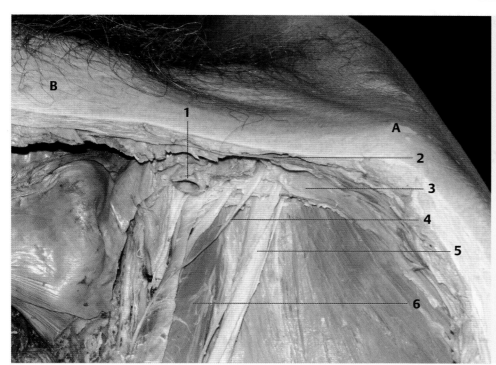

**Fig. 10.3** Cranial view of the right inguinal region. Note that the fascia lata and the iliac fascia have to be penetrated to block the femoral nerve ("double-click").
1 Femoral artery
2 Fascia lata
3 Iliac fascia with iliopectineal arc
4 Genitofemoral nerve
5 Femoral nerve
6 Psoas major
A Anterior superior iliac spine
B Symphysis

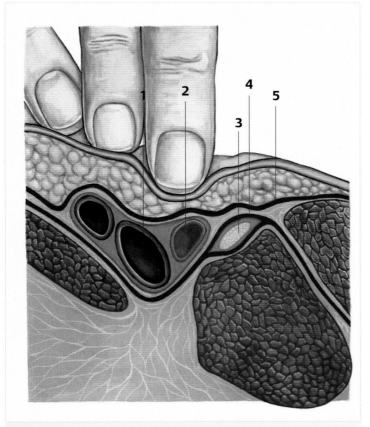

**Fig. 10.4** Cranial view of the right inguinal region. Note that the fascia lata and the iliac fascia have to be penetrated to block the femoral nerve ("double-click," see also ▶ Fig. 10.3).
1 Femoral vein
2 Femoral artery
3 Femoral nerve
4 Iliac fascia
5 Fascia lata

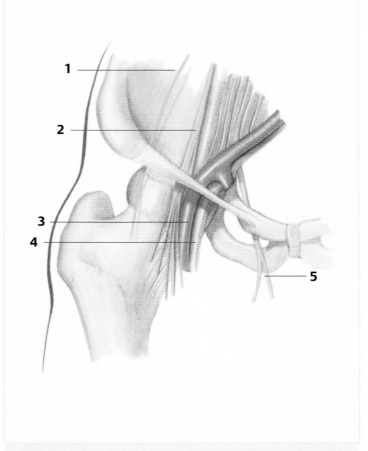

**Fig. 10.5** Anatomical overview of the inguinal region: note IVAN (from Inside: Vein, Artery, Nerve).
1 Lateral cutaneous nerve of the thigh
2 Femoral nerve
3 Femoral artery
4 Femoral vein
5 Obturator nerve

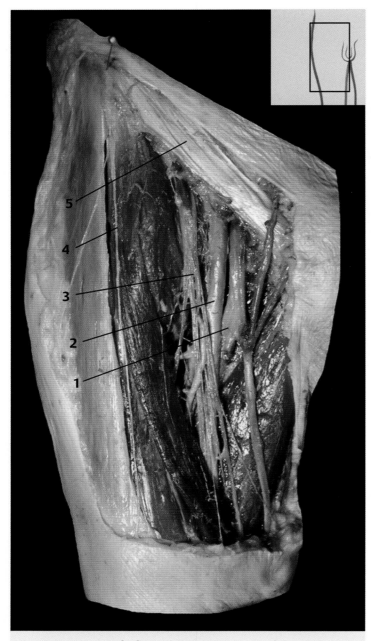

**Fig. 10.6** Overview of a femoral trigone: note IVAN (from Inside: Vein, Artery and Nerve). The femoral nerve soon branches out in a fanlike shape. The needle corresponds to the anterior superior iliac spine.
1 Femoral vein
2 Femoral artery
3 Femoral nerve
4 Lateral cutaneous nerve of the thigh
5 Inguinal ligament

# 10.2 Femoral Nerve Block ▶

The inguinal paravascular lumbar plexus block was described in 1973 by Winnie (Winnie et al 1973) as a so-called 3-in-1 block. However anesthesia of the obturator nerve was not proven and is also not likely given the anatomical situation. The technique is therefore called femoral nerve block.

## 10.2.1 Needle Approach
### Landmarks

▶ **Anterior superior iliac spine, pubic tubercle.** The anterior superior iliac spine and the pubic tubercle are marked and joined by a line. This connecting line corresponds to the inguinal ligament. The classical puncture site described is 1 cm below the inguinal ligament and about 1.5 cm lateral to the femoral artery (note: IVAN = from Inside: Vein, Artery, Nerve; ▶ Fig. 10.5 and ▶ Fig. 10.6).

Divergence from the original technique is recommended, selecting the injection site about 1 cm below the inguinal crease, that is, markedly further distally (▶ Fig. 10.7 and ▶ Fig. 10.8).

### Position

The patient lies supine and the leg is slightly abducted and externally rotated. In difficult anatomical situations, a flat pad can be placed under the patient's buttocks in order to show the topography of the inguinal region better.

### Method

The landmarks are marked and the femoral artery is palpated. If the artery cannot be palpated, a vascular Doppler probe can be used for orientation.

After skin disinfection and intracutaneous or superficial subcutaneous local anesthesia about 3 cm (Härtel 1916, Moore 1969) below the inguinal ligament (or 1 cm below the inguinal crease) and about 1.5 cm lateral to the artery, the skin is incised with a small lancet. The needle is then advanced cranially and dorsally at an angle of 30° to the skin and parallel to the artery until the tough resistance of the fascia lata is felt. If a short beveled needle is used, the bevel direction should be parallel to the artery. The resistance is overcome by slightly increasing pressure (▶ Fig. 10.9 and ▶ Fig. 10.10).

While cautiously advancing the needle further, there is often a second "loss of resistance" when the tip of the needle passes through the iliac fascia (so-called "double-click"). The end of the needle should then be lowered before advancing the needle further proximally parallel to the artery under peripheral nerve stimulation (PNS).

> **Practical Note**
>
> Contractions in the quadriceps femoris muscle and "dancing" of the patella indicate that the tip of the needle is in the correct position in the immediate vicinity of the femoral nerve.

Following negative aspiration, 20 to 40 mL of a medium-acting or long-acting local anesthetic is injected. Digital pressure distal to the needle can promote distribution of the local anesthetic in cranial direction (▶ Fig. 10.11, ▶ Fig. 10.12, ▶ Fig. 10.13).

If a continuous technique is planned, a flexible 20G catheter is advanced approximately 3 to 5 cm beyond the tip of the needle

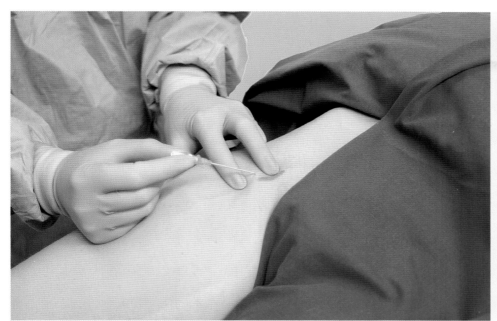

**Fig. 10.7** When index and middle finger are on the femoral artery, the puncture site is exactly at the level of the distal phalanx. Right thigh.

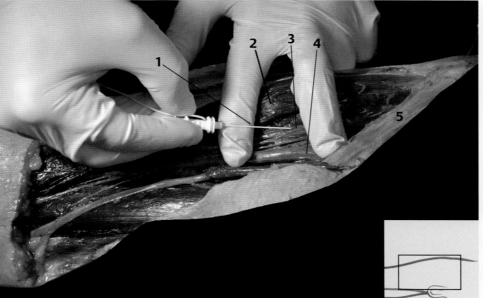

**Fig. 10.8** Recommended puncture site for femoral nerve block.
1 Puncture site
2 Sartorius muscle
3 Femoral nerve
4 Femoral artery
5 Inguinal ligament

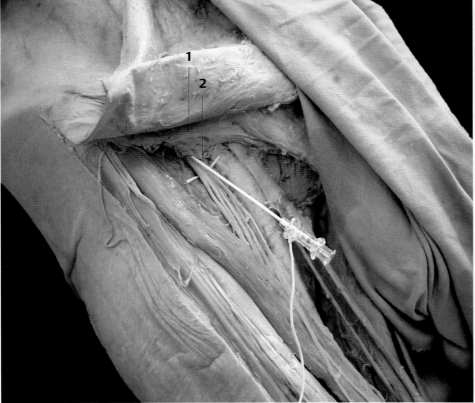

**Fig. 10.9** Needle approach to the femoral nerve. Fascia lata and iliac fascia must be penetrated. Right inguinal region:
1 Fascia lata
2 Iliac fascia with iliopectineal arc

161

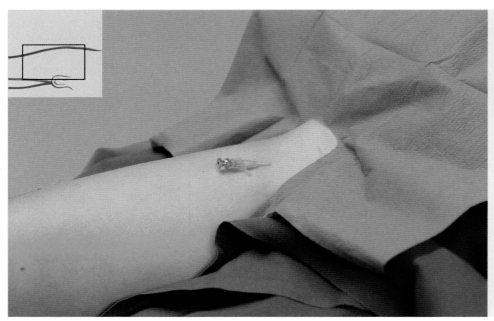

Fig. 10.10 Needle approach for femoral nerve block. The needle is advanced proximally in the surrounding sheath using electrostimulation. It must not be forced against resistance. If the response is lost, it can be useful to direct the needle tip somewhat anteriorly by lowering the hub of the needle. Right thigh.

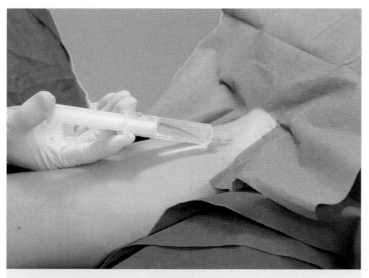

Fig. 10.11 After aspiration, 30 to 40 mL of local anesthetic is injected slowly and with repeated aspiration. Digital compression distal to the needle can be helpful. Right inguinal region.

after injection of the local anesthetic. Before connecting the catheter to a bacterial filter, the catheter should be aspirated again to exclude an intravascular position. Checking the position using ultrasound makes it possible to correct the position by withdrawing the catheter if spread is insufficient in the target region (▶ Fig. 10.14).

## Local Anesthetic, Dosages

Initially: 30 mL of a 1% (10 mg/mL) medium-acting local anesthetic (e.g., mepivacaine, prilocaine) or a long-acting local anesthetic (e.g., ropivacaine 0.75% [7.5 mg/mL])

Continuous block: 8 to 10 mL/h ropivacaine 0.2–0.375% (2–3.75 mg/mL)

Combination block with the sciatic nerve: see below

## 10.2.2 Needle Approach with Ultrasound

Linear transducer: 10 to 12 MHz
Needle: 6 cm

### Nerve Localization

Finding the femoral nerve appears to be difficult for beginners. It is always located in the inguinal region close (lateral) to the femoral artery in a triangle formed by the femoral artery (medially), the iliopsoas muscle (laterally), and the iliac fascia/fascia lata (anteriorly). The femoral nerve has stronger anisotropic behavior than other nerves, making it important to have the correct angle of the transducer (Soong et al 2005). Because they have similar reflective properties, it often cannot be clearly distinguished from the surrounding fatty tissue until after the local anesthetic is injected (▶ Fig. 10.18). ▶

> **Practical Note**
>
> The femoral nerve can be best visualized somewhat proximal to the origin of the deep femoral artery from the femoral artery at the level of the inguinal ligament in the short axis.

It is usually an oval hyperechoic structure lying on the iliopsoas muscle lateral to the femoral artery (▶ Fig. 10.15). Further distally in the region of the origin of the deep femoral artery, the nerve soon begins to divide into its branches, so that even after injection of local anesthetic, the compact structure of a single nerve is no longer seen, but individual branches (▶ Fig. 10.16). The nerve is covered by the fascia lata and iliac fascia. ▶ Lymph nodes are visible above the fascia in some patients (▶ Fig. 10.17).

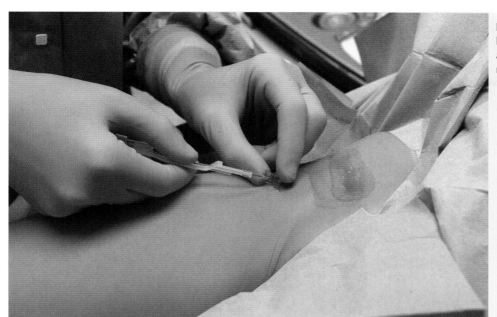

**Fig. 10.12** Introduction of a flexible catheter by the needle. The catheter should not be advanced more than 3 to 4 cm beyond the needle tip.

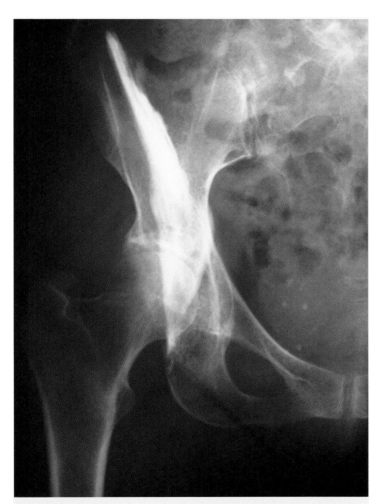

**Fig. 10.13** Spread of local anesthetic, shown radiologically using contrast medium. Note the lateral spread. Contrary to the idea of a 3-in-1 block, there is not necessarily central spread toward the lumbar plexus.

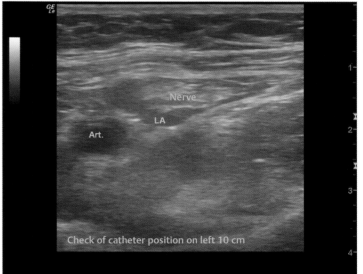

**Fig. 10.14** Check of the position of a femoral nerve catheter using ultrasound (the local anesthetic injected through the catheter spreads around the femoral nerve).

## Needle Approach

Needle insertion can be made out of plane from caudal to cranial (► Fig. 10.15 ▶) or in plane from lateral to medial (► Fig. 10.16 and ► Fig. 10.18 ▶).

► **Out-of-plane approach.**

In an out-of-plane needle approach, especially when using a rather blunt needle, it can be observed that the fascia lata and iliac fascia are initially compressed by the tip of the needle before the fascia are penetrated (▶). At the lateral edge of the femoral nerve is the motor segment, which is primarily responsible for innervation of the quadriceps muscle. The medial part contains the motor cords of the sartorius muscle (Anns et al 2011). Successful anesthesia generally occurs in single-shot blocks regardless of the puncture site (medial or lateral) and thus of the response (quadriceps or sartorius when a nerve stimulator is also used) when the local anesthetic spreads around the nerve (Anns et al 2011).

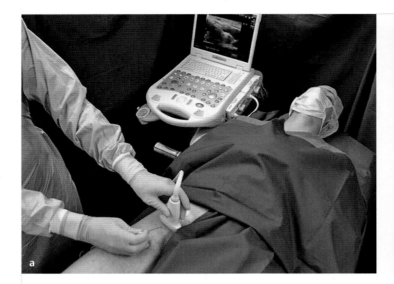

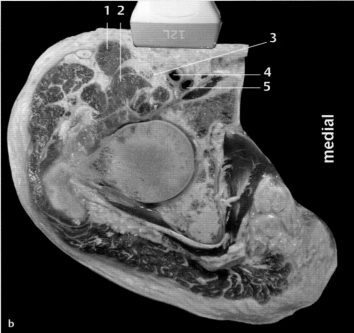

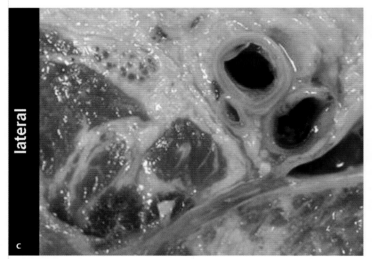

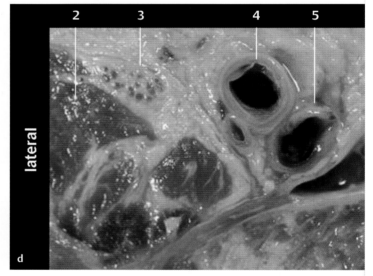

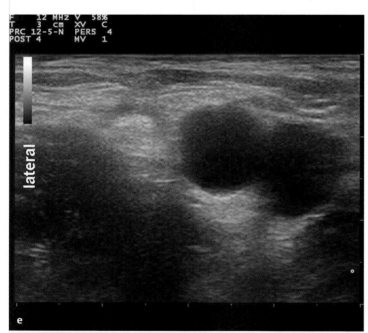

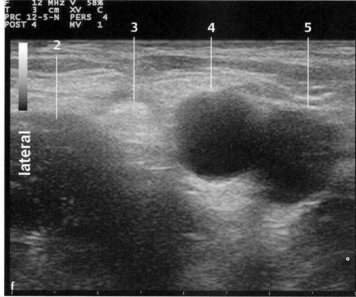

**Fig. 10.15** Visualization of the femoral nerve using ultrasound immediately proximal to the origin of the deep femoral artery from the femoral artery (approximately at the level of the inguinal ligament, short axis).

a Clinical setting.
b Anatomical overview.
c Enlargement of b.
d Identical to c, labeled.
e Ultrasound image corresponding to c.
f Identical to e, labeled.

1 Sartorius muscle
2 Iliopsoas muscle
3 Femoral nerve
4 Femoral artery
5 Femoral vein

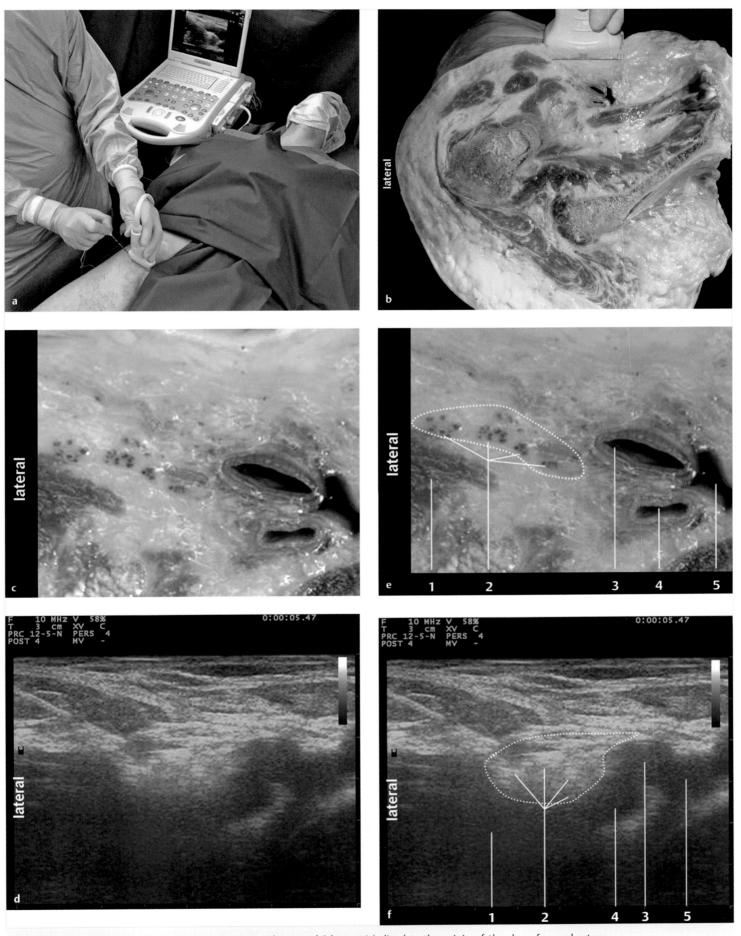

**Fig. 10.16** Visualization of the femoral nerve using ultrasound (short axis) distal to the origin of the deep femoral artery.
a Clinical setting (in plane).
b Anatomical overview.
c Enlargement of b.
d Ultrasound image corresponding to c.
e Identical to c, labeled.
f Identical to d, labeled.

1 Iliopsoas muscle
2 Femoral nerve
3 Femoral artery
4 Deep femoral artery
5 Femoral vein

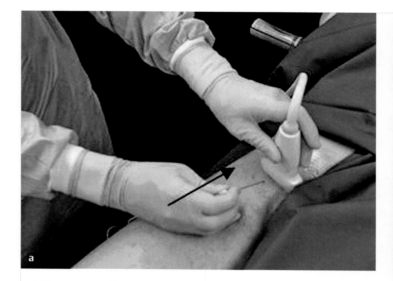

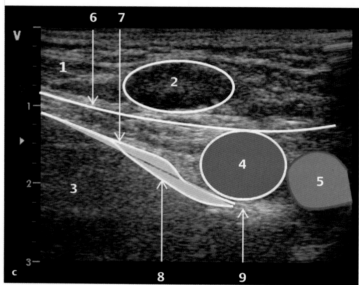

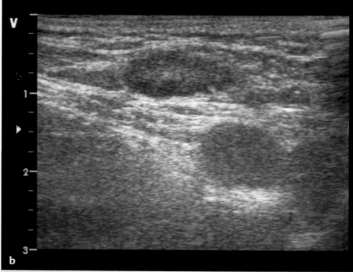

Fig. 10.17 Femoral nerve, right inguinal region with lymph nodes.
a Clinical setting.
b Ultrasound image, unlabeled.
c Ultrasound image, labeled.
Right femoral nerve block.
→, View to the acoustic window
1 Subcutaneous fat
2 Lymph nodes
3 Iliopsoas muscle
4 Femoral artery
5 Femoral vein
6 Fascia lata
7 Iliac fascia
8 Femoral nerve
9 Artifact (posterior enhancement)

▶ **In-plane approach.**

In the in-plane technique, as described above, the femoral nerve is visualized along with the femoral artery in the short axis. Then the nerve is found in plane from lateral (▶ Fig. 10.19).

The local anesthetic must spread under the iliac fascia. The entire nerve is either pressed down—that is, the local anesthetic spreads only directly above the nerve—or the nerve is completely surrounded by the local anesthetic (▶ Fig. 10.18). Somewhat more distally, at the level of the branch of the deep femoral artery, the femoral artery is already divided into its individual branches, which can be seen in the fluid after injection (▶ Fig. 10.19).

## Catheter Placement

A catheter can be placed both out of plane and in plane (Niazi et al 2009, Aveline et al 2010, Wang et al 2010), although our own experience using the in-plane approach has shown that advancing the catheter more than 2 cm beyond the tip of the needle is not recommended, as it leads to an incorrect position. ▶

### Practical Note

The spread of local anesthetic through the catheter should be checked by ultrasound; sometimes withdrawing the catheter allows spread in the correct space.

### Tips and Tricks

- The light-colored structure posterior to the femoral artery caused by acoustic enhancement should not be mistaken for the femoral nerve (▶ Fig. 10.15, ▶ Fig. 10.16, ▶ Fig. 10.18)!
- The nerve stimulator is useful.
- The needle should not be inserted too far distally where the nerve has already separated into its terminal branches. Visualization with ultrasound (short axis) should be immediately proximal to the bifurcation of the femoral artery.
- The femoral nerve can also be visualized in the long axis (▶ Fig. 10.20).
- Szücs et al (2014) suggest that there is no advantage in attempting to deposit the local anesthetic circumferential to the femoral nerve (versus depositing it above/superficial to the nerve).

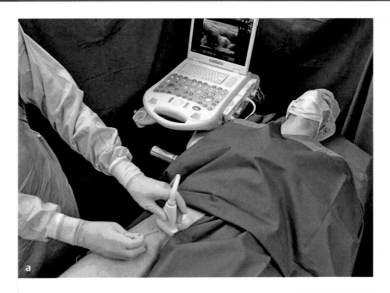

**Fig. 10.18** Right femoral nerve block.
**a** Clinical setting.
**b** Before injection of local anesthetic (unlabeled).
**c** Before injection of local anesthetic (labeled).
**d** After injection of local anesthetic (unlabeled).
**e** After injection of local anesthetic (labeled).
1 Iliac fascia
2 Femoral nerve
3 Iliopsoas muscle
4 Femoral artery

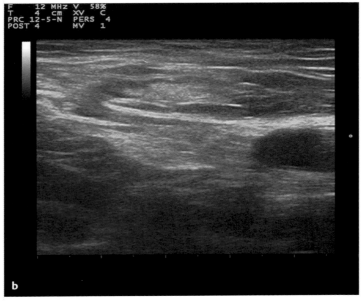

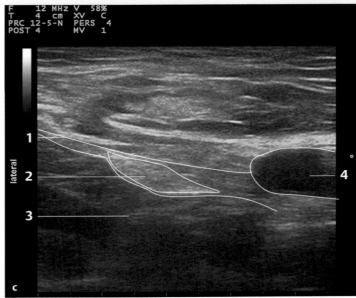

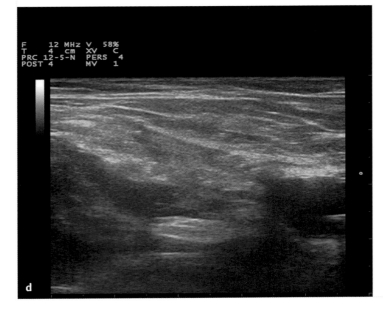

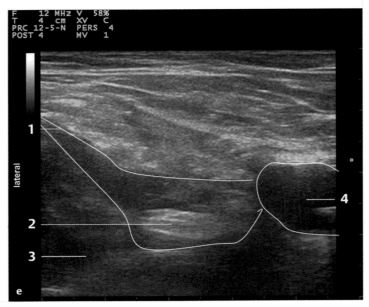

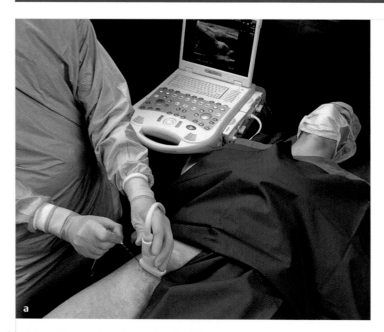

**Fig. 10.19** Right femoral nerve block (in-plane technique) at the level of the bifurcation of the femoral artery.

**a** Clinical setting, direction of needle.

**b** Ultrasound image before injection of local anesthetic (unlabeled).

**c** Ultrasound image before injection of local anesthetic (labeled).

**d** Ultrasound image after injection of 15 mL local anesthetic (unlabeled).

**e** Ultrasound image after injection of 15 mL local anesthetic (labeled).

1 Sartorius muscle

2 Iliopsoas muscle

3 Femoral nerve (some branches embedded in fatty tissue, see also ▶ Fig. 10.17)

4 Deep femoral artery

5 Femoral artery

White arrows: needle (SonoPlex, Pajunk GmbH)

Comment: Even after the injection of liquid, in this region the femoral nerve is no longer visualized as a single nerve because it has already separated into individual branches.

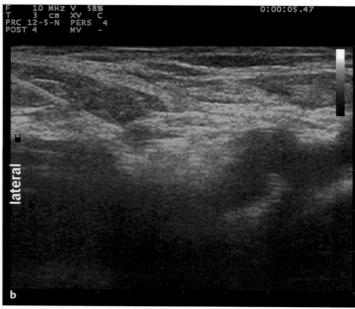

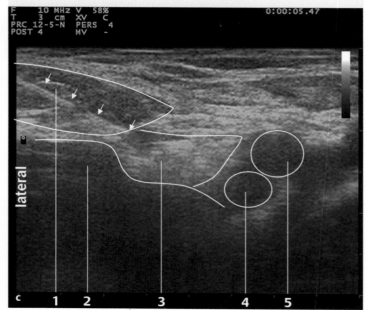

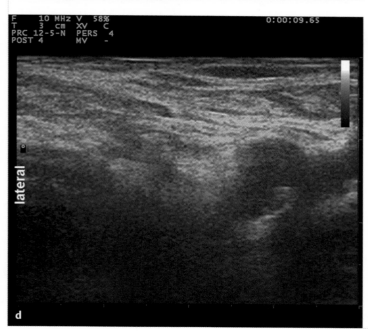

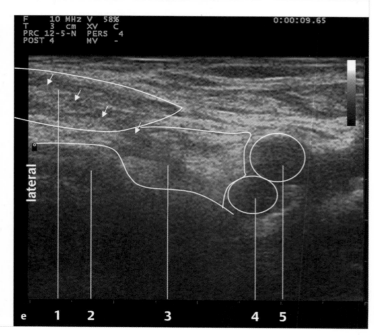

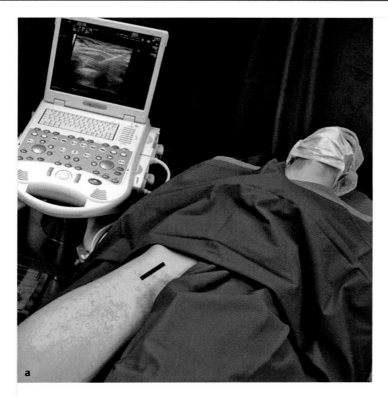

Fig. 10.20 Visualization of the femoral nerve in the long axis after injecting a few milliliters of local anesthetic.
a Clinical setting indicating the position of the transducer (black mark indicates the position of the linear transducer).
b Ultrasound image, unlabeled.
c Ultrasound image, labeled.
1 Femoral nerve
Arrows: needle (SonoPlex needle, Pajunk GmbH)

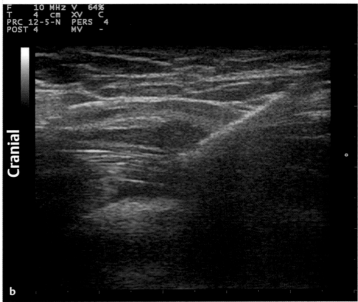

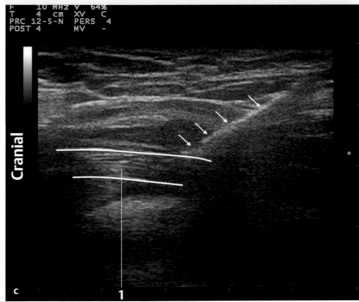

## 10.3 Sensory and Motor Effects

The femoral nerve provides the *sensory* innervation of the front of the thigh and is involved in the innervation of the hip, knee, and femur. It is the motor supply to the knee extensors and hip flexors. The saphenous nerve is the sensory terminal branch of the femoral nerve and innervates the inside of the lower leg. The anesthesia can include the great toe in some cases (Clara 1959).

## 10.4 Indications and Contraindications

### 10.4.1 Indications

- In combination with a block of the sciatic nerve (sacral plexus), all operations on the leg can be performed. For more complex

procedures on the knee (total knee replacement), additional obturator nerve block is necessary, see Chapter 13.4.
- Wound management and skin grafts on the anterior and lateral thigh and on the inside of the lower leg.
- Pain therapy after operations on the knee (e.g., arthroscopic operations, anterior cruciate ligament repair, knee replacement, etc.) and pain reduction after hip operations or thigh amputation.
- Pain therapy—for example, in femoral shaft fracture (Tobias 1994); patellar fracture; painless positioning for spinal anesthesia (e.g., before surgery of femoral neck fractures; mobilization; physiotherapy).

### 10.4.2 Contraindications

- General contraindications (see Chapter 20.2).
- Tumor in the groin (relative: painful lymph nodes in the groin).
- Previous inguinal vascular surgery (relative).

# 10.5 Complications, Side Effects, Method-Specific Problems

Vascular puncture with subsequent hematoma is possible. Femoral nerve lesions have been described in case reports.

## 10.5.1 Method-Specific Problems

- Identification of the perineural space is possible in principle without a nerve stimulator only using the loss-of-resistance technique. However, the nerve stimulator should not be omitted, as the femoral nerve is primarily a motor nerve and therefore paresthesia is not produced in every case in the event of (unintentional) puncture of the nerve (Urmey 1997). A proven alternative is to perform it under ultrasound guidance.
- The femoral nerve is separated from the artery by the iliopectineal arc (see ▶ Fig. 10.2 and ▶ Fig. 10.4). A transarterial technique, such as that described for the brachial plexus, is therefore not possible (Urmey 1997, Rosenquist and Lederhaas 1999).
- The advice to observe so-called dancing of the patella must be relativized according to the study by Anns (Anns et al 2011). A response of the Sartorius muscle (medial thigh) had no statistically significant different effect on the quality of anesthesia compared with a response of the quadriceps.
- The classical technique was described in 1924 by Labat. This technique also describes the insertion site at the inguinal ligament. In autopsy studies, the more favorable position of the tip of the needle was found for needle insertion at the level of the inguinal crease. Compared to an insertion site in the region of the inguinal ligament, the femoral nerve here is wider and much closer below the fascia lata (Vloka et al 1999; see ▶ Fig. 10.8). Needle insertion somewhat distal to the inguinal crease is therefore recommended and not, as in the classical technique of femoral nerve block, at the level of the inguinal ligament.
- The quality of anesthesia is not improved by advancing the catheter further forward and/or using greater injection volume than stated (Singelyn et al 1996; ▶ Fig. 10.21).
- The anesthesia may, in a few cases, include the great toe through the saphenous nerve (sensory terminal branch of the femoral nerve) (Clara 1959).
- Persistent pain in the region of the knee with otherwise complete anesthesia on the front of the thigh and a good motor block of the hip flexors and knee extensors can indicate insufficient obturator nerve block (Paul 1999).

# 10.6 Remarks on the Technique

Cranial to the inguinal ligament, the femoral nerve passes in a fascial sheath that is formed posterolaterally by the iliac fascia, medially by the psoas fascia, and anteriorly by the transversalis fascia. When it passes under the inguinal ligament, the nerve begins to split underneath and soon comes closer to the surface, dividing into its terminal branches. Immediately below the inguinal ligament, the femoral nerve is separated from the artery by the iliopectineal arch, which now forms side fascial sheath that continues to surround the medial part of the nerve, which is composed posterolaterally of the merged iliopsoas fascia and anteriorly of the fascia lata.

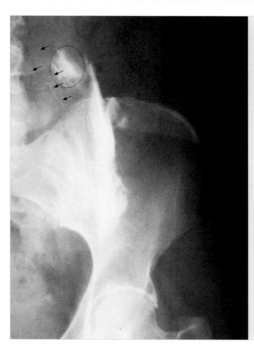

Fig. 10.21 Advancing the catheter too far may lead to looping and incorrect catheter position.
Arrows: Catheter
Oval: Diffuse spread of contrast injected through the catheter

Winnie postulated in 1973 that this fascial sheath should be understood as a sheath surrounding the nerve plexus throughout, from the proximal psoas compartment to its distal branching. According to Winnie, this fascial tube can be "filled" with local anesthetic by an appropriate injection technique not only from above as a psoas compartment block but also from the groin.

According to Winnie, the femoral, obturator, and lateral cutaneous nerves of the lumbar plexus should be reached with 20 mL of local anesthetic. This technique is also described as the anterior approach to the lumbar plexus (Hahn et al 1996). Winnie called the method the "3-in-1 technique" (Winnie et al 1973, 1974).

Winnie's classic concept is currently under discussion on the basis of recent information. The shared and continuous fascial sheath he described was not always found in anatomical studies. In particular, there is doubt whether the obturator nerve is reached at all with this block (Cauhèpe et al 1989; Kozlov et al 1991; Dupré 1996; Ritter 1995; Capdevilla et al 1998; ▶ Fig. 10.22, ▶ Fig. 10.23, ▶ Fig. 10.24).

Lang found in a prospective study that when the Winnie technique was used, the femoral nerve was anesthetized in 81% and the lateral cutaneous nerve of the thigh in 96%, but that the obturator nerve was blocked in only 4% of cases (Lang et al 1993).

The area of sensory innervation of this nerve on the inside of the thigh is very inconstant and is not suitable for investigation (Bergmann 1994). Demonstration of the degree to which the obturator nerve is involved in the block is therefore very difficult.

Paul and Drechsler (1993) found a completely anesthetized area of skin in only 5% of cases in isolated obturator nerve blocks despite the fact that there was obvious motor block of the adductors. On the basis of these observations, the obturator nerve appears to be of subordinate importance for the innervation of the knee in most cases. That would explain the very effective use of the so-called 3-in-1 technique, even if this probably leads only to a "2-in-1 block" (Rosenquist and Lederhaas 1999). The extent and significance of block of the lateral cutaneous nerve of the thigh have not yet been conclusively elucidated.

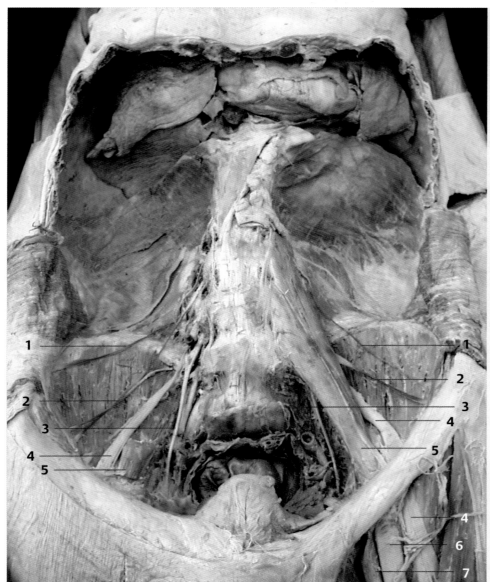

Fig. 10.22 Lumbar plexus with femoral nerve and obturator nerve. In femoral nerve block, the psoas major muscle (largely removed on the right) usually prevents spread of the local anesthetic to the obturator nerve in femoral nerve block.
1 Ilioinguinal nerve
2 Lateral cutaneous nerve of the thigh
3 Obturator nerve
4 Femoral nerve
5 Psoas major muscle (mostly removed on the right)
6 Femoral artery
7 Femoral vein

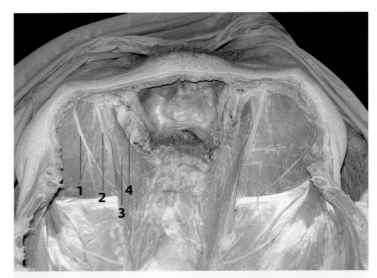

Fig. 10.23 Cranial view of the retroperitoneal region. The psoas major muscle prevents spread of the local anesthetic to the obturator nerve in femoral nerve block.
1 Lateral cutaneous nerve of the thigh
2 Femoral nerve
3 Psoas major muscle
4 Obturator nerve

► **Needle insertion site.**

In the technique described by Winnie, the insertion site selected was 1 cm below the inguinal ligament with the needle directed vertically toward the nerve. At this point, the femoral nerve is still relatively deep. Löfström mentions a depth of 3.5 to 4 cm (Löfström 1980). For this reason, Härtel (1916) and later Moore (1976) recommended an insertion site 2 to 3 cm further distal. In its further course, the nerve very quickly becomes more superficial and divides.

Vloka et al (1999) found that an insertion site at the level of the inguinal crease and directly lateral to the artery led most frequently (71%) to contact between the needle and the nerve. The nerve was significantly wider at this point (1.4 cm vs. 0.98 cm) and was closer to the fascia lata (0.68 cm vs. 2.64 cm) than at the level of the inguinal ligament (Vloka et al 1999).

Because of the branching of the nerve, however, an insertion site even further distally might be problematic and might also make placement of a catheter more difficult (Urmey 1997).

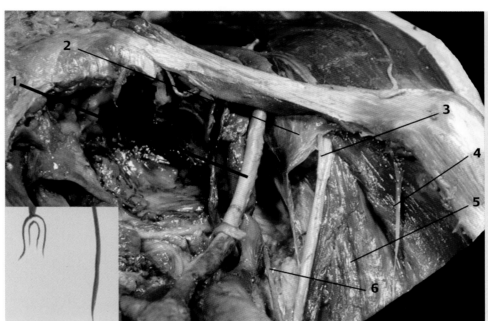

Fig. 10.24 Right vascular and muscular space, cranial view. The psoas fascia is a clear divider between the femoral nerve and the obturator nerve.
1 External iliac artery
2 Psoas fascia
3 Femoral nerve
4 Lateral cutaneous nerve of the thigh
5 Iliacus muscle
6 Obturator nerve

### Practical Note

Good anatomical orientation is possible even without producing paresthesia. The "double click," being a loss of resistance that can be felt on penetrating the fascia lata and the iliac fascia, especially when short-bevel needles are used, is a very reliable indication that the tip of the needle is in the correct position.

► **Peripheral nerve stimulation.** Whether the success rate can be improved by PNS during femoral nerve block is controversial. However, as the femoral nerve in the majority of cases has motor fibers, an intraneural injection might remain unnoticed on the basis of absent paresthesia if the nerve is approached too closely. With pure motor neurons, a disproportionate incidence of intraneural injection can be anticipated (Gentili and Wargnier 1993, Urmey 1997, Graf and Martin 2001). For safety reasons, the use of PNS or ultrasound is strongly recommended.

► **Indications.** The indications for inguinal paravascular femoral nerve block for intraoperative anesthesia are very limited.

Femoral nerve block, when performed on admission to hospital in the case of femoral neck or femoral shaft fractures, can allow pain-free examination and also administration of spinal anesthesia for surgery. Complete analgesia in the hip cannot be achieved as the hip is also supplied by the sacral plexus, but a clear reduction in pain is obtained (Esteve et al 1990, Fournier et al 1998).

► **Femoral nerve block and spinal anesthesia.** A combination of spinal anesthesia and femoral nerve block in transurethral operations on the bladder wall to eliminate the obturator reflex seldom leads to the desired effect. By blocking the obturator nerve, contractions of the adductor muscles due to unintentional stimulation by electroresection should be prevented. However, the femoral nerve block not only leads to an inadequate obturator nerve block but is also cranial to the site of stimulation. In order to obtain an effective block of the obturator nerve for this purpose, a selective obturator nerve block must be performed distal to the bladder.

► **Femoral nerve block and sciatic nerve block.** An inguinal perivascular femoral nerve block can be combined very successfully with sciatic nerve block for operations on the leg (Sprotte 1981, Kaiser et al 1986, Geiger et al 1989, 1995, Anke-Moller et al 1990, Elmas and Atanassoff 1993, Mackenzie 1997).

For complex surgery requiring a thigh tourniquet and operations on the knee, where dorsal parts of the joint are also involved, combination with a proximal sciatic nerve block is always necessary. A total of 60 mL of a 1% (10 mg/mL) medium-acting amide is recommended (Büttner and Meier 1999; Meier and Büttner 2009). A mixture of 0.375% (3.75 mg/mL) ropivacaine or bupivacaine with 1% (10 mg/mL) mepivacaine (30 mL of each), for example, can also be used (Marhofer et al 2000a, 2000b).

► **Psoas block.** For complex knee operations using only regional anesthesia, an additional obturator nerve block is required if a femoral nerve block combined with a sciatic block is performed. A comparison of psoas block and femoral nerve block for these indications (total knee replacement) shows that the psoas block is the method with better quality of anesthesia, but higher risks.

For postoperative pain therapy after major knee surgery, the femoral nerve catheter and continuous psoas block have been shown to have a comparable quality of anesthesia.

### Practical Note

Due to the low risk, the femoral nerve catheter is preferable for solely postoperative pain therapy (Morin 2006).

► **Mobilization.** It should be taken into consideration when the risks of the procedure are explained to the patient and when instructions are given to the ward that (continuous) regional anesthesia for complex procedures on the lower limb requires special attention for mobilization (risk of falls; Illfeld et al 2010).

▶ **Continuous pain therapy.** As continuous pain therapy, femoral nerve block provides sufficient analgesia for operations on the femur and patella and reduces pain in operations on the hip or knee. For rehabilitation after knee operations, continuous femoral nerve block provides effective pain relief and leads to shorter hospitalization and better functional results compared to general anesthesia (Capdevila et al 1999, Chelly et al 2001, Hebl et al 2005). The continuous femoral nerve block combined with a sciatic nerve block is as effective as an epidural infusion for postoperative pain control and rehabilitation course (Al-Zahrani et al 2014).

# References

Al-Zahrani T, Doais KS, Aljassir F, Alshaygy I, Albishi W, Terkawi AS. Randomized clinical trial of continuous femoral nerve block combined with sciatic nerve block versus epidural analgesia for unilateral total knee arthroplasty. J Arthroplasty 2014: Epub ahead of print

Anke-Moller E, Dahl JB, Spangsberg NLM et al. Inguinal paravascular block (three-in-one block). Ugeskr Laeger 1990; 152: 1655–658

Anns JP, Chen EW, Nirkavan N, McCartney CJ, Awad IT. A comparison of sartorius versus quadriceps stimulation for femoral nerve block: a prospective randomized double-blind controlled trial. Anesth Analg 2011; 112: 725–731

Aveline C, Le Roux A, Le Hetet H, Vautier P, Cognet F, Bonnet F. Postoperative efficacies of femoral nerve catheters sited using ultrasound combined with neurostimulation compared with neurostimulation alone for total knee arthroplasty. Eur J Anaesthesiol 2010; 27: 978–984

Bergmann RA. Compendium of Human Anatomic Variations. Munich: Urban and Schwarzenberg; 1994: 143–147

Büttner J, Meier G. Kontinuierliche periphere Techniken zur Regionalanästhesie und Schmerztherapie—Obere und untere Extremität. Bremen: Uni-Med; 1999

Capdevila X, Biboulet P, Bouregba M, Barthelet Y, Rubenovitch J, d'Athis F. Comparison of the three-in-one and fascia iliaca compartment blocks in adults: clinical and radiographic analysis. Anesth Analg 1998; 86: 1039–1044

Capdevila X, Barthelet Y, Biboulet P, Ryckwaert Y, Rubenovitch J, d'Athis F. Effects of perioperative analgesic technique on the surgical outcome and duration of rehabilitation after major knee surgery. Anesthesiology 1999; 91: 8–15

Cauhèpe C, Oliver M, Colombani R, Railhac N. [The "3-in-1" block: myth or reality?] [Article in French] Ann Fr Anesth Reanim 1989; 8: 376–378

Chelly JE, Greger J, Gebhard R et al. Continuous femoral blocks improve recovery and outcome of patients undergoing total knee arthroplasty. J Arthroplasty 2001; 16: 436–445

Clara M. Das Nervensystem des Menschen. 3rd ed. Leipzig: Barth; 1959

Dupré LJ. Three-in-one block or femoral nerve block. What should be done and how? [Article in French] Ann Fr Anesth Rea nim 1996; 15: 1099–1101

Elmas C, Atanassoff PG. Combined inguinal paravascular (3-in-1) and sciatic nerve blocks for lower limb surgery. Reg Anesth 199 3; 18: 88–92

Estève M, Veillette Y, Ecoffey C, Orhant EE. [Continuous block of the femoral nerve after surgery of the knee: pharmacokinetics of bupivacaine] [Article in French] Ann Fr Anesth Reanim 1990; 9: 322–325

Fournier R, Van Gessel E, Gaggero G, Boccovi S, Forster A, Gamulin Z. Postoperative analgesia with "3-in-1" femoral nerve block after prosthetic hip surgery. Can J Anaesth 1998; 45: 34–38

Geiger P, Weindler M, Wollinsky KH, et al. Met-Hb-Spiegel bei kombiniertem Ischiadicus/3-in-1-Block mit alleiniger Verwendung von Prilocain im Vergleich zu einer Prilocain-Bupivacain-Kombination. Innsbruck: Zentraleuropäischer Anästhesiekongress; 1989

Geiger P, Moßbrucker H, Gelowicz-Maurer M, et al. Postoperative analgesia with 3-in-1—or psoas-compartment-catheter—are there differences in efficiency? Prague: XIV Annual ESRA Congress (special abstract issue); 1995: 68

Gentili ME, Wargnier JP. Peripheral nerve damage and regional anaesthesia. Br J Anaesth 1993; 70: 594

Graf BM, Martin E. Peripheral nerve block. An overview of new developments in an old technique. Anaesthesist 2001; 50: 312–322

Hahn MB, McQuillan PM, Sheplock GJ. Regional anesthesia: an atlas of anatomy and techniques. St. Louis: Mosby; 1996

Härtel F. Die Lokalanästhesie. Stuttgart: Enke; 1916

Hebl JR, Kopp SL, Ali MH et al. A comprehensive anesthesia protocol that emphasizes peripheral nerve blockade for total knee and total hip arthroplasty. J Bone Joint Surg Am 2005; 87 Suppl 2: 63–70

Ilfeld BM, Duke KB, Donohue MC. The association between lower extremity continuous peripheral nerve blocks and patient falls after knee and hip arthroplasty. Anesth Analg 2010; 111: 1552–1554

Kaiser H, Niesel HC, Klimpel L, Menge M. Technik und Indikationen der kontinuierlichen 3-in-1-Blockade. In: Hempelmann G, Biscoping J, eds. Regionalanästhesiologische Aspekte I. Kontinuierliche Verfahren der Regionalanästhesie. Wedel: Astra; 1986: 83–94

Kozlov SP, Shatrov AI, Svetlov VA. [The inguinal paravascular technique of lumbar plexus block—anatomical pretests were unsuccessful] [Article in Russian] Anesteziol Reanimatol 1991; 5: 37–39

Labat G. Regional anesthesia: Its technique and clinical application. Philadelphia: Saunders; 1924: 45

Lang SA, Yip RW, Chang PC, Gerard MA. The femoral 3-in-1 block revisited. J Clin Anesth 1993; 5: 292–296

Löfström B. Blockaden der peripheren Nerven des Beines. In: Eriksson E, ed. Atlas der Lokalanästhesie. 2nd ed. Berlin: Springer; 1980:101–115

Mackenzie JW. 3-in-1 Block via femoral nerve sheath cannula: a simple method of pain relief for fractured neck of femur. Int Monitor Reg Anesth 1997; 9: 91

Marhofer P, Nasel C, Sitzwohl C, Kapral S. Magnetic resonance imaging of the distribution of local anesthetic during the three-in-one block. Anesth Analg 2000a; 90: 119–124

Marhofer P, Oismüller C, Faryniak B, Sitzwohl C, Mayer N, Kapral S. Three-in-one blocks with ropivacaine: evaluation of sensory onset time and quality of sensory block. Anesth Analg 2000b; 90: 125–128

Meier G, Büttner J. Kompendium Regionalanästhesie. Munich: Arcis; 2009

Moore DC. Lesions of the peripheral nerves. In: Moore DC, ed. Complications of Regional Anesthesia. Philadelphia: Davis; 1969: 112–118

Moore DC. Regional Block: Block of the Sciatic and Femoral Nerves. Springfield: Thomas; 1976: 275–299

Morin AM. Regional anaesthesia and analgesia for total knee replacement. Article in German Anasthesiol Intensivmed Notfallmed Schmerzther 2006; 41: 498–505

Niazi AU, Prasad A, Ramlogan R, Chan VWS. Methods to ease placement of stimulating catheters during in-plane ultrasound-guided femoral nerve block. Reg Anesth Pain Med 2009; 34: 380–381

Paul W, Drechsler HJ. Clinical efficacy and radiological representation of continuous 3-in-1 block placed by the Seldinger technique. Int Monitor Reg Anesth 1993; 4: 531–32

Paul W. Die kontinuierliche Blockade des N. femoralis. In: Mehrkens HH, Büttner J, ed. Kontinuierliche periphere Leitungsblockaden. Munich: Arcis; 1999: 49–58

Platzer W. Color Atlas of Human Anatomy Vol 1. Locomotor System. 7th edition. Stuttgart: Thieme; 2014

Ritter JW. Femoral nerve "sheath" for inguinal paravascular lumbar plexus block is not found in human cadavers. J Clin Anesth 1995; 7: 470–473

Rosenquist RW, Lederhaas G. Femoral and lateral femoral cutaneous nerve block. Tech Reg Anesth Pain Manage 1999; 3: 33–38

Singelyn FJ, Gouverneur JMA, Goossens F, van Roy C. During continuous "3-in-1" block a high position of the catheter increases the success rate of the technique. Int Monitor Reg Anesth 1996; (A)8: 105

Soong J, Schafhalter-Zoppoth I, Gray AT. The importance of transducer angle to ultrasound visibility of the femoral nerve. Reg Anesth Pain Med 2005; 30: 505

Sprotte G. Die inguinale Blockade des Plexus lumbalis als Analgesie-Verfahren in der prä- und postoperativen Traumatologie und Orthopädie. Region Anästh 1981; 4: 39–41

Szűcs S, Morau D, Sultan SF, Iohom G, Shorten G. A comparison of three techniques (local anesthetic deposited circumferential to vs. above vs. below the nerve) for ultrasound guided femoral nerve block. BMC Anesthesiol 2014; 14: 6

Tobias JD. Continuous femoral nerve block to provide analgesia following femur fracture in a paediatric ICU population. Anaesth Intensive Care 1994; 22: 616–618

Urmey WF. Femoral nerve block for the management of postoperative pain. Tech Reg Anesth Pain Manage 1997; 1: 88–92

Vloka JD, Hadzić A, Drobnik L, Ernest A, Reiss W, Thys DM. Anatomical landmarks for femoral nerve block: a comparison of four needle insertion sites. Anesth Analg 1999; 89: 1467–1470

Wang AZ, Gu L, Zhou QH, Ni WZ, Jiang W. Ultrasound-guided continuous femoral nerve block for analgesia after total knee arthroplasty: catheter perpendicular to the nerve versus catheter parallel to the nerve. Reg Anesth Pain Med 2010; 35: 127–131

Winnie AP, Ramamurthy S, Durrani Z. The inguinal paravascular technic of lumbar plexus anesthesia: the "3-in-1 block." Anesth Analg 1973; 52: 989–996

Winnie AP, Ramamurthy S, Durrani Z, Radonjic R. Plexus blocks for lower extremity surgery. New answers to old problems. Anesth Rev 1974; 11–16

Woodburne RT. The lower limb. In: Woodburne RT, ed. Essentials of Human Anatomy. 7th ed. New York: Oxford University Press; 1983: 557–571

# 11 Proximal Sciatic Nerve Block

## 11.1 Anatomical Overview

The sacral plexus can be divided into three parts:
• Pudendal plexus
• Coccygeal plexus
• Sciatic plexus

The sacral plexus is not subdivided in all anatomy textbooks. However, as the division is useful from the clinical aspect, it is used as a basis here.

### 11.1.1 Sciatic Plexus

The sciatic plexus derives its roots from part of the anterior ramus of the fourth lumbar nerve and from the entire anterior ramus of the fifth lumbar nerve, which together form the lumbosacral trunk, along with the anterior rami of the first and second and part of the third sacral nerves. The anterior ramus of the first sacral nerve is not only the biggest branch of the lumbosacral plexus but the biggest anterior ramus overall.

All of the roots of the plexus converge from their exit sites toward the greater sciatic foramen so that the plexus forms a triangular sheet, the apex of which points toward the infrapiriform foramen where the sciatic nerve emerges (▶ Fig. 11.1). The nerve plexus lies for the most part on the piriformis muscle and is covered toward the pelvis by the parietal peritoneum and the tissues lying below it that form the parietal pelvic fascia and branches of the internal iliac artery. The articular branches that supply parts of the hip joint capsule and the periosteal branches that innervate the periosteum of the sciatic tuber, greater trochanter, and lesser trochanter also come from the sciatic plexus.

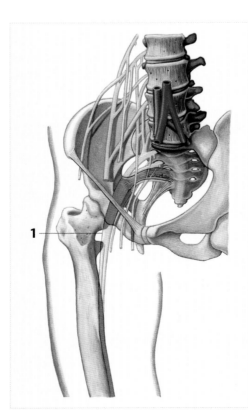

**Fig. 11.1** Course of the sciatic nerve, main nerve of the sacral plexus.
1 Sciatic nerve

## 11.1.2 Sciatic Nerve (L4–S3)

The sciatic nerve derives its fibers from all the roots of the sacral plexus. It is the biggest and longest nerve in the body, it supplies the widest area, and at the same time it has the greatest resistance among all the nerve cords, with a tear strength of 91.5 kg (!). Excessive stretching can even tear the nerve trunk from its roots in the spinal cord. The roots of the sciatic nerve unite into the trunk immediately before the greater sciatic foramen at the lower border of the piriformis (▶ Fig. 11.2).

The sciatic nerve consists of two components, the common fibular nerve (synonym: common peroneal nerve) and the tibial nerve, which are surrounded in the lesser pelvis and thigh by a shared connective-tissue sheath and therefore have the appearance of a single nerve trunk. The division into the two branches can occur at varying levels (▶ Fig. 11.3 and ▶ Fig. 11.4).

At dissection, the nerve can almost always be separated into its two divisions as far as the hip region, even if they run in a common sheath (Ericksen et al 2002).

The sciatic nerve usually leaves the true pelvis (lesser pelvis) through the infrapiriform foramen as a 1.4 cm (up to 3 cm) wide and 0.4 to 0.5 cm (up to 0.9 cm) thick nerve cord (▶ Fig. 11.3 and ▶ Fig. 11.4) and enters the gluteal region. It divides into the tibial nerve and the common fibular nerve at the latest where it enters the popliteal fossa.

The sciatic nerve provides motor innervation through its tibial division to all of the flexor muscles of the thigh (with the exception of the short head of the biceps femoris) and the lower leg and with its fibular division it innervates the short head of the biceps femoris and the fibular muscles and all the extensors in the lower leg and foot. It provides sensory innervation through both divisions to the skin of the lower leg and foot.

> **Practical Note**
>
> If the trunk of the sciatic nerve is paralyzed, external rotation of the thigh and knee flexion are greatly impaired. Complete anesthesia leads to the corresponding impairment. Because of the unopposed extensor action of the quadriceps muscle, the leg behaves like a stilt. The foot is unstable at the ankle and can no longer be dorsiflexed (foot drop).

### 11.1.3 Posterior Cutaneous Nerve of the Thigh (S1–S3)

The posterior cutaneous nerve of the thigh, which is the sensory supply to the posterior aspect of the thigh, leaves the pelvis together with the sciatic nerve and the inferior gluteal nerve through the infrapiriform foramen. The nerve lies medial to the sciatic nerve and reaches the posterior surface of the thigh under the gluteus maximus muscle. There it lies subfascially, but close to the fascia lata, through which it passes at varying levels. The distribution of the posterior cutaneous nerve of the thigh is variable and extends from the distal third of the buttocks as far as the distal boundary of the popliteal fossa.

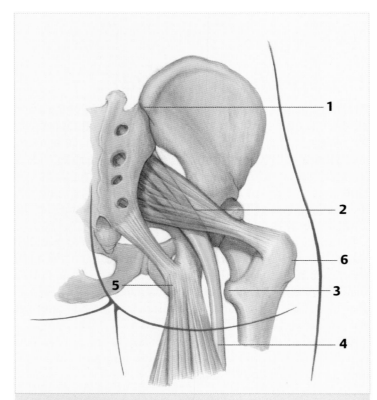

**Fig. 11.2** After emerging from the lesser pelvis through the infrapiriform foramen, the sciatic nerve, covered by the gluteal muscles, runs peripherally midway between the greater trochanter and the ischial tuberosity, behind and medial to the lesser trochanter. The three palpable bony points (posterior superior iliac spine, greater trochanter, and ischial tuberosity) are used for orientation in all dorsal techniques of proximal sciatic nerve block.
1 Posterior superior iliac spine
2 Piriformis muscle
3 Lesser trochanter
4 Sciatic nerve
5 Ischial tuberosity
6 Greater trochanter

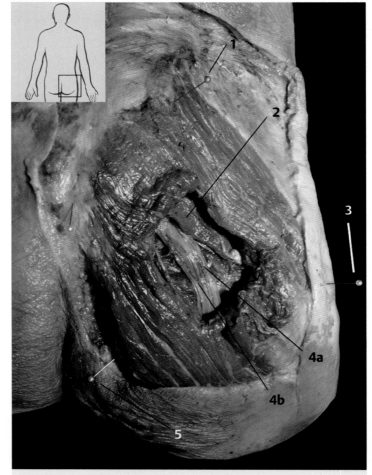

**Fig. 11.3** Exit of the sciatic nerve from the infrapiriform foramen in a fenestrated gluteus maximus muscle.
1 Needle is in the posterior superior iliac spine
2 Piriformis muscle
3 Needle is in the furthest lateral part of the greater trochanter
4a Fibular part of the sciatic nerve
4b Tibial part of the sciatic nerve
5 Needle is in the ischial tuberosity

## Overview of the Nerves of the Sciatic Plexus

The superior gluteal nerve and the inferior gluteal nerve along with the posterior cutaneous nerve of the thigh and the sciatic nerve belong to the sciatic plexus.

Only the sciatic nerve (tibial nerve, common fibular nerve) and the posterior cutaneous nerve of the thigh are important for anesthesia and analgesia of the leg.

## 11.1.4 Periosteal Innervation

### Relevant Facts for Anesthesia and Pain Therapy

The periosteum of the femur is supplied posteriorly by the sciatic nerve in the upper third, by the obturator nerve in the middle third, and in the distal third by the sciatic nerve laterally and by the femoral and obturator nerves medially.

Innervation of the knee is provided anteriorly by branches of the femoral nerve and sciatic nerve and posteriorly by parts of the sciatic nerve, the obturator nerve, and the saphenous nerve.

The periosteum of the tibia and fibula apart from the lateral head of the tibia and the head of the fibula (common fibular nerve) is supplied by the tibial nerve (important for lower leg amputations, fractures).

The ankle receives its sensory supply from the tibial nerve and sural nerve.

The periosteum of the tarsal bones is innervated by the sural nerve and parts of the tibial nerve, the metatarsals, and the phalanges by the deep fibular nerve and the terminal branches of the tibial nerve (Wagner 1994).

## 11.2 Anterior Proximal Sciatic Nerve Block (with Patient in Supine Position) ▷

### 11.2.1 Technique of Anterior Sciatic Nerve Block

The classical technique of anterior sciatic nerve block was described in 1963 by G.P. Beck (Beck 1963). The technique was

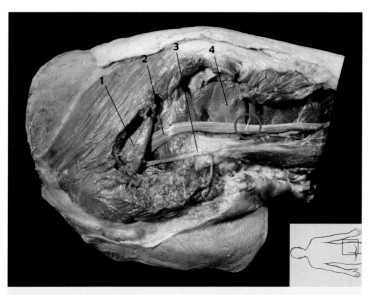

**Fig. 11.4** The red circle marks the penetrating needle in an anterior sciatic nerve block.
1 Piriformis muscle
2 Sciatic nerve
3 Posterior cutaneous nerve of the thigh
4 Quadratus femoris muscle

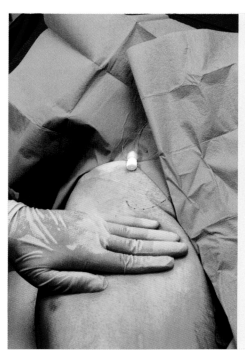

**Fig. 11.5** In practice, it has proved effective not to measure distances to find the insertion site for the anterior sciatic nerve block. Orientation is a good hand's breadth below the inguinal crease or below the insertion site for a femoral nerve block. Right thigh, caudal view.

modified by Meier (Meier 1998) to simplify the procedure and allow placement of a catheter.

## Anterior Block of the Sciatic Nerve (according to Beck, Classical Technique)

### Landmarks

Inguinal crease, gap between the rectus femoris and sartorius muscles. (Note: We have dispensed with the extensive description of orientation with various landmarks and lines, as the method described below has been proven for years.)

### Position

The patient lies supine with the leg to be anesthetized extended.

### Procedure

The puncture site is approximately 10 cm (hand breadth) below the inguinal crease (▶ Fig. 11.5).

The puncture site is the muscle gap between the rectus femoris and the sartorius. In this muscle gap, vertical pressure is exerted on the femur with two fingers, and the bone is used as an abutment ("two-finger grasp"; ▶ Fig. 11.6, ▶ Fig. 11.7, ▶ Fig. 11.8). The blood vessels are pushed medially by this maneuver and the likelihood of accidental vascular puncture is reduced (▶ Fig. 11.7, ▶ Fig. 11.8, ▶ Fig. 11.9, ▶ Fig. 11.10). A 15-cm needle is then advanced at an angle of 75 to 85° to the skin in cranial, posterior and slightly lateral direction (▶ Fig. 11.8 and ▶ Fig. 11.10). When a cranial direction is maintained, the sciatic nerve is reached further proximal by a few centimeters, depending on the angle of insertion; if the nerve is reached more tangentially, it is easier to

advance an indwelling catheter (▶ Fig. 11.11). For ultrasound visualization, a curved array transducer is recommended owing to the depth (▶ Fig. 11.12, Chapter 11.2.5). The sciatic nerve can be reached well using this technique.

Branches of the femoral nerve are often stimulated after the needle is advanced a few centimeters. The position of the needle tip is corrected (usually laterally) until no further response can be detected from the quadriceps femoris muscle and it is then advanced further. Stimulation is initially with a current of 0.8 to 1.0 mA. After 6 to 10 cm, the adductor fascia is reached, which is often signaled by an obvious loss of resistance. The needle is advanced further until a motor response is produced in one of the two divisions of the sciatic nerve (fibular nerve, dorsiflexion: tibial nerve, plantar flexion; ▶ Fig. 11.13).

> **Practical Note**
>
> The correct position of the needle is indicated by a response in the foot. If there is a response in the ischiocrural muscles, the needle must be withdrawn significantly and corrected laterally ("below the femur") (▶ Fig. 11.14, ▶ Fig. 11.15, ▶ Fig. 11.16). Then 30 mL of a medium-acting or long-acting local anesthetic is injected.

- In the continuous technique, following injection of the local anesthetic, a 20G catheter is advanced 4 cm proximally by the needle (▶ Fig. 11.17 and ▶ Fig. 11.18). Short, mild resistance can occur when the catheter tip reaches the end of the needle (▶ Fig. 11.17), but this is normally easily overcome, and the catheter can then be advanced smoothly.

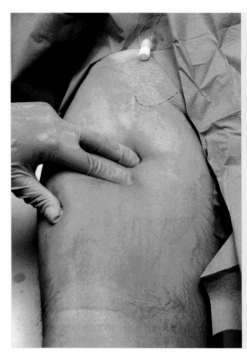

Fig. 11.6 Two-finger grasp for identifying the muscle gap between rectus femoris and sartorius muscles (right thigh, seen from above). This grasp will also push the blood vessels medially.

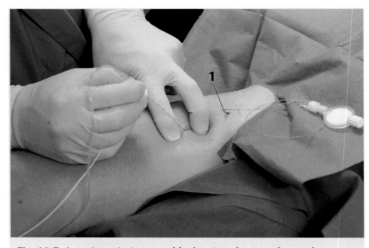

Fig. 11.7 Anterior sciatic nerve block using the muscle gap between rectus femoris and sartorius muscles for orientation. The puncture site is a good hand's breadth below the puncture site for femoral nerve block. Note the cranial and slightly lateral needle direction ("below the femur") and the two-finger grasp in the muscle gap, which pushes the blood vessels medially. Right thigh.
1 Femoral nerve catheter

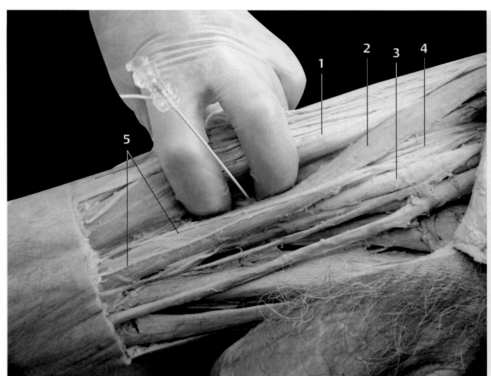

Fig. 11.8 Anterior sciatic nerve block using the muscle gap between rectus femoris and sartorius muscles for orientation. The insertion site is a good hand's breadth below the insertion site for femoral nerve block. Note the "two-finger grasp" in the muscle gap that pushes the vessels medially. When the needle is inserted under nerve stimulation, there is occasionally a response in the anterior part of the thigh in the quadriceps muscle after about 2 to 4 cm through stimulation of branches of the femoral nerve.
1 Rectus femoris muscle
2 Sartorius muscle
3 Femoral artery
4 Femoral nerve
5 Fibers of the femoral nerve

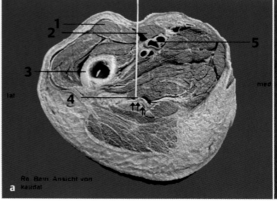
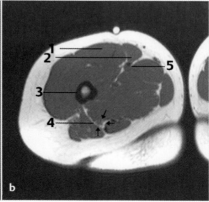

Fig. 11.9 Anterior sciatic nerve block using the muscle gap between rectus femoris and sartorius for orientation: anatomical cross-section and MRI at the level of the puncture.
1 Rectus femoris muscle
2 Sartorius muscle
3 Femur
4 Sciatic nerve
5 Blood vessels
a Right leg, seen from below.
b MR image, right thigh.

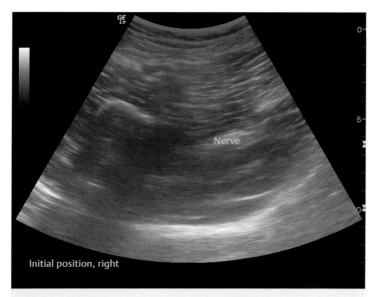

Fig. 11.10 Anterior sciatic nerve block: visualization of the nerve using ultrasound. The curved array transducer is usually used due to the penetration depth.

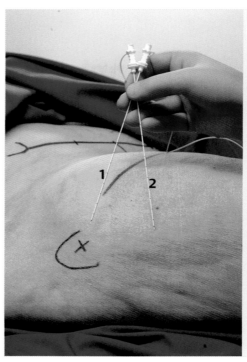

Fig. 11.12 Anterior proximal sciatic nerve block (lateral view). When the needle is directed cranially, the sciatic nerve is reached a few centimeters further proximal, depending on the needle angle. A more tangential approach to the nerve makes advancement of a catheter easier. Right thigh, lateral view.
1 Cranial needle direction
2 Purely sagittal needle direction

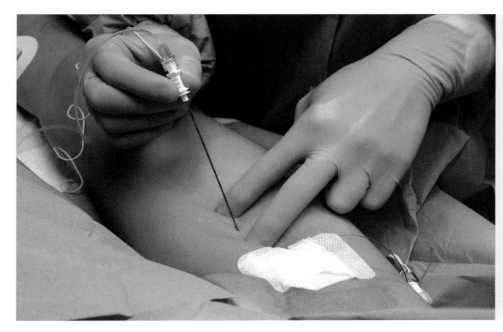

Fig. 11.11 Two-finger grasp to identify the muscle gap between the rectus femoris and sartorius muscles. The vessels are pushed medially. Right thigh, cranial view.

- The technique should be performed with peripheral nerve stimulation.
- If sciatic nerve block is combined with a femoral nerve block, anesthetizing the femoral nerve first is useful as this leads to anesthesia of the anterior thigh and helps to improve patient comfort (▶ Fig. 11.17).
- The technique can also be performed in obese patients (▶ Fig. 11.19 and ▶ Fig. 11.20).

## 11.2.2 Indications and Contraindications (in Combination with Femoral Nerve Block)

### Indications

- Operations on the knee, lower leg, or foot (e.g., knee replacement, tibial head osteotomy, arthrodesis, lateral ligament suture, forefoot operation).

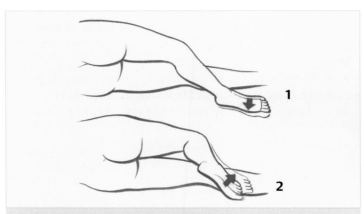

**Fig. 11.13** The correct muscle response for all proximal sciatic nerve blocks should be seen in the foot. Either the (medially located) tibial part (plantar flexors) or the (laterally located) fibular part (dorsiflexors) is stimulated. In the Labat and Mansour techniques, a response by the ischiocrural muscles (thigh flexors or "hamstring muscles") can also be regarded as a correct response.
1 Response of tibial part of the sciatic nerve: plantar flexion
2 Response of fibular part of the sciatic nerve: dorsiflexion

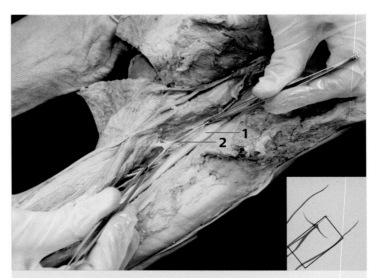

**Fig. 11.14** If the ischiocrural muscles (thigh flexors) are stimulated during anterior sciatic nerve block, the needle tip is too far medial; it must be corrected lateral to the sciatic nerve. To do this, the needle should be withdrawn a few centimeters and then the tip of the needle advanced more laterally ("below the femur") by turning the needle hub medially. The correct response in anterior sciatic nerve blocks should always be sought in the foot (fibular or tibial division of the sciatic nerve).
1 Sciatic nerve
2 Motor branches to the ischiocrural muscles

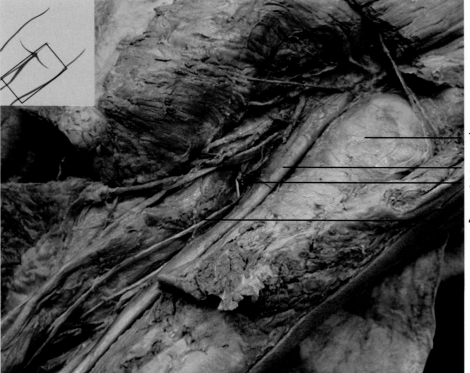

**Fig. 11.15** Visualization of the motor branches of the sciatic nerve, which supply the ischiocrural muscles and run medial to the sciatic nerve, here with anteriorly advanced needle. Right thigh, posterior view.
1 Greater trochanter
2 Sciatic nerve
3 Needle tip
4 Motor branches to the ischiocrural muscles

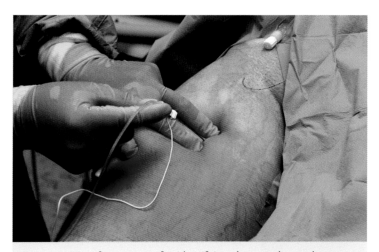

- Reposition of fractures in the lower leg and foot area.
- Amputations in the thigh (► Fig. 11.21), lower leg, and foot.
- Regional sympathetic block (e.g., perfusion disorders, wound healing disorders, CRPS 1).
- Pain therapy (e.g., postoperative, achillodynia, oligoarthritis).
- Postoperative pain therapy after total knee replacement, particularly when there is incomplete extension in the knee joint (► Fig. 11.22).
- Traumatology (e.g., pain-free positioning for diagnostic investigation).

**Fig. 11.16** Two-finger grasp for identifying the muscle gap between rectus femoris and sartorius muscles. This grasp will also push the blood vessels medially. When the ischiocrural muscles (hamstring muscles) are stimulated, the needle must be withdrawn and the tip of the needle advanced laterally by also moving the needle hub medially. Right thigh, seen from above.

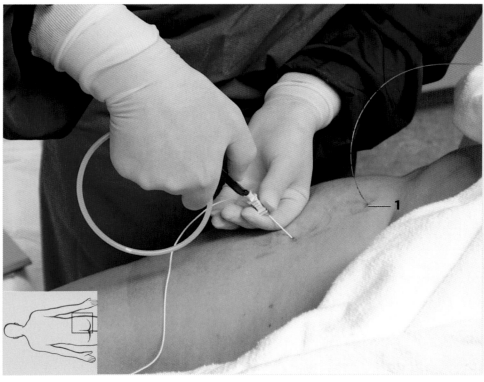

**Fig. 11.17** Advancing an indwelling sciatic catheter. Using a cranial needle direction, the catheter can usually be advanced easily after overcoming the slight resistance when the catheter tip has reached the end of the needle. 1 Femoral nerve catheter in situ

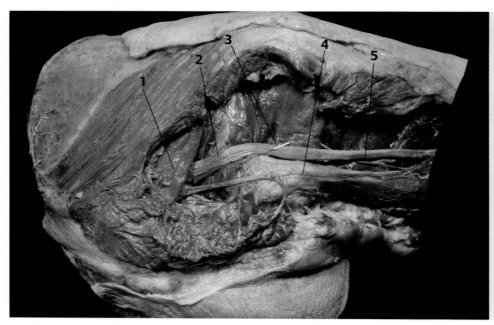

**Fig. 11.18** Anterior sciatic nerve block with needle introduced and catheter advanced cranially.
1 Piriformis muscle
2 Sciatic nerve
3 Needle with catheter
4 Posterior cutaneous nerve of the thigh
5 Branches of the ischiocrural muscle group

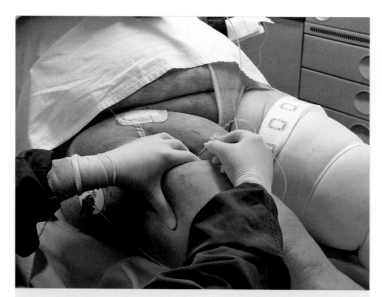

**Fig. 11.19** Anterior sciatic nerve block is possible even in obese patients, in whom the sciatic nerve can be expected at a depth of 13 to 15 cm. Note the hand grasp!

## Contraindications

- General contraindications (see Chapter 20.2)
- Special contraindications: none

## 11.2.3 Side Effects and Complications

There are no known special complications of sciatic nerve block. There have been few reports of side effects. Major complications including late sequelae are very rare. Dysesthesia for 1 to 3 days, which resolved spontaneously, has been described.

## 11.2.4 Remarks on the Technique

In Beck's classical anterior technique (Beck 1963) the sciatic nerve is reached relatively distally. For this reason, anesthesia of the posterior cutaneous nerve of the thigh is often inadequate, which may cause problems in patients requiring a tourniquet at the thigh. In addition, with the Beck technique the sciatic nerve may be difficult to locate. With the modified technique, directing the needle at an angle of 75° to the skin causes needle contact with the sciatic nerve 3 to 4 cm more proximally; therefore both the sciatic nerve and the posterior cutaneous nerve of the thigh are reached (Meier 1999a).

The diameter of the sciatic nerve, the largest nerve in the body, is impressive. In anatomical studies only part of the nerve was stained after injection of 10 mL of methylene blue through the catheter (Meier 1999a; ▶ Fig. 11.23).

### Tips and Tricks

- The leg should be in neutral position.
- Digital support ("two-finger grasp") markedly reduces the risk of vascular puncture and the skin–nerve distance is shortened considerably (Meier 1999b).
- In contrast to the Beck classical anterior technique, the Meier approach is about 1 to 1.5 cm further medial and distal so that contact with the periosteum of the femur is avoided (Meier 1999a).
- The course of the deep blood vessels can also be established with a Doppler probe (Büttner and Meier 1999).
- Using the Meier approach, the tip of the needle reaches the nerve 3 to 4 cm more proximal than with the technique described by Beck. The posterior cutaneous nerve of the thigh can therefore also be anesthetized (Meier 1999b).
- If no stimulation response is produced, the needle should be withdrawn and corrected laterally (Meier 2001).
- The catheter can be advanced more smoothly if the local anesthetic has been injected beforehand.
- Advancing the catheter more than 4 cm beyond the tip of the needle has no advantages (▶ Fig. 11.24).
- No change in patient position is required when the technique is combined with a femoral nerve block.
- The onset of the block (as indicated by corresponding sympathetic block) can be checked through the rise in plantar temperature using a skin thermometer (Büttner and Meier 1999).

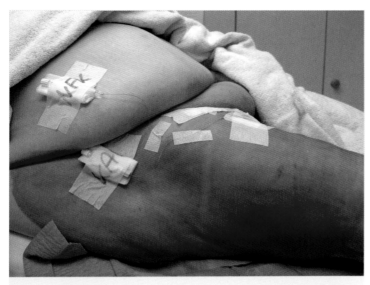

**Fig. 11.20** Obese patients in particular benefit from the combination of a femoral nerve catheter and a sciatic nerve catheter: nerve block prior to total knee replacement.

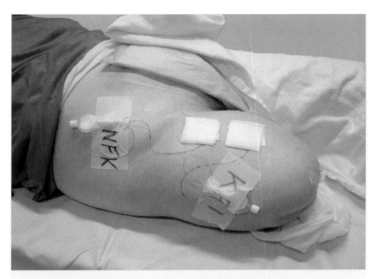

**Fig. 11.21** Planned thigh amputation, operation on the thigh stump, phantom and/or stump pain are proper indications for continuous proximal sciatic nerve block. The patient can control the needle passage by giving phantom information about the response to the nerve stimulator ("the foot is now moving downward"). Ultrasound-guided puncture can be helpful here.

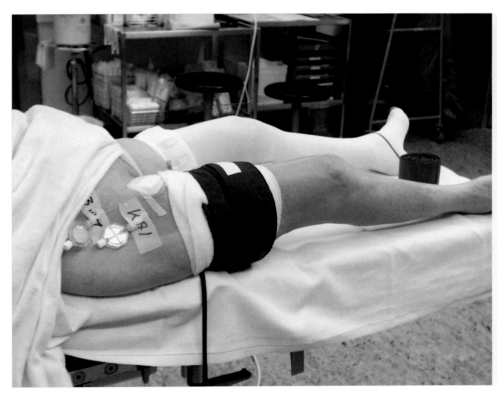

**Fig. 11.22** Particularly when extension of the knee is prevented, continuous block of the sciatic nerve in conjunction with a femoral nerve block is of great importance to achieve good postoperative mobility after insertion of a total knee replacement. KAI: continuous anterior sciatic nerve block; "3-in-1" femoral nerve block.

**Practical Note**

To achieve complete anesthesia of the sciatic nerve, at least 20 mL of a local anesthetic should be injected. When positioning the patient, it should be ensured that the leg to be anesthetized is in neutral position. Bone contact is not necessary and the stimulating needle can be advanced past the femur (lesser trochanter) much more easily when the leg is in neutral position.

The distance from the skin of the anterior thigh to the sciatic nerve is around 6 to 10 cm in adults when the needle is directed vertically. With the needle directed cranially, the nerve is reached after 8 to 12 cm, and sometimes only after 13 to 15 cm in muscular or obese patients (Brown 1996, Chelly et al 1997, Bridenbaugh and Wedel 1998, Ericksen et al 2002). Paresthesia should be avoided.

During stimulation, note that contractions of gluteus maximus or tensor fasciae latae do not represent an adequate response. The vicinity of the sciatic nerve is indicated by a response in the area supplied by the nerve (hamstring muscles, triceps surae, tibialis anterior, fibular group; Wagner and Missler 1987, Kaiser et al 1990, Wagner 1994).

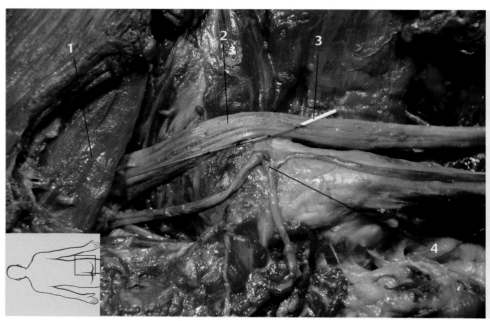

Fig. 11.23 Anterior sciatic nerve block with the approaching needle and the catheter advanced too far.
1 Piriformis muscle
2 Sciatic nerve
3 Needle with catheter
4 Posterior cutaneous nerve of the thigh and inferior clunial nerves

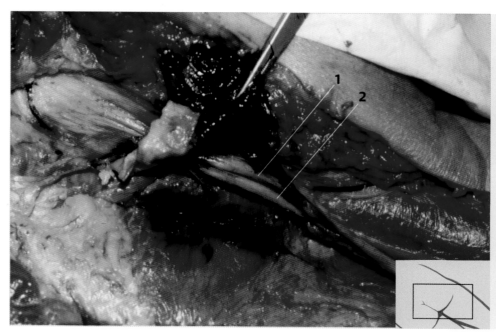

Fig. 11.24 Our studies with dye (methylene blue) in non-preserved cadavers have shown that a minimum volume of 20 mL is required to block the entire sciatic nerve. Right gluteal region, posterior view after a volume of 10 ml of dye.
1 Sciatic nerve: fibular division, surrounded by dye
2 Sciatic nerve: tibial division, not surrounded by dye

The motor response should be optimized so that plantar flexion (tibial nerve) or dorsiflexion (common fibular nerve) is produced in the foot.

In a study by Neuburger et al (2001), the stimulated muscle group (whether innervated by the tibial nerve or fibular nerve) had no effect on the block result. With correct stimulation (below 0.5 mA), a success rate over 95% can be achieved (Niesel 1994, Chelly et al 1999).

> **Practical Note**
>
> Performing the block with an immobile needle technique is beneficial as it enables aspiration to exclude vascular puncture and accidental intravascular injection of local anesthetic (Winnie 1975, Büttner and Meier 1999).

For anesthesia, 30 mL of a medium-acting or long-acting local anesthetic of adequate concentration should be injected (Wagner and Taeger 1988, Bridenbaugh and Wedel 1998, Chelly and Delaunay 1999; ▶ Fig. 11.25). In combination with a lumbar plexus block (psoas or so-called "3-in-1 block"), a further 30 to 40 mL of local anesthetic is required. When complete anesthesia of the leg is required, the combination of an anterior sciatic nerve block with femoral nerve block is a good alternative, as both blocks can be performed in the same sterile field without a change in position or repeated disinfection (▶ Fig. 11.7 and ▶ Fig. 11.10).

The femoral nerve block should be performed before the sciatic nerve block. This allows a largely pain-free anterior proximal sciatic nerve block to be performed.

▶ **Catheter.** A catheter for continuous anesthesia or analgesia can be placed (Meier 1999a) because the sciatic nerve is surrounded by a fascial sheath from its emergence from the infrapiriform foramen until it enters the popliteal fossa (Clara 1959, Benninghoff and Goerttler 1975). Advancing the catheter more than 4 to

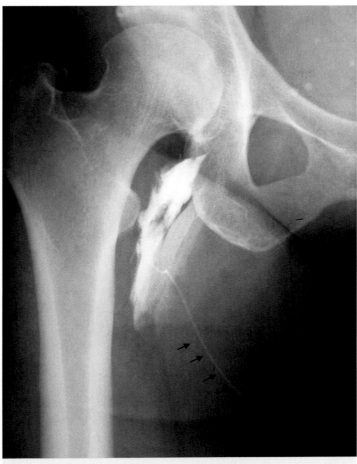

**Fig. 11.25** Spread of the local anesthetic after anterior sciatic nerve block (contrast was added to the local anesthetic).
→ Catheter

5 cm can lead to deviation of the catheter into the true pelvis (lesser pelvis) and should be avoided (see ▶ Fig. 11.24).

In a study by Meier (1999b) of 85 patients, the catheter was kept in situ for an average of 4 days (up to a maximum of 8 days). No infections were observed at the puncture site. No side effects, complications, or neurological deficits were found.

▶ **Continuous anterior sciatic nerve block.** Pain therapy through a continuous anterior sciatic nerve block can be provided with 6 mL/h of ropivacaine 0.33% (3.3 mg/mL) or bolus injections of 20 mL of ropivacaine 0.2 to 0.375% (2–3.75 mg/mL) every 6 to 8 hours (Meier 2001). The maximum dose of ropivacaine should not exceed 37.5 mg/h. Büttner and Meier (1999) reviewed continuous pain therapy with ropivacaine in clinical practice, which was performed without complications in over 6,000 peripheral catheters.

## Summary

The anterior technique allows block of the sciatic nerve with the patient in supine position. No change of position is required. The anesthesia can therefore also be performed, for example, in the presence of vertebral fractures, fractures of the pelvis or long bones, and also in the case of obesity, chronic polyarthritis, and other positioning problems. If a femoral nerve block is performed before the anterior sciatic nerve block and periosteal contact is

avoided, the technique can be performed with little pain. The modified technique according to Meier enables anesthesia that includes the posterior cutaneous nerve of the thigh. A catheter can be placed readily without the potential risks seen with transgluteal or parasacral sciatic nerve block (Chapter 11.5 and Chapter 11.6). As a continuous technique, the procedure can be used for postoperative pain therapy after major surgery on the knee, lower leg, and foot, and for the treatment of pain syndromes distal to the knee and for regional sympathetic block.

## 11.2.5 Anterior Proximal Sciatic Nerve Block Using Ultrasound

Curved array: 5 to 2 MHz, linear multifrequency broadband transducer with phased-array technique
Penetration depth: 10 to 20 cm
Needle: 8 to 15 cm

### Ultrasound Orientation

The sciatic nerve is visualized on the anterior proximal technique in supine position at the inside of the thigh 8 to 10 cm distal to the inguinal fold at the level of the lesser trochanter or slightly distal to it. The leg is abducted and rotated externally.

The following structures are sought:
- The femur as a convex hyperechoic line with an acoustic shadow behind it
- The femoral vessels (femoral artery and deep femoral artery)

Medial to and below the femoral arteries is the adductor muscle group, the largest muscle of which is the adductor magnus. The adductors originate at the femur. The sciatic nerve is in the layer between the adductor magnus and the gluteus maximus (▶ Fig. 11.26). The sciatic nerve is hyperechoic here and has a round to oval shape (1.66 ± 0.68 cm maximum diameter) and can be visualized at a depth of 6.21 ± 0.68 cm below the surface of the skin (Chan et al 2006).

### Needle Insertion

The approach can be out of plane (▶ Fig. 11.27) or in plane (▶ Fig. 11.28). ▶

▶ **Out-of-plane approach.** In an out-of-plane approach the nerve is set in the center of the acoustic field and the needle is inserted about 1 cm distal to the transducer at the smallest possible angle (steep) to the transducer (▶ Fig. 11.27). The tip of the needle should be lateral or medial to the nerve.

▶ **In-plane approach.** The in-plane approach can be made from lateral to medial (▶ Fig. 11.28) or from medial to lateral in the acoustic window.

▶ **Volume.** Approximately 20 mL local anesthetic.

### Catheter Placement

A catheter can be placed; the out-of-plane technique is preferable because the catheter can be advanced more easily.

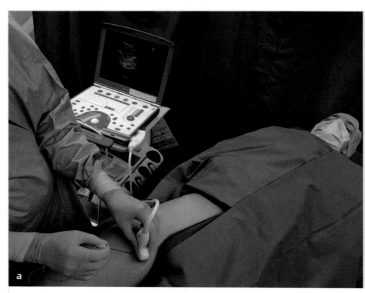

**Fig. 11.26** Anatomical cross-section of the proximal third of the thigh in the region of the anterior puncture of the sciatic nerve under ultrasound guidance. Enlargement, see ▶ Fig. 11.27.
**a** Clinical setting.
**b** Anatomical cross-section.
**c** Anatomical cross-section (labeled).
1 Vastus medialis muscle
2 Sartorius muscle
3 Femoral and deep femoral arteries
4 Gracilis muscle
5 Adductor longus muscle
6 Adductor magnus muscle
7 Semimembranosus muscle
8 Semitendinosus muscle
9 Biceps femoris muscle
10 Gluteus maximus muscle
11 Sciatic nerve
12 Femur

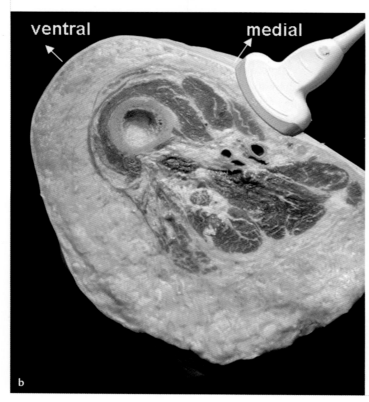

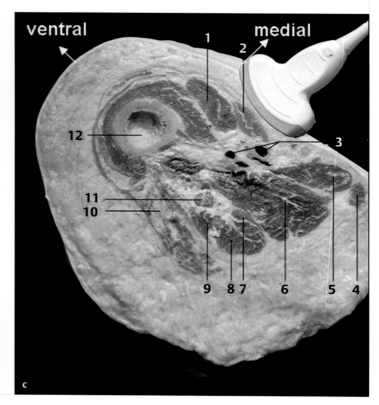

## Tips and Tricks

- Due to the depth, the sciatic nerve is often difficult to visualize. The nerve lies in the space between the adductor magnus and gluteus maximus.
- A second hyperechoic structure that can be easily mistaken for the sciatic nerve is a tendinous structure of the adductor magnus (▶ Fig. 11.27).
- The structure assumed to be the sciatic nerve must be preserved when the transducer is advanced cranially and caudally to be certain that it is the nerve.
- A click is occasionally felt when the back of the adductor magnus is penetrated (Tsui and Özelsel 2008).
- The ultrasound-guided anterior block has the same success rate as posterior techniques, but requires less time in total, as the patient does not have to be repositioned (Ota et al 2009). The anterior technique is preferable, especially in combination with a femoral nerve block.
- Tsui and Özelsel (2008) recommend visualizing the sciatic nerve in the long axis (▶ Fig. 11.29). After visualizing the sciatic nerve with the probe in the gap between the sartorius and the rectus femoris in the short axis, the transducer is rotated 90° to the long axis without losing sight of the target structure. The sciatic nerve now appears as a cablelike structure (▶ Fig. 11.29 and ▶ Fig. 11.30). This technique ensures that the nerve has been correctly identified in the short axis. The puncture can be made in plane when the nerve is visualized in the long axis.
- A linear transducer can also be used for slim patients (▶ Fig. 11.30).

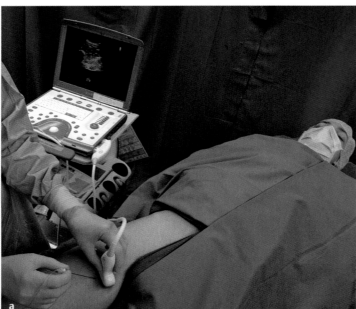

**Fig. 11.27** Anatomical cross-section of the anterior sciatic nerve block with corresponding ultrasound image (enlargement of ▶ Fig. 11.26).
**a** Clinical setting (out-of-plane technique).
**b** Anatomical section (unlabeled).
**c** Anatomical section (labeled).
**d** Ultrasound image corresponding to b.
**e** Ultrasound image corresponding to c.
1 Vastus medialis muscle
2 Sartorius muscle
3 Femoral/deep femoral arteries
5 Adductor longus muscle
6 Adductor magnus muscle
7 Semimembranosus muscle
8 Semitendinosus muscle
9 Biceps femoris muscle
10 Gluteus maximus muscle
11 Sciatic nerve
12 Femur
* Tendon of the adductor magnus

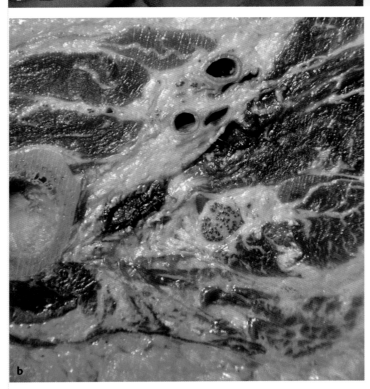

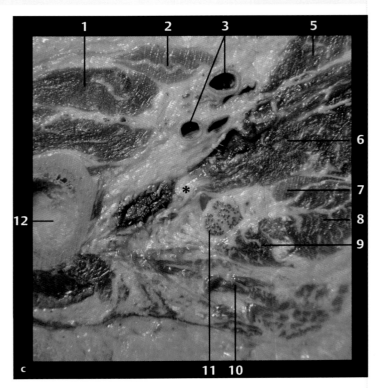

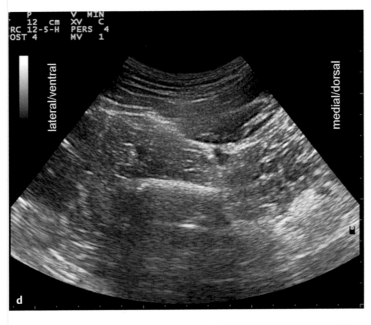

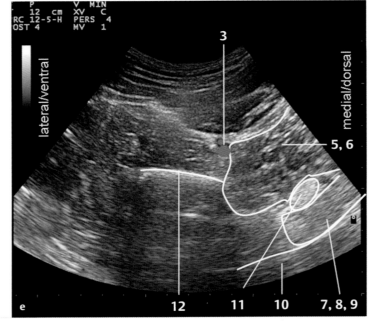

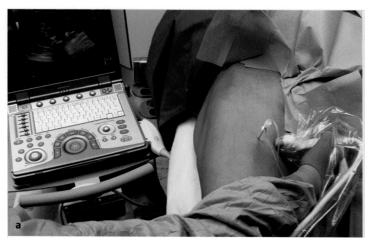

**Fig. 11.28** Anterior sciatic nerve block with the in-plane technique (visualization in the short axis).
**a** Clinical setting.
**b** Ultrasound image (unlabeled).
**c** Ultrasound image (labeled).
1 Femoral/deep femoral arteries
2 Adductor muscles
3 Sciatic nerve
4 Femur

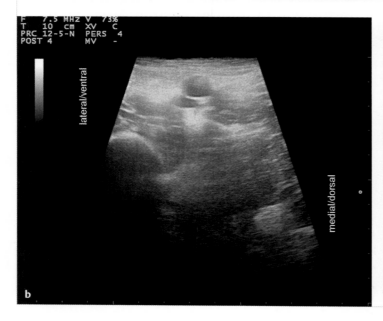

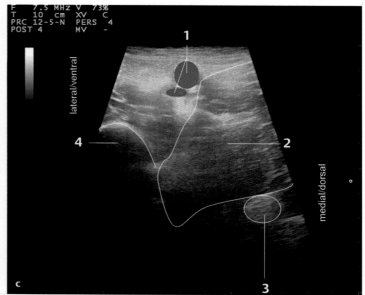

## 11.3 Posterior Proximal Sciatic Nerve Block (in Supine Position) ▶

### 11.3.1 Technique

The subgluteal technique was first implemented in 1975 as a single-shot technique (Raj et al 1975), but it can also be easily performed as a continuous technique.

The sciatic nerve leaves the pelvis through the greater sciatic foramen and passes to the thigh between the greater trochanter and the ischial tuberosity. When the limb is flexed at the hip, the sciatic nerve is stretched and passes relatively superficially under the gluteus maximus muscle through the groove between the greater trochanter and ischial tuberosity (▶ Fig. 11.31 and ▶ Fig. 11.32).

### Landmarks

The anatomical landmarks of the greater trochanter and ischial tuberosity are joined by a line. The middle of this line is the needle insertion site.

### Position

The patient lies supine. The limb to be blocked is flexed maximally at the hip (90–120°) and 90° at the knee. The sciatic nerve runs extended and relatively superficially under the gluteus maximus through the "trough" between the greater trochanter and ischial tuberosity (▶ Fig. 11.31 and ▶ Fig. 11.32).

### Needle Approach

A needle 10 to 15 cm long is connected to a nerve stimulator and advanced proximally vertical to the skin. The vicinity of the sciatic nerve is reached after 5 to 10 cm. When there is a motor response in the foot (plantar flexion or dorsiflexion), 30 mL of a medium-acting or long-acting local anesthetic is injected.

▶ **Continuous technique.** The catheter is advanced 4 to 5 cm proximally following the injection (▶ Fig. 11.33).

### 11.3.2 Indications and Contraindications

See also anterior technique.

### 11.3.3 Side Effects and Complications

There are no known special side effects or complications.

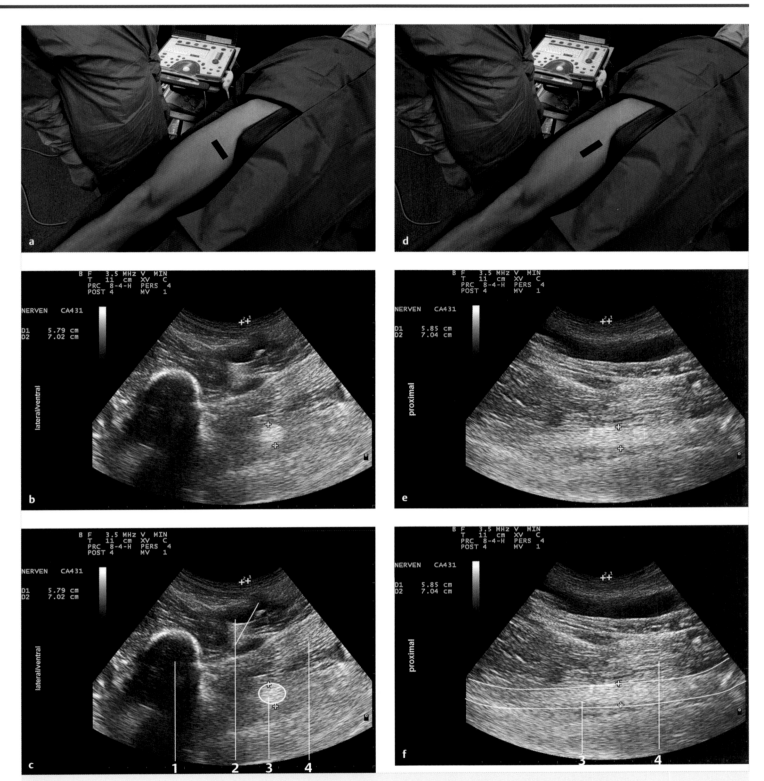

**Fig. 11.29** Visualization of the proximal sciatic nerve in the short (**a–c**) and long (**d–f**) axis with a curved-array transducer.

1 Femur
2 Femoral artery and deep femoral artery
3 Sciatic nerve
4 Adductor magnus muscle

The black bar indicates the position of the transducer.
Note the depths measured that indicate an identical depth of the identified structure in the short and long axis.

**a** Position of the transducer in the short axis.
**b** Ultrasound image of the sciatic nerve in the short axis (unlabeled).
**c** Ultrasound image of the sciatic nerve in the short axis (labeled).
**d** Position of the transducer in the long axis.
**e** Ultrasound image of the sciatic nerve in the long axis (unlabeled).
**f** Ultrasound image of the sciatic nerve in the long axis (labeled).

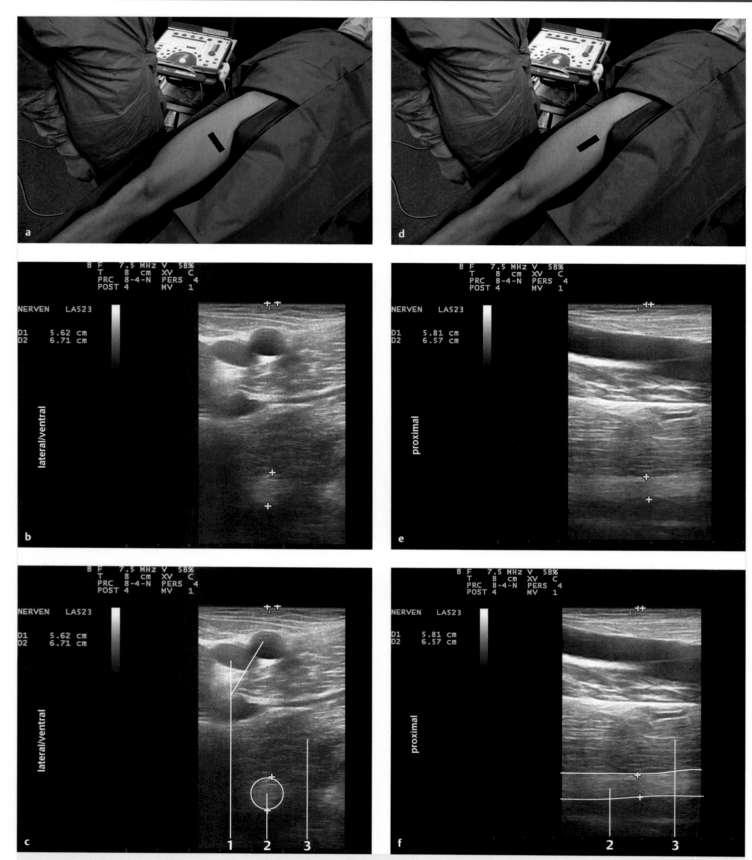

**Fig. 11.30** Visualization of the proximal sciatic nerve in the short (**a–c**) and long (**d–f**) axis with a linear transducer.
**a** Position of the transducer in the short axis.
**b** Ultrasound image of the sciatic nerve in the short axis (unlabeled).
**c** Ultrasound image of the sciatic nerve in the short axis (labeled).
1 Femoral artery and deep femoral artery
2 Sciatic nerve
3 Adductor magnus muscle

Note the depths measured that indicate an identical depth of the identified structure in the short and long axis.
**d** Position of the transducer in the long axis.
**e** Ultrasound image of the sciatic nerve in the long axis (unlabeled).
**f** Ultrasound image of the sciatic nerve in the long axis (labeled).

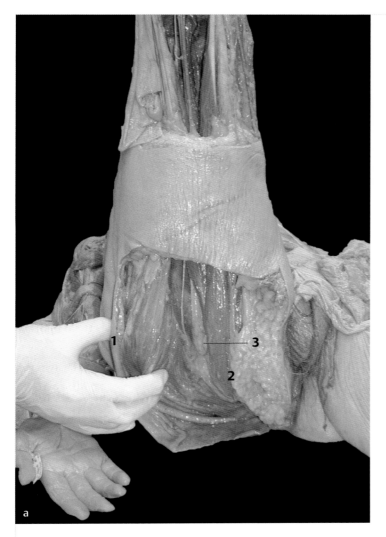

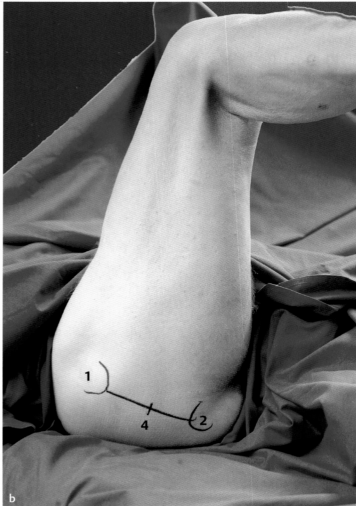

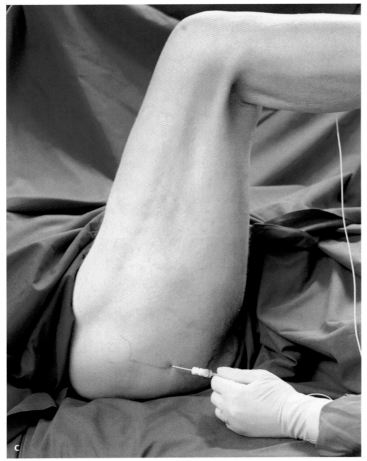

**Fig. 11.31** Subgluteal sciatic nerve block, Raj technique. The nerve runs midway between the greater trochanter and ischial tuberosity. The patient lies supine, the leg is flexed at a right angle at the hip and knee.
**a** Anatomy.
**b** Model.
**c** After puncture.
1 Greater trochanter
2 Ischial tuberosity
3 Sciatic nerve
4 Needle insertion site

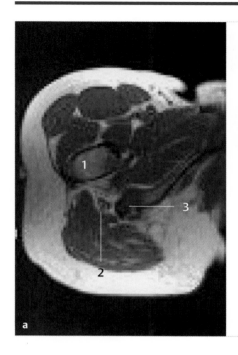

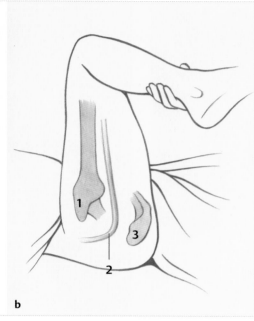

**Fig. 11.32** Subgluteal (proximal) sciatic nerve block, Raj technique. The line connecting the greater trochanter and ischial tuberosity is halved. The midpoint marks the puncture site. The needle is advanced in cranial direction vertical to the skin surface. After about 5 (max. 10) cm, the correct needle position is indicated by a response in the foot.
1 Greater trochanter
2 Sciatic nerve
3 Ischial tuberosity

---

**Tips and Tricks**

- The leg to be anesthetized can be placed in a stirrup (lithotomy position, ▶ Fig. 11.33; Meier and Büttner 2001).
- The technique is a good alternative to the anterior technique (Meier and Heinrich 1995). If the anterior technique proves problematic, it can be performed with the patient in supine position.
- The technique is well suited for placing a catheter.
- The technique can be performed under ultrasound guidance with minor modifications (Chapter 11.3.5). The position of the catheter can also be checked by ultrasound (▶ Fig. 11.34).

## 11.3.4 Remarks on the Technique

The advantage of this technique is the shorter distance to the sciatic nerve. The disadvantage is the necessity of changing the position of the leg to be blocked, as the leg has to be held and the change in position can cause pain, for example, in the case of fractures. Provided the patient is not troubled by pain, the leg to be anesthetized can be elevated in a stirrup. Studies of a large enough number of cases to allow a scientific evaluation of the technique are lacking.

For anesthesia, 30 mL of prilocaine 1% (10 mg/mL) or mepivacaine 1% (10 mg/mL) or a combination of a medium-acting with a long-acting local anesthetic; for example, 20 mL of mepivacaine 1% (10 mg/mL) with 10 mL ropivacaine 0.75% (7.5 mg/mL). An onset of 15 to 30 minutes from the time of injection must be allowed before the operation can commence (Meier and Heinrich 1995).

Experience shows that a catheter can be placed readily and without problems because of the direction of the needle (Meier and Büttner 2001). If a continuous technique is planned, the catheter should be advanced 4 to 5 cm proximally through the stimulation needle after injection of the local anesthetic. (Comment: the catheter is also very well tolerated subsequently by the patient when sitting.)

## Summary

Subgluteal sciatic nerve block is an easily performed technique with few complications. Its advantage is the relatively short distance to the sciatic nerve. The method is suitable as an alternative to anterior block, provided the leg to be anesthetized can be adequately positioned without pain.

## 11.3.5 Posterior Proximal Sciatic Nerve Block (in Supine Position) with Ultrasound

Curved array: 5 to 2 MHz, linear transducer 7.5 MHz
Penetration depth: 5 to 15 cm
Needle: 7 to 12 cm

### Scanning Technique

The patient lies supine, the leg is positioned in a stirrup or positioning device so that it is possible to follow the sciatic nerve from the popliteal to the infragluteal region. The sciatic nerve lies in the infragluteal region on the biceps femoris or crosses it from medial to lateral. The skin–nerve distance in the infragluteal region, which is 3 to 4 cm here, becomes shorter further distally, and in the middle of the thigh again reaches an average skin–nerve distance of 3.4 cm (Bruhn et al 2008, Moayeri et al 2010). A connecting line from the ischial tuberosity to the head of the fibula divides the gluteal fold just where the sciatic nerve runs. The sciatic nerve is visualized in this region as a flat to slightly oval hyperechoic structure; further distally it becomes rounder.

With the exception of positioning depending on the puncture site, this ultrasound-guided block technique is equivalent to the ultrasound-guided infragluteal or proximal block in lateral position (see Chapter 11.5).

### Needle Approach

The needle can be inserted out of plane (▶ Fig. 11.35) or in plane (▶ Fig. 11.36 ▶).

▶ **Volume.** Approximately 20 mL local anesthetic.

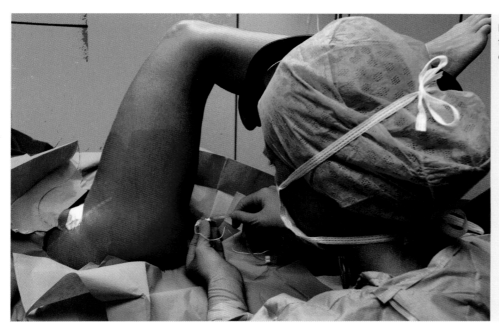

**Fig. 11.33** Subgluteal sciatic nerve block, Raj technique. A catheter can be advanced without difficulty.

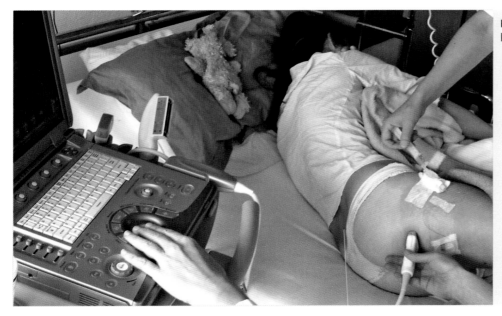

**Fig. 11.34** Check of the position of the indwelling sciatic nerve catheter (see Chapter 1).

## Catheter Placement

A catheter can be placed in both the in-plane and the out-of-plane techniques.

# 11.4 Proximal Lateral Sciatic Nerve Block (with Patient in Supine Position) ▶

## 11.4.1 Technique

### Landmarks

Greater trochanter, ischial tuberosity.

### Position

The patient lies supine with the leg to be anesthetized in neutral position. A small pad is placed under the popliteal fossa so that the greater trochanter is moved slightly forward.

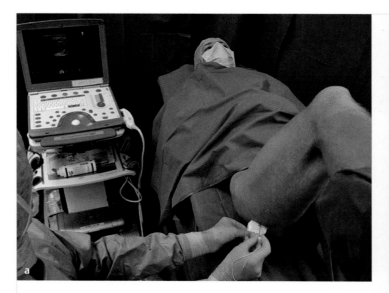

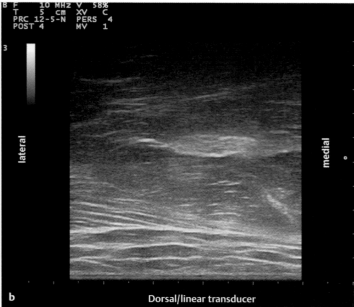

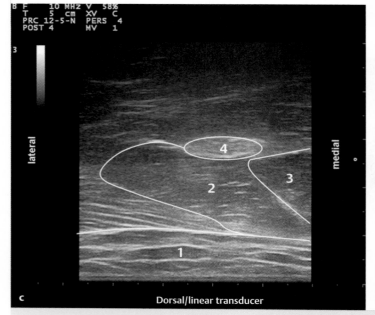

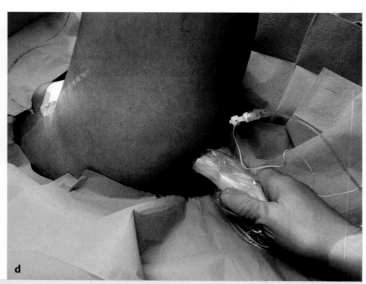

**Fig. 11.35** Subgluteal (proximal) puncture of the sciatic nerve in supine position (ultrasound image "upside down," skin level is at the bottom of the ultrasound image!). Note the hyperechoic structure between the biceps femoris and semitendinosus muscles (see text).

a Clinical setting.

b Ultrasound image (unlabeled).

c Ultrasound image (labeled).

d Clinical setting.

1 Subcutaneous fat tissue

2 Biceps femoris muscle

3 Semitendinosus muscle

4 Sciatic nerve

## Procedure

The needle insertion site for the lateral approach to proximal sciatic nerve block is 3 to 5 cm distal to the most prominent lateral part of the greater trochanter. The skin is entered at the level of the posterior border of the femur and the needle is directed dorsally (15–30°) and cranially; the response must be in the foot, as in anterior sciatic nerve block (▶ Fig. 11.37, ▶ Fig. 11.38, ▶ Fig. 11.39). Muscular contractions on the back of the thigh are frequent (Gligorijevic 2000). The sciatic nerve is reached after 8 to 12 cm (▶ Fig. 11.40) and the correct position of the needle tip in the vicinity of the nerve is confirmed by a motor response in the foot region (dorsiflexion or plantar flexion). After careful aspiration, 20 to 30 mL of a medium-acting or long-acting local anesthetic is injected.

## 11.4.2 Indications, Contraindications, Complications, Side Effects

(See under anterior sciatic nerve block.)

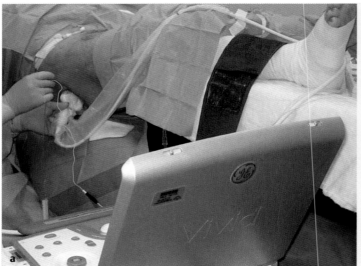

**Fig. 11.36** Subgluteal (proximal) puncture of the sciatic nerve in supine position: in-plane technique. (Ultrasound image "upside down," skin level at the bottom of the ultrasound image!). Obese patient, curved array 5 to 2 MHz.
**a** Clinical setting.
**b** Ultrasound image before injection of local anesthetic (unlabeled).
**c** Ultrasound image before injection of local anesthetic (labeled).
**d** Ultrasound image after injection of local anesthetic (unlabeled).
**e** Ultrasound image after injection of local anesthetic (labeled).
1 Sciatic nerve
2 Border with local anesthetic around the nerve
Arrows: needle

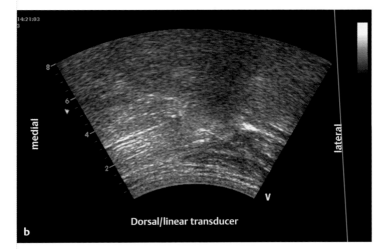

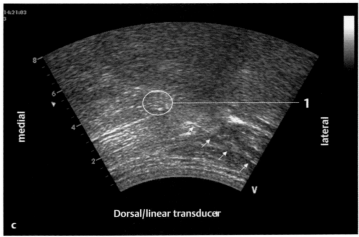

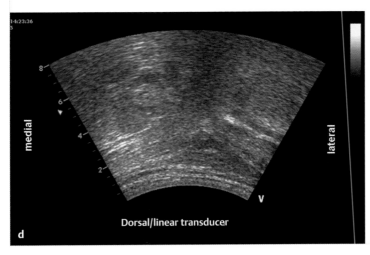

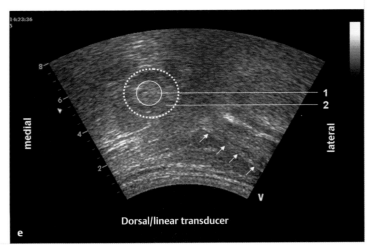

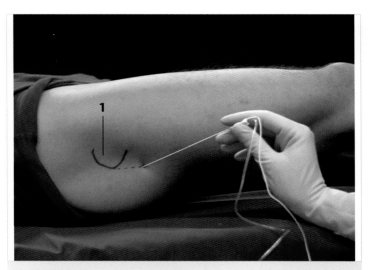

Fig. 11.37 The insertion site for the lateral approach to the proximal sciatic nerve block is 3 to 5 cm distal to the most prominent lateral part of the greater trochanter. The needle enters at the level of the posterior border of the femur and is directed dorsally (15–30°) and cranially; as in anterior sciatic nerve block, the stimulation response must be in the foot.
1 Greater trochanter

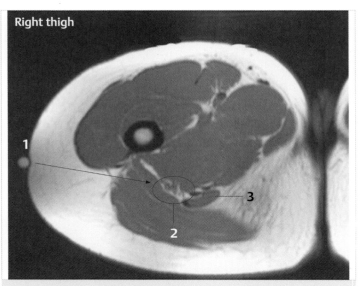

Right thigh

Fig. 11.38 Lateral approach to the proximal sciatic nerve: note the somewhat dorsal needle direction in the MR image, which is necessary for contacting the sciatic nerve.
1 Nitro capsule marking the insertion site
2 Sciatic nerve
3 Ischial tuberosity

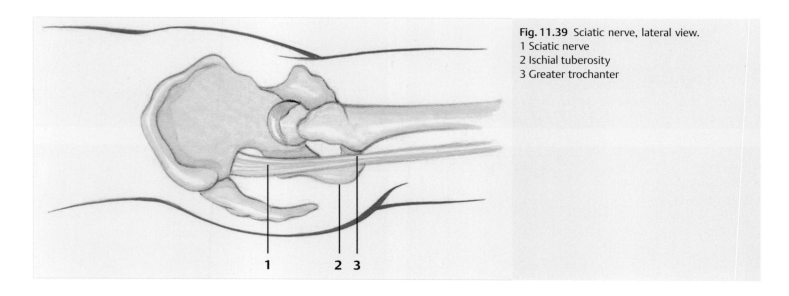

Fig. 11.39 Sciatic nerve, lateral view.
1 Sciatic nerve
2 Ischial tuberosity
3 Greater trochanter

### Tips and Tricks

- The patient should be positioned as close to the edge of the positioning table as possible. This makes the procedure easier to perform and facilitates maintaining sterile conditions.
- If no motor response is produced, the needle should be withdrawn and corrected in the anterior direction when it is advanced again.
- The common fibular nerve is stimulated first with the described needle direction. The motor response with this technique is therefore usually dorsiflexion of the foot initially.

## 11.4.3 Remarks on the Technique

Guardini reported a success rate of 95% for lateral sciatic nerve block (Guardini et al 1985). The method can be performed without changing the patient's position. The procedure is unsuitable for patients with fractures of the neck of the femur, hematoma in this region, or previous total hip replacement on the side to be anesthetized (anatomical orientation may be impaired). At the level at which the sciatic nerve is reached, the nerve runs together with the inferior gluteal artery behind the quadratus femoris. The artery is medial to the sciatic nerve. The posterior cutaneous nerve of the thigh, which usually separates from the sciatic nerve further medially and superficially, is sometimes not blocked sufficiently and pain can then occur on the back of the thigh during operation with a thigh tourniquet.

## Summary

Lateral proximal sciatic nerve block in combination with lumbar plexus anesthesia is suitable for operations on the knee and lower leg. Anatomical orientation can present problems when the thigh is of large circumference.

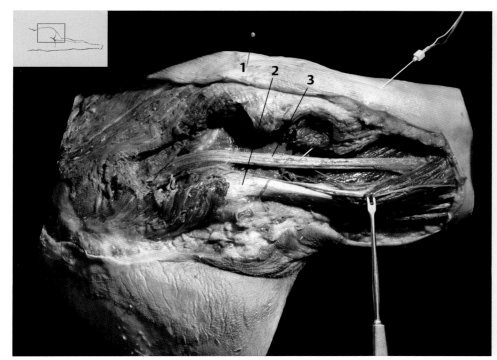

**Fig. 11.40** Lateral sciatic nerve block.
1 Greater trochanter
2 Ischiocrural group
3 Sciatic nerve

## 11.5 Proximal Sciatic Nerve Block (with Patient Lying on Side) ▶

The posterior transgluteal technique of sciatic nerve block was first described in 1924 by Labat. The most important supplement to the method was the addition of another landmark by Winnie (Winnie 1975; ▶ Fig. 11.42).

The gluteal region is a triangle, the apex of which is formed by the posterior superior iliac spine, the medial corner by the ischial tuberosity, and the lateral corner by the greater trochanter (▶ Fig. 11.41). The two sides and the base of the triangle form three orientation lines:

• Spine–tuberosity line
• Spine–trochanter line
• Tuberosity–trochanter line

These lines are the basis of anatomical orientation in all proximal posterior techniques of sciatic nerve block.

### 11.5.1 Techniques of Posterior Transgluteal Sciatic Nerve Block

#### Posterior Transgluteal Sciatic Nerve Block according to Labat (Classical Technique)

The posterior Labat technique is called the standard technique and is performed with the patient lying on his or her side. The procedure can be combined particularly well with a psoas block as the patient's position does not have to be changed.

### Landmarks

Posterior superior iliac spine, greater trochanter.

### Position

The patient lies on his or her side with the side to be blocked uppermost. The leg underneath can be extended, and the leg to be blocked is flexed about 30 to 40° at the hip and about 70° at the knee. The posterior superior iliac spine and greater trochanter are sought as anatomical landmarks, marked, and joined by a line (▶ Fig. 11.42).

### Procedure

The midpoint of the line connecting the spine and the trochanter is marked; a line is then drawn caudally from the midpoint at a right angle and the puncture site is marked after 4 (max. 5) cm (▶ Fig. 11.42). As an additional aid to orientation, a line can be drawn joining the greater trochanter and the sacral hiatus (Winnie 1975). This line generally intersects the previously drawn perpendicular to the spine–trochanter line at the established puncture site (▶ Fig. 11.42).

The needle is advanced vertically to the skin surface (▶ Fig. 11.43 and ▶ Fig. 11.44). An immobile needle technique enables aspiration (▶ Fig. 11.45). On bone contact, the skin–bone distance is recorded and the needle is then withdrawn sufficiently to allow correction of its position when it is advanced again. The needle should not be advanced further than the measured skin–bone distance so as to exclude puncture of the lesser pelvis.

The needle direction is corrected in a fan pattern along the Labat line until a distal motor response is visible in the sciatic nerve area (tibial nerve, common fibular nerve). The nerve is reached after 7.5 to 15 cm (Chelly and Delaunay 1999). Then 30 to 40 mL of a medium-acting or long-acting local anesthetic of adequate concentration is injected.

A continuous technique can also be performed from the same insertion site with modification of the needle direction. In this case, the direction of the needle is not perpendicular to the skin but is directed toward the middle third between the ischial tuberosity and the greater trochanter where the sciatic nerve passes from the gluteal region to the back of the thigh (▶ Fig. 11.46, ▶ Fig. 11.47, ▶ Fig. 11.48). The nerve is reached after about 8 to 12 cm at an angle of around 45° to the skin.

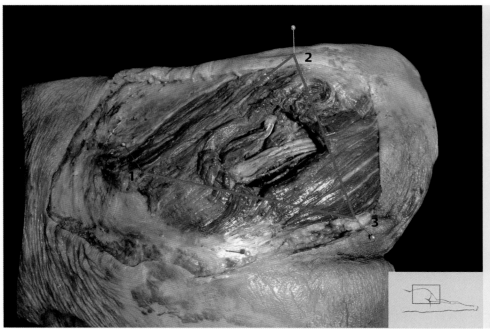

**Fig. 11.41** Right leg, posterior view.
1 Posterior superior iliac spine
2 Greater trochanter
3 Ischial tuberosity

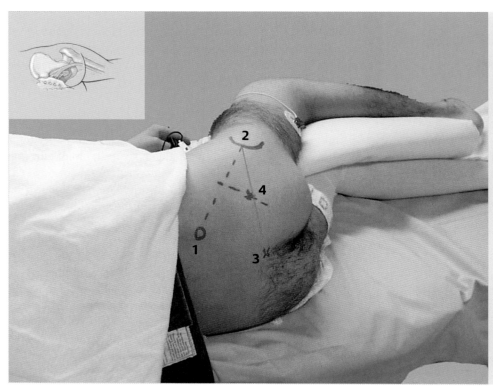

**Fig. 11.42** Posterior sciatic nerve block, Labat technique. The injection site is 4 to 5 cm caudal to the perpendicular through the midpoint of the line between the posterior superior iliac spine and the greater trochanter. A connecting line between the sacral hiatus and the greater trochanter intersects this perpendicular at the injection site. The leg to be blocked is positioned so that the shaft of the femur lies in the continuation of the tuberosity trochanter line.
1 Posterior superior iliac spine
2 Greater trochanter
3 Sacral hiatus
4 Injection site

## Posterior (Transgluteal) Continuous Sciatic Nerve Block

### Landmarks

Posterior superior iliac spine, greater trochanter, ischial tuberosity.

The landmarks are established by the spine–tuberosity line and the tuberosity–trochanter line (Rongstad et al 1996, Polino et al 2000). The spine–tuberosity line is the line from the posterior superior iliac spine to the ischial tuberosity. The infrapiriform foramen is in the middle of this line. The midpoint of the spine–tuberosity line marks the insertion site. The tuberosity–trochanter line is the line from the ischial tuberosity to the greater trochanter and divided into three parts. The sciatic nerve runs between the inner and middle thirds (▶ Fig. 11.49, ▶ Fig. 11.50, ▶ Fig. 11.51).

### Position

The patient lies on his or her side with the side to be blocked uppermost. The leg underneath is extended, and the leg to be blocked is flexed about 30 to 40° at the hip and about 70° at the knee.

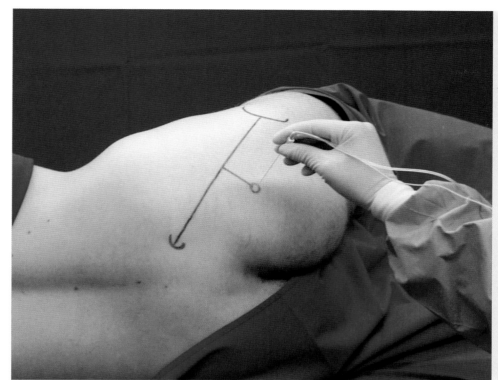

**Fig. 11.43** Posterior sciatic nerve block, Labat technique. The puncture is made perpendicular to the skin surface. The nerve is reached after 7.5 to 12 cm. The stimulation response should be in the foot, but with this approach a response in the ischiocrural muscles (thigh flexors or "hamstring muscles") can also be regarded as adequate. A response in the gluteal muscles, which is often produced when the needle is advanced, is not adequate: the needle must be advanced further.

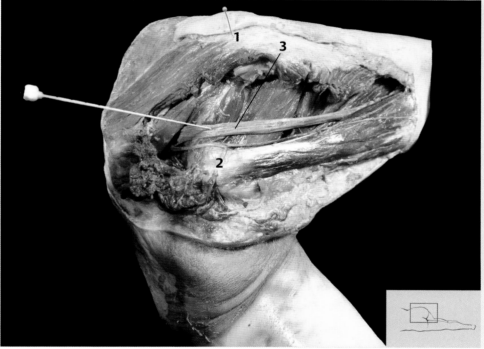

**Fig. 11.44** Posterior sciatic nerve block, Labat technique. The needle is inserted perpendicular to the skin surface.
1 Greater trochanter
2 Ischial tuberosity
3 Sciatic nerve

## Procedure

A needle is advanced at an angle of around 45° to the skin in the direction of the junction of the inner and middle thirds of the tuberosity–trochanter line. It reaches the sciatic nerve after 10 to 12 cm. If the direction of the needle has to be corrected, this should be done medially. A response in the foot indicates that the tip of the needle is in the correct position; 20 to 30 mL of a medium-acting or long-acting local anesthetic is injected. The tangential approach of the needle to the sciatic nerve enables placement of a catheter (▶ Fig. 11.52). The catheter is advanced 3 to 5 cm caudally beyond the needle tip.

## 11.5.2 Indications and Contraindications

### Indications for a Proximal Posterior Sciatic Nerve Block

(in combination with a psoas block)
- Operations on the knee, lower leg, or foot (including tourniquet at the thigh during, e.g., total knee replacement, tibial head osteotomy, arthrodesis, lateral ligament suture, forefoot operations)
- Repositioning of fractures of the lower leg and foot
- Amputation in the thigh, lower leg, and foot

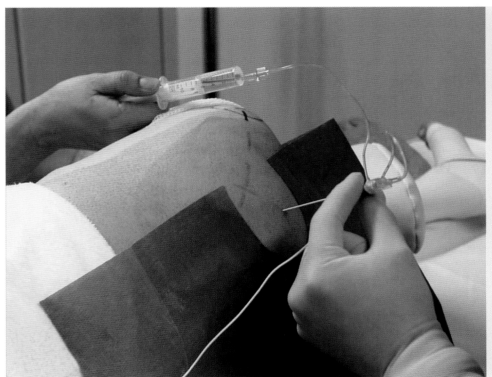

**Fig. 11.45** Posterior sciatic nerve block, Labat technique. The needle is inserted perpendicular to the skin surface. The nerve is reached after 7.5 to 12 cm. Aspiration must be performed at regular intervals during injection of the local anesthetic to exclude intravascular injection.

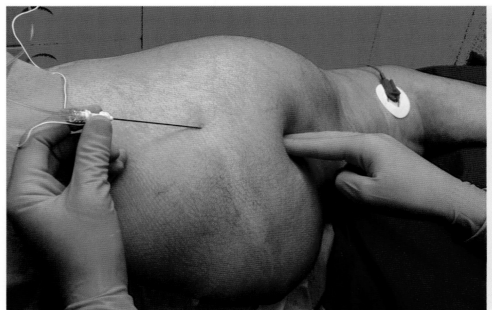

**Fig. 11.46** Needle direction for continuous posterior sciatic nerve block.

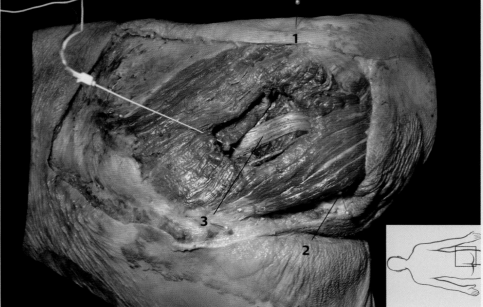

**Fig. 11.47** Continuous posterior sciatic nerve block.
1 Greater trochanter
2 Ischial tuberosity
3 Sciatic nerve

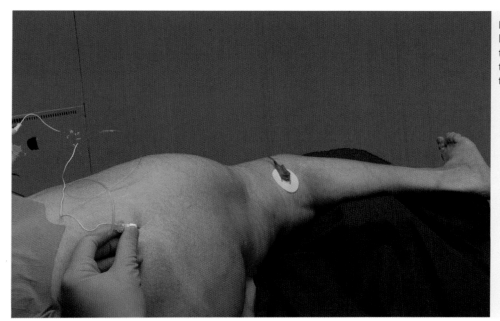

**Fig. 11.48** Continuous posterior sciatic nerve block. The tip of the needle should be directed to follow the course of the sciatic nerve toward the middle third of the line between the ischial tuberosity and greater trochanter.

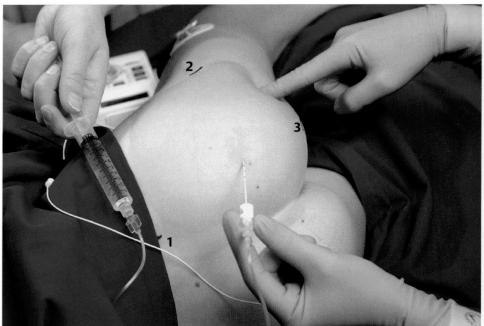

**Fig. 11.49** Posterior continuous technique to block the sciatic nerve (as modified by Meier, Bauereis): The insertion site is the middle of the spine-tuberosity line; the needle should be directed to follow the course of the sciatic nerve, i.e., toward the middle of the line between the ischial tuberosity and the greater trochanter. In this way, a tangential approach to the nerve is achieved, which enables the catheter to be advanced easily.
1 Posterior superior iliac spine
2 Greater trochanter
3 Ischial tuberosity

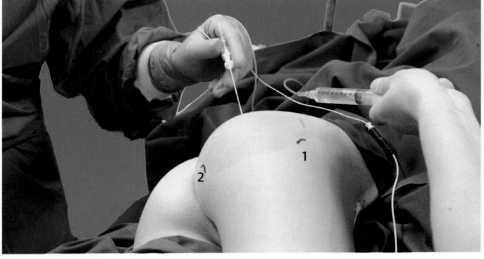

**Fig. 11.50** As in ▶ Fig. 11.49, posteroinferior view.
1 Greater trochanter
2 Ischial tuberosity

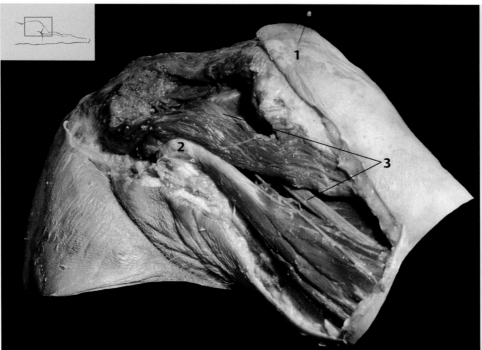

**Fig. 11.51** Posterior continuous technique to block the sciatic nerve.
1 Greater trochanter
2 Ischial tuberosity
3 Sciatic nerve

- Regional sympathetic block (perfusion disorders, wound healing disorders, CRPS 1)
- Pain therapy (e.g., postoperative, achillodynia, oligoarthritis)
- Traumatology (e.g., pain-free positioning for diagnostic investigations)

## Contraindications

- General contraindications (see Chapter 20.2)
- Coagulation disorders

## 11.5.3 Complications and Side Effects

Very little has been reported regarding complications or side effects. Major complications and late sequelae are regarded as very rare.

### Tips and Tricks

- Combination with a psoas block enables sufficient anesthesia of the entire leg.
- As the posterior cutaneous nerve of the thigh is usually also anesthetized, the technique ensures that a thigh tourniquet will be well tolerated.
- The method should be performed with a nerve stimulator. In contrast to sciatic nerve blocks performed with the patient supine, a response in the ischiocrural muscles is here also regarded as adequate.
- This block can be performed under ultrasound guidance, but is limited by the distance to the nerve. The position of the catheter can also be checked using ultrasound.
- A motor response of the gluteus maximus muscle must not be misinterpretd as the right answer to the nerve stimulation. The adequate motor response is in the lower leg and foot region.
- Large vessels can be punctured, but this can be avoided by the use of a Doppler probe or ultrasound.
- To establish the onset of the block, the rise in plantar temperature can be measured with a surface thermometer.

## 11.5.4 Remarks on the Technique

The transgluteal technique of sciatic nerve block ensures good to very good quality of anesthesia. Practically the whole sacral plexus can be blocked. However, complete sacral plexus anesthesia also means that the inferior gluteal nerve and pudendal nerve are anesthetized (Wagner 1994, Mansour and Bennetts 1996). This leads to hypoesthesia in the perineal region and possibly also to urinary retention. Impairment of bladder function should therefore be watched for.

### Caution

With the Labat technique, misplacement of the needle into the lesser pelvis is a possibility. Blood vessels can also be accidentally punctured, particularly the inferior gluteal artery (Wagner 1994, Meier 2001; ▶ Fig. 11.53).

The inferior gluteal artery, the largest artery from the internal iliac artery, runs 1 to 2 cm medial to the line from the puncture site using the proximal technique in the lateral position (▶ Fig. 11.54). The length of the perpendicular line showing the puncture site should therefore not exceed 4 cm.

### Note

The block should always be performed with peripheral nerve stimulation and/or ultrasound.

The motor response to nerve stimulation must be in the lower leg and foot. Whether the stimulated muscle group (tibial nerve or common fibular nerve) has an influence on the result of the block is controversial. In contrast to sciatic nerve blocks performed in supine position, a response of the ischiocrural muscles is here regarded as adequate.

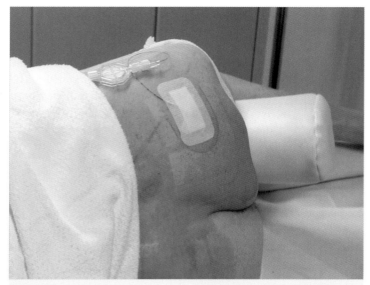

Fig. 11.52 Indwelling catheter in situ in a posterior sciatic nerve block.

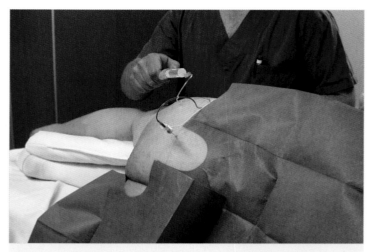

Fig. 11.53 With the Labat technique, puncture too far medially should be avoided, as the blood vessels are found here. A distance of 4 to 5 cm from the spine–trochanter line should not be exceeded. Bloody aspiration ensues after vascular puncture.

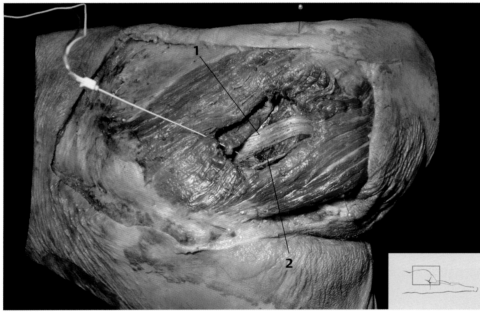

Fig. 11.54 Using the Labat technique, needle puncture too far medially should be avoided as blood vessels pass here.
1 Sciatic nerve
2 Inferior gluteal vessels

Sciatic nerve block as a selective anesthesia for surgery is indicated in just a few situations (e.g., foot surgery). When using a thigh tourniquet, it must be combined with a lumbar plexus block. In this case, a combination of the psoas block and the posterior technique is most rational, as the patient's position does not have to be changed. If an operation is performed with a calf tourniquet, a saphenous nerve block provides adequate supplementary anesthesia.

When two block techniques are combined (lumbar plexus and sacral plexus), 60 mL of a local anesthetic of adequate concentration is usually necessary (▶ Fig. 11.55 and ▶ Fig. 11.56).

▶ **Disadvantage of the Labat technique.** A disadvantage of the Labat technique is the direction of the stimulation needle vertical to the course of the nerve, which means that a catheter often cannot be advanced or can be advanced only with difficulty.

▶ **Catheter placement.** For smoother catheter placement, the needle direction must be changed. The recommended procedure

is to determine the direction using the spine–tuberosity line and the tuberosity–trochanter line. This is a technique that is easy to follow in clinical practice and has been performed many times (Meier 1999b). The needle should be directed to the middle third between the ischial tuberosity and the greater trochanter. Unlike the continuous parasacral technique of sciatic nerve block (see Chapter 11.6), there is no danger of perforating vessels and organs of the lesser pelvis.

### Practical note

Catheter placement is always useful when pain lasting longer than 24 hours can be anticipated or if long-term sympathetic block is desired. This applies, for example, to total knee replacement.

Particularly if there has been a flexion contracture previously, this operation can be associated with very severe postoperative pain in the posterior region of the knee. As the sciatic nerve has a

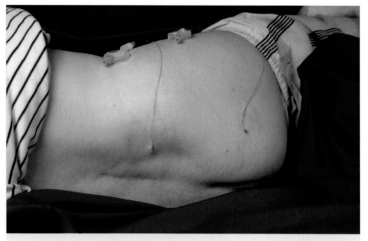

**Fig. 11.55** Posterior sciatic nerve catheter in situ in combination with a psoas catheter.

large proportion of sympathetic fibers, it is rational to use the continuous sciatic nerve block for therapeutic and diagnostic sympathetic block (Smith and Siggins 1988).

The onset of the block can be checked by measuring the increase in plantar temperature with a skin thermometer. The rise in temperature occurs after a few minutes and in the absence of previous vascular disease can nearly reach core body temperature when the sympathetic block is complete.

## Summary

Transgluteal sciatic nerve block has been a highly effective standard anesthesia for decades. In combination with psoas block, for example (see Chapter 9), the method provides complete anesthesia of the leg. A disadvantage is the need for a change in patient position. Complications are very rare.

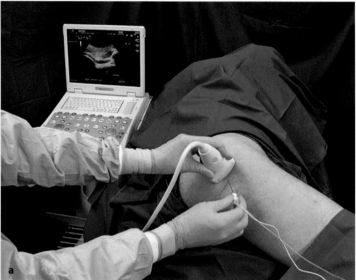

**Fig. 11.56** Visualization of the sciatic nerve in the "subgluteal space" (tuberosity–trochanter line) right. See further detail in ▶ Fig. 11.57.
**a** Clinical setting.
**b** Anatomical section.
1 Greater trochanter
2 Sciatic nerve
3 Quadratus femoris muscle
4 Ischial tuberosity
5 Gluteus maximus muscle

## 11.5.5 Proximal Sciatic Nerve Block (in Lateral Position) with Ultrasound

Curved array: 5 to 2 MHz, linear transducer 7.5 MHz
Penetration depth: 5 to 15 cm
Needle: 7 to 12 cm

### Scanning Technique

The proximal sciatic nerve can be visualized transgluteally or subgluteally at several levels ▶ with patients lying on their side. In the subgluteal region, the ischial tuberosity and the greater trochanter (tuberosity–trochanter line) are clear landmarks for finding the nerve using ultrasound (Karmakar et al 2007). This approach is also called transgluteal (Kapral 2007).

A sector transducer is preferred because of the better overview. In slim patients, a linear transducer can also be used. The transducer is set on the tuberosity–trochanter line so that medial to the ischial tuberosity and lateral to the greater trochanter a structure considered typical for bones (hyperechoic line with acoustic shadow behind it) can be seen (▶ Fig. 11.56 ▶).

Between the bony structures, the sciatic nerve appears as a flat, oval hyperechoic structure. It can often not be clearly distinguished from the surrounding fat tissue due to similar reflective properties. The sciatic nerve lies in front of the quadratus femoris, which runs from the greater trochanter to the ischial tuberosity. The nerve is covered by the gluteus maximus. The space between these two muscles at the level of the tuberosity–trochanter line is known as the subgluteal space. A branch of the inferior gluteal artery also passes through this space. This is a small artery medial and posterior to the sciatic nerve (▶ Fig. 11.57). There is little danger of puncturing this artery; however, it can be easily visualized with a Doppler probe and this can be used for additional orientation.

In this region, the nerve is an average of 3.34 ± 0.85 cm below the skin (Chan et al 2006) and is 1.57 ± 0.17 cm wide.

### Needle Approach

The needle insertion can be made out of plane or in plane ▶.

▶ **Volume.** Approximately 20 to 30 mL local anesthetic.

### Catheter Placement

A catheter can be placed in both the in-plane and the out-of-plane technique.

> **Tips and Tricks**
>
> - When the subgluteal space is penetrated, a "click" can often be felt (Karmakar et al 2007).
> - Use of a nerve stimulator (dual guidance) can be helpful.
> - If it is difficult to visualize, the nerve can be sought distally and followed in proximal direction to the subgluteal region.
> - It can be helpful to visualize the nerve in the long axis (very thin, wide nerve).
> - If the nerve cannot be visualized, an attempt can be made to detect the typical structure of the quadratus femoris. The subgluteal space is located above the muscle. The nerve can often be distinguished better after injecting a few milliliters of fluid.

## 11.5.6 Infragluteal Block of the Sciatic Nerve in Lateral Position with Ultrasound

Curved array: 5 to 2 MHz, linear transducer 7.5 MHz
Penetration depth: 5 to 15 cm
Needle: 7 to 12 cm

### Scanning Technique

The infragluteal region is in the area of the gluteal fold. The sciatic nerve can be found in this region in supine position with the leg positioned high (see Chapter 11.3) and in prone or lateral position (▶ Fig. 11.58). It lies anterior to the long head of the biceps femoris. The skin–nerve distance is 3 to 4 cm in the infragluteal region, becomes shorter further distally, and in the middle of the thigh again reaches an average skin–nerve distance of 3.4 cm (Bruhn et al 2008, Moayeri et al 2010).

The sciatic nerve is visualized in this region as a flat to slightly oval hyperechoic structure (▶ Fig. 11.59); further distally it becomes rounder ▶. Bruhn et al (2009) describe an unchanging hyperechoic line at the medial border of the biceps femoris in the area 2 to 10 cm distal to the gluteal fold, which runs posterior to anterior directly toward the sciatic nerve (▶ Fig. 11.58). The line represents tendinous segments of the biceps femoris that maintain an unchanged position relative to the sciatic nerve (▶ Fig. 11.60). To identify this hyperechoic line, the biceps femoris is scanned from lateral to medial. The *first* hyperechoic structure running from posterior to anterior with a slight shift in lateral direction is caused by the tendinous segments in or at the medial border of the biceps femoris. The sciatic nerve is located at its posterior end.

### Needle Approach

The needle insertion can be made in the short axis out of plane or in plane.

▶ **Out-of-plane approach.**
In the out-of-plane approach, the nerve is set in the center of the acoustic window in the short axis and the needle is inserted about 1 cm distal or proximal to the transducer at the smallest angle possible (steep) to the transducer (▶ Fig. 11.58 ▶).

▶ **In-plane approach.** The in-plane approach in the short axis can be made from lateral to medial or from medial to lateral in the acoustic window.

▶ **Volume.** Approximately 20 mL local anesthetic (▶ Fig. 11.61).

### Catheter Placement

A catheter can be placed; the out-of-plane technique (short axis) is preferable. A long axis view and in-plane insertion of the needle is recommended by Tammam (2013).

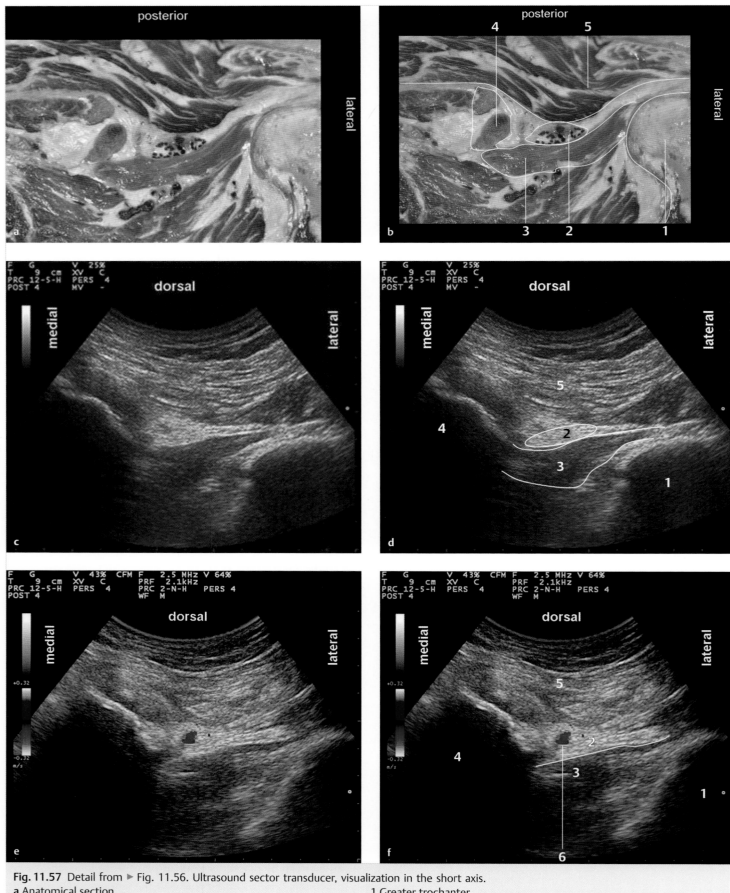

**Fig. 11.57** Detail from ▶ Fig. 11.56. Ultrasound sector transducer, visualization in the short axis.

a Anatomical section.
b Anatomical section (labeled).
c Ultrasound image corresponding to a (unlabeled).
d Ultrasound image corresponding to b (labeled).
e Ultrasound image with Doppler (CFM, color flow mode; unlabeled).
f Ultrasound image with Doppler (CFM; labeled).

1 Greater trochanter
2 Sciatic nerve
3 Quadratus femoris muscle
4 Ischial tuberosity
5 Gluteus maximus muscle
6 Branch of the inferior gluteal artery

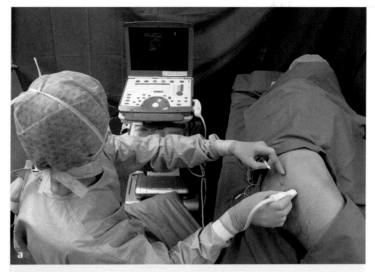

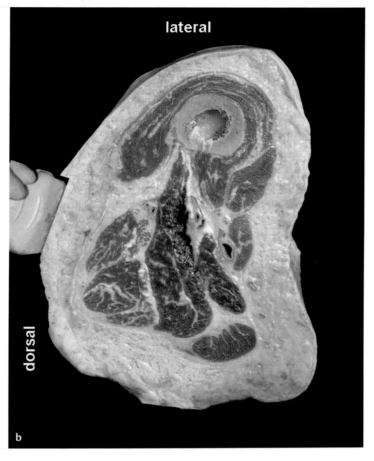

**Fig. 11.58** Puncture of the right proximal sciatic nerve in the infragluteal region in lateral position. For detail, see ▶ Fig. 11.59.
**a** Clinical setting.
**b** Anatomical section.

---

**Tips and Tricks**

- A linear transducer can be used for slim patients.
- Additional use of the nerve stimulator is recommended, especially when visualization is poor.
- Visualization in the long axis (▶ Fig. 11.62) can be combined with the in-plane technique.

# 11.6 Parasacral Sciatic Nerve Block (Mansour Technique) ▶

## 11.6.1 Technique

This technique was described by Mansour in 1996 (Mansour and Bennetts 1996) and is an alternative to the "classical" posterior sciatic nerve block. Since the greater trochanter is not needed for anatomical orientation, this method is suitable for patients with a total hip replacement on the side to be anesthetized.

## Landmarks

Posterior superior iliac spine, ischial tuberosity.

## Position

The patient lies on his or her side with the leg to be anesthetized uppermost. The leg underneath can be extended, and the leg to be blocked is flexed about 30 to 40° at the hip and about 70° at the knee (▶ Fig. 11.63).

## Procedure

The posterior superior iliac spine and the ischial tuberosity are identified and joined by a line. The puncture site is 6 cm caudal to the posterior superior iliac spine on this line (▶ Fig. 11.63, ▶ Fig. 11.64, ▶ Fig. 11.65).

A needle 10 to 15 cm long is advanced in sagittal direction (perpendicular to the skin) until the motor response is seen in the foot, at a current of 0.5 mA and a pulse duration of 0.1 ms at a depth of 10 to 15 cm in the vicinity of the sciatic nerve (▶ Fig. 11.63). Then 30 mL of a medium-acting or long-acting local anesthetic is injected. A continuous technique can also be performed from the insertion site in the Mansour technique by changing the needle direction toward the middle third of the line between the greater trochanter and the ischial tuberosity. The catheter is advanced 4 to 5 cm caudally through the needle (▶ Fig. 11.65).

## 11.6.2 Indications and Contraindications

(See 11.5.2)

## 11.6.3 Side Effects and Complications

(See 11.5.3)

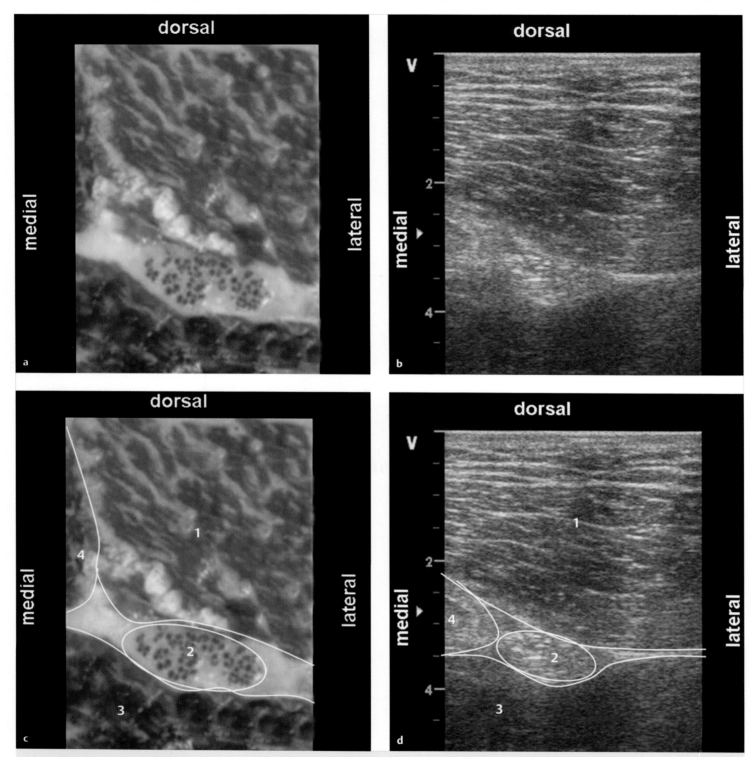

**Fig. 11.59** Puncture of the right proximal sciatic nerve in the infragluteal region in lateral position (close-up of the anatomical overview in ▶ Fig. 11.58 with the corresponding ultrasound image).
**a** Anatomical section.
**b** Ultrasound image corresponding to a (unlabeled).
**c** Anatomical section (labeled).
**d** Ultrasound image corresponding to c (labeled).

1 Biceps femoris muscle
2 Sciatic nerve
3 Adductor magnus muscle
4 Semitendinosus muscle

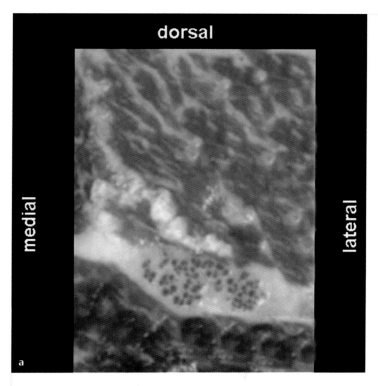

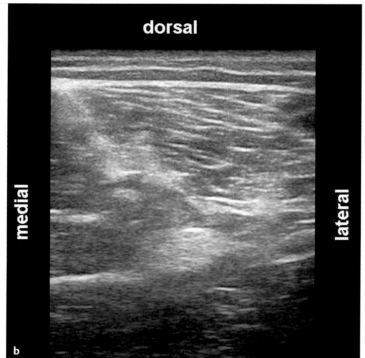

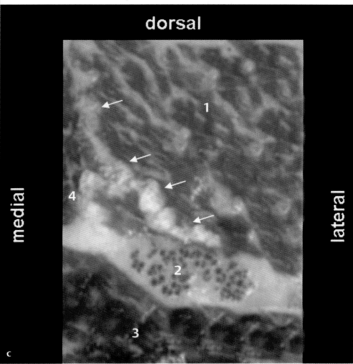

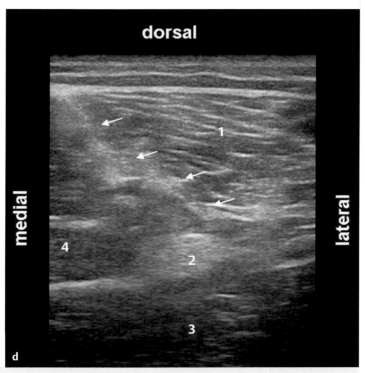

**Fig. 11.60** Tendon of the long head of the biceps femoris as landmark for finding the sciatic nerve in the infragluteal region.

a Anatomical section.
b Ultrasound image corresponding to **a** (unlabeled).
c Anatomical section (labeled).
d Ultrasound image corresponding to **c** (labeled).

1 Biceps femoris muscle
2 Sciatic nerve
3 Adductor magnus muscle
4 Semitendinosus muscle

Arrows: Tendon of the biceps femoris, which appears in ultrasound as a hyperechoic line from posterior to anterior with a slight lateral shift and can be used as a landmark for finding the sciatic nerve (Bruhn et al 2009).

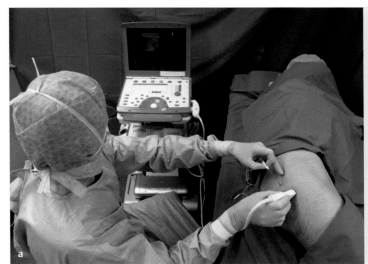

**Fig. 11.61** Puncture of the right proximal sciatic nerve in the infragluteal region in lateral position (close-up of the anatomical overview with corresponding ultrasound image) after injection of local anesthetic.
**a** Clinical setting.
**b** Ultrasound image (unlabeled).
**c** Ultrasound image (labeled).
1 Biceps femoris muscle
2 Sciatic nerve
3 Adductor magnus muscle
4 Semitendinosus muscle
Arrow: Tip of the needle in local anesthetic

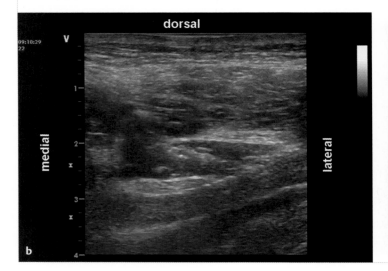

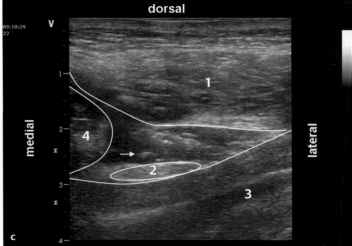

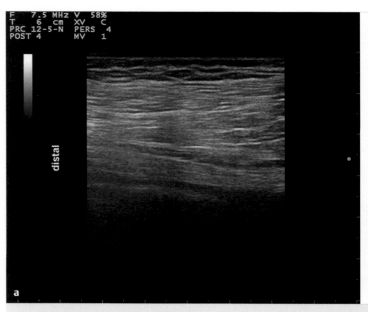

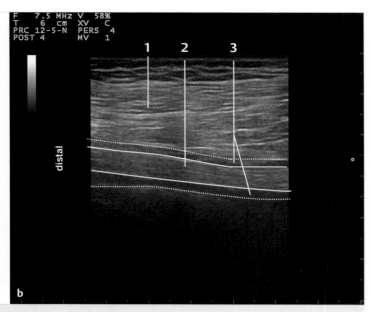

**Fig. 11.62** Puncture of the right proximal sciatic nerve in the infragluteal region in lateral position (close-up of the anatomical overview with corresponding ultrasound image) after injection of local anesthetic. Visualization of the sciatic nerve in the long axis (here after injecting local anesthetic).
**a** Ultrasound image (unlabeled).
**b** Ultrasound image (labeled).
1 Biceps femoris muscle
2 Sciatic nerve (long axis)
3 Local anesthetic

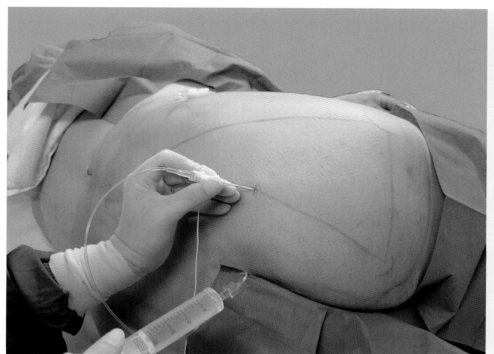

**Fig. 11.63** Posterior sciatic nerve block, Mansour technique. The needle is inserted in sagittal direction and the nerve is reached after about 10 cm. The leg does not have to be flexed at the hip for this technique.

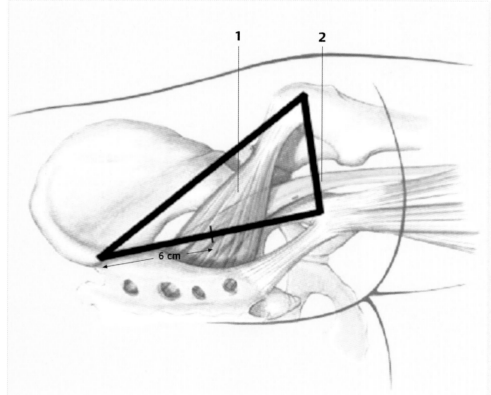

**Fig. 11.64** Posterior sciatic nerve block according to the Mansour technique is oriented by the spine–tuberosity line. The insertion site is located 6 cm distal to the posterior superior iliac spine. The nerve is reached so far proximally that block of the entire sacral plexus results.
1 Piriformis muscle
2 Sciatic nerve

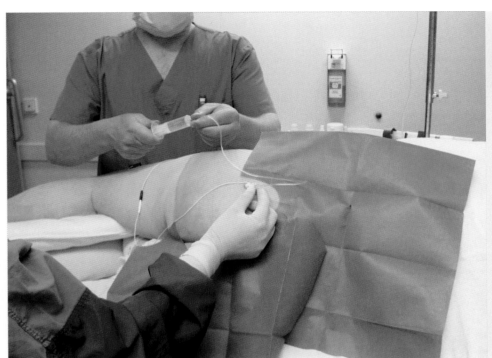

Fig. 11.65 A continuous technique can also be performed from the Mansour insertion site by lowering the needle hub and altering the needle direction toward the middle third between the greater trochanter and ischial tuberosity.

**Tips and Tricks**

- As the greater trochanter is not required for anatomical orientation, the technique is suitable for patients with a total hip replacement on the side to be anesthetized.
- If there is no response at a needle depth of up to 10 cm, the needle direction should be corrected 5 to 10° distally (Meier 2001).
- If there is contact with the bone during the procedure, the needle should be withdrawn and advanced again 1 to 2 cm further distally on the spine–tuberosity line (Morris et al 1997, Morris and Lang 1999).
- The onset of all sciatic nerve block techniques can be tested by checking the rise in plantar temperature using a skin thermometer (Büttner and Meier 1999).

## 11.6.4 Remarks on the Technique

In parasacral anesthesia of the sciatic nerve, the nerve is reached so far proximally that block of the entire sacral plexus occurs. Morris and Lang assume that the obturator nerve is also anesthetized due to its anatomical vicinity. In their view the parasacral block of the sciatic nerve together with a so-called "3-in-1 block" will cause complete anesthesia of the leg (Morris and Lang 1997). However, as the technique is performed in the lateral position, combination of parasacral sciatic nerve block with psoas block is more useful, as a change of patient position is not necessary.

## Summary

Parasacral anesthesia of the sciatic nerve is easy to learn and has a high success rate (Ripart et al 2005). The technique is performed with the patient in lateral position and is suitable for patients who can be positioned in this way without pain.

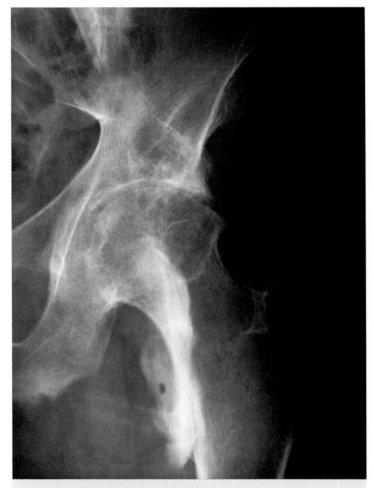

Fig. 11.66 Injection of contrast through a posterior sciatic nerve catheter: note the spread along the course of the nerve in the middle third between the ischial tuberosity and greater trochanter. The course behind the lesser trochanter is also worth noting (see also anterior sciatic nerve block, Beck technique, 11.2.4).

The anatomical orientation can be difficult in obese patients. Catheter placement is easily performed (► Fig. 11.66) and the analgesia is effective. For adequate anesthesia, 20 to 30 mL of a medium-acting or long-acting local anesthetic should be injected. Ropivacaine 0.33% (3.3 mg/mL) 6 mL/h or 20 mL of ropivacaine 0.2 to 0.375% (2–3.75 mg/mL) every 6 to 8 hours is suitable for a continuous block.

## 11.6.5 Parasacral Sciatic Nerve Block with Ultrasound

A promising parasacral ultrasound-guided technique to block the sciatic nerve with clear landmarks has been described by Bendtsen et al (2011).

## References

Beck GP. Anterior approach to sciatic nerve block. Anesthesiology 1963; 24: 222–224

Bendtsen TF, Lönnqvist PA, Jepsen KV, Petersen M, Knudsen L, Børglum J. Preliminary results of a new ultrasound-guided approach to block the sacral plexus: the parasacral parallel shift. Br J Anaesth 2011; 107: 278–280

Benninghoff A, Goerttler K. Lehrbuch der Anatomie des Menschen. 11th ed. Munich: Urban & Schwarzenberg; 1975

Bridenbaugh PhO, Wedel DJ. The lower extremity. In: Cousins MJ, Bridenbaugh PhO, eds. Neural Blockade in Clinical Anesthesia and Management of Pain. 3rd ed. Philadelphia: Lippincott-Raven; 1998: 373–409

Brown DL. Regional Anesthesia and Analgesia. Philadelphia: Saunders; 1996: 279–288

Bruhn J, Van Geffen GJ, Gielen MJ, Scheffer GJ. Visualization of the course of the sciatic nerve in adult volunteers by ultrasonography. Acta Anaesthesiol Scand 2008; 52: 1298–1302

Bruhn J, Moayeri N, Groen GJ et al. Soft tissue landmark for ultrasound identification of the sciatic nerve in the infragluteal region: the tendon of the long head of the biceps femoris muscle. Acta Anaesthesiol Scand 2009; 53: 921–925

Büttner J, Meier G. Kontinuierliche periphere Techniken zur Regionalanästhesie und Schmerztherapie–Obere und untere Extremität. Bremen: Uni-Med; 1999

Chan VWS, Nova H, Abbas S, McCartney CJ, Perlas A, Xu DQ. Ultrasound examination and localization of the sciatic nerve: a volunteer study. Anesthesiology 2006; 104: 309–314, discussion 5A

Chelly JE, Greger J, Howart G. Simple anterior approach for sciatic blockade. Reg Anesth 1997; 22: 114

Chelly JE, Delaunay L. A new anterior approach to the sciatic nerve block. Anesthesiology 1999; 91: 1655–1660

Chelly JE, Delaunay L, Matuszczak M, Hagberg C. Sciatic nerve blocks. Tech Reg Anesth Pain Manage 1999; 3: 39–46

Clara M. Das Nervensystem des Menschen. 3rd ed. Leipzig: Barth; 1959

Ericksen ML, Swenson JD, Pace NL. The anatomic relationship of the sciatic nerve to the lesser trochanter: implications for anterior sciatic nerve block. Anesth Analg 2002; 95: 1071–1074

Gligorijevic P. Lower extremity blocks for day surgery. Tech Reg Anesth Pain Manage 2000; 4: 30–37

Guardini R, Waldron BA, Wallace WA. Sciatic nerve block: a new lateral approach. Acta Anaesthesiol Scand 1985; 29: 515–519

Kaiser H, Niesel HC, Hans V. Fundamentals and requirements of peripheral electric nerve stimulation. A contribution to the improvement of safety standards in regional anesthesia. Reg Anaesth 1990; 13: 143–147

Kapral S. Regionalanästhesie, Periphere Blockaden. In: Grau T, ed. Ultraschall in der Anästhesie und Intensivmedizin. Lehrbuch der Ultraschalldiagnostik. Cologne: Deutscher Ärzte-Verlag; 2007: 245–282

Karmakar MK, Kwok WH, Ho AM, Tsang K, Chui PT, Gin T. Ultrasound-guided sciatic nerve block: description of a new approach at the subgluteal space. Br J Anaesth 2007; 98: 390–395

Labat G. Regional Anesthesia: Its Technique and Clinical Application. Philadelphia: Saunders; 1924: 45

Mansour NY, Bennetts FE. An observational study of combined continuous lumbar plexus and single-shot sciatic nerve blocks for post-knee surgery analgesia. Reg Anesth 1996; 21: 287–291

Meier G, Heinrich Ch. Sciatic Nerve Block: A Comparison of three different Techniques. 24th Central European Congress on Anesthesiology. Bologna: Monduzzi; 1995: 509–512

Meier G et al. Schmerztherapie mit Ischiadikuskathetern—anatomische Voraussetzungen. Schmerz 1998; 13: 75

Meier G. Der kontinuierliche anteriore Ischiadicuskatheter (KAI). In: Mehrkens HH, Büttner J, ed. Kontinuierliche periphere Leitungsblockaden. Munich: Arcis; 1999a; 47–48

Meier G. Technik der kontinuierlichen anterioren Ischiadicusblockade (KAI). In: Büttner J, Meier G, ed. Kontinuierliche periphere Techniken zur Regionalanästhesie und Schmerztherapie—Obere und untere Extremität. Bremen: Uni-Med; 1999b; 132–137

Meier G. Peripheral nerve block of the lower extremities. [Article in German] Anaesthesist 2001; 50: 536–557, quiz 557, 559

Meier G, Büttner J. Regionalanästhesie–Kompendium der peripheren Blockaden. Munich: Arcis; 2001

Moayeri N, van Geffen GJ, Bruhn J, Chan VW, Groen GJ. Correlation among ultrasound, cross-sectional anatomy, and histology of the sciatic nerve: a review. Reg Anesth Pain Med 2010; 35: 442–449

Morris GF, Lang SA. Continuous parasacral sciatic nerve block: two case reports. Reg Anesth 1997; 22: 469–472

Morris GF, Lang SA, Dust WN, Van der Wal M. The parasacral sciatic nerve block. Reg Anesth 1997; 22: 100–104

Morris GF, Lang SA. Innovations in lower extremity blockade. Tech Reg Anesth Pain Manage 1999; 3: 9–18

Neuburger M, Rotzinger M, Kaiser H. Electric nerve stimulation in relation to impulse strength. A quantitative study of the distance of the electrode point to the nerve. [Article in German] Anaesthesist 2001; 50: 181–186

Niesel HCh, ed. Regionalanästhesie, Lokalanästhesie, regionale Schmerztherapie. Stuttgart: Thieme; 1994

Ota J, Sakura S, Hara K, Saito Y. Ultrasound-guided anterior approach to sciatic nerve block: a comparison with the posterior approach. Anesth Analg 2009; 108: 660–665

Polino F, Castro A, Bello R et al. Postoperative analgesia by continuous 3-in-1-blockade in total hip arthroplasty. Int Monitor Reg Anesth 2000; 12: 245

Raj PP, Parks RI, Watson TD, Jenkins MT. A new single-position supine approach to sciatic-femoral nerve block. Anesth Analg 1975; 54: 489–493

Ripart J, Cuvillon P, Nouvellon E, Gaertner E, Eledjam JJ. Parasacral approach to block the sciatic nerve: a 400-case survey. Reg Anesth Pain Med 2005; 30: 193–197

Rongstad K, Mann RA, Prieskorn D, Nichelson S, Horton G. Popliteal sciatic nerve block for postoperative analgesia. Foot Ankle Int 1996; 17: 378–382

Smith BE, Siggins. Low volume, high concentration block of the sciatic nerve. Anaesthesia 1988; 43: 8–11

Tammam TF. Ultrasound-guided infragluteal sciatic nerve block: a comparison between four different techniques. Acta Anaesthesiol Scand 2013; 57: 243–248

Tsui BCH, Özelsel TJP. Ultrasound-guided anterior sciatic nerve block using a longitudinal approach: "expanding the view." Reg Anesth Pain Med 2008; 33: 275–276

Wagner F, Missler B. Combined 3-in-1 sciatic block. Prilocaine 500 mg vs. 650 mg. [Article in German] Anaesthesist 1 987; 46: 195–200

Wagner F, Taeger L. Combined sciatic/3-in-1 block. III. Prilocaine 1% versus mepivacaine 1%. [Article in German] Reg Anaesth 1988; 11: 61–64

Wagner F. Beinnervenblockaden In: Niesel HC, ed. Regionalanästhesie, Lokalanästhesie, regionale Schmerztherapie. Stuttgart: Thieme; 1994: 417–521

Winnie AP. Regional anesthesia. Surg Clin North Am 1975; 55: 861–892

# 12 Blocks at the Knee

## 12.1 Anatomical Overview

The sciatic nerve (L4–S3) consists of two components, the common fibular nerve (synonym: common peroneal nerve) and the tibial nerve, which are surrounded in the lesser pelvis and thigh by a common connective-tissue sheath and therefore give the impression of a single nerve trunk. The level at which the division into the two branches can take place varies. The common connective-tissue sheath ends at the latest on entry to the popliteal fossa and the nerve divides into the tibial nerve and the common fibular nerve (▶ Fig. 12.1).

▶ **Common fibular nerve.** The common fibular nerve (L4–S2) divides below the popliteal fossa into the deep fibular nerve and the superficial fibular nerve. The deep fibular nerve innervates the extensor muscles of the lower leg and foot. The superficial fibular nerve supplies the muscles of the fibular group. The tibial nerve (L4–S3) is responsible for the motor supply of the toe and foot flexors.

▶ **Tibial nerve.** The tibial nerve innervates the skin of the lateral lower leg and the sole of the foot and, after joining the communicating branch of the fibular nerve to form the sural nerve, it supplies the lateral border of the heel and foot. The dorsum of the foot is innervated by the superficial fibular nerve, apart from the area between the great toe and second toe (deep fibular nerve).

## 12.2 Classical Popliteal Block, Posterior Approach

### 12.2.1 Technique

**Landmarks and Position**

Popliteal fossa, popliteal crease.

The patient lies prone. With the knee extended, puncture is performed at the level of the popliteal crease or slightly cranial to it (▶ Fig. 12.2). The tibial nerve is found about 1 cm lateral to the artery. It is situated at a depth of 1 to 3 cm. To block the common fibular nerve from the same insertion site, the needle is withdrawn under the skin and advanced again further laterally toward the head of the fibula. After around 3 to 4 cm a response will be obtained from the nerve.

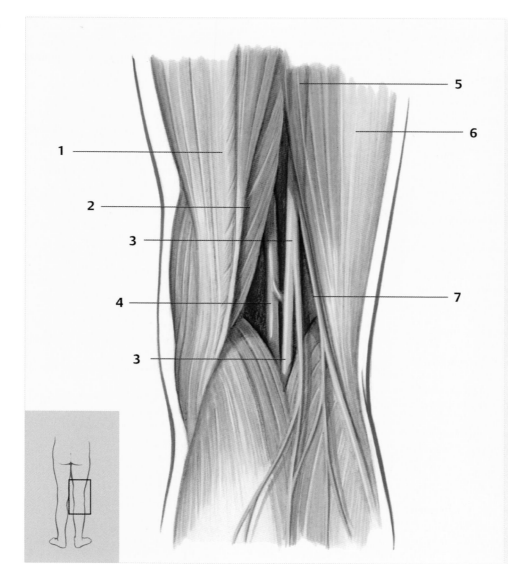

**Fig. 12.1** The sciatic nerve, which often divides very proximally into the tibial nerve and common fibular nerve, leaves the common sheath that surrounds the two divisions at the latest on entering the popliteal fossa (about 8–10 cm above the popliteal crease), and the tibial nerve and common fibular nerves separate here. In order to block both divisions of the sciatic nerve in the region of the popliteal fossa with one injection, this must be performed at least 8 to 10 cm above the popliteal crease. A continuous technique can also be performed here without difficulty. A complete block distal to the knee requires an additional block of the saphenous nerve, a main branch of the femoral nerve that provides sensory innervation of the medial lower leg.
1 Semitendinosus muscle
2 Semimembranosus muscle
3 Tibial nerve
4 Popliteal artery
5 Sciatic nerve (covered by muscle)
6 Biceps femoris muscle
7 Common fibular nerve

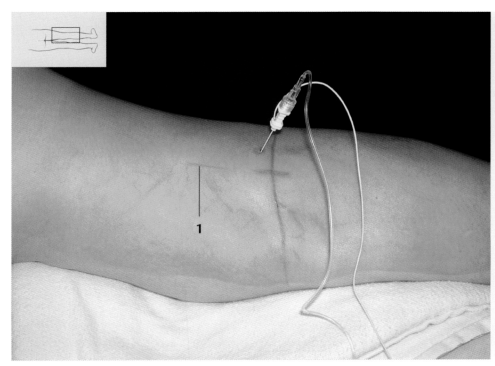

1

**Fig. 12.2** Popliteal block (classical technique). The classical "popliteal block" is performed in the popliteal crease where the tibial nerve and fibular nerve are already separated, so that the two nerves may have to be found and blocked individually to obtain a complete block of the lower leg (see Chapter 12.3.5). Right popliteal fossa, posteromedial view.
1 Popliteal artery

## 12.2.2 Remarks on the Technique

**Definition**

Anesthesia of the sciatic nerve or of its two divisions (fibular nerve and tibial nerve) in the region of the popliteal fossa, known as popliteal block or "knee block," has often been described. It is a highly effective technique and is easily performed without problems.

▶ **Disadvantage.** The disadvantage of the classical popliteal block in the popliteal fossa or slightly more cranial is the necessity of finding two nerves separately in order to be able to anesthetize the entire foot. The fibular and tibial nerves can be separately blocked in the popliteal fossa or somewhat proximal to it from one puncture site because of the close vicinity of the two nerves. This requires a change in the direction of the needle for selective stimulation of the two nerves.

▶ **Double injection technique.** The double injection technique should be a quick procedure, as the risk of intraneural injection increases with the time required (Gligorijevic 2000).

**Practical Note**

Administration of the local anesthetic after finding the first nerve can result in partial anesthesia of the second nerve, even before it has been localized, because of its proximity. This prevents both an adequate response by the nerve stimulator and the patient's warning of paresthesia due to inadvertent intraneural injection of the local anesthetic.

The double injection technique leads to a short onset period and an effective block (Bailey et al 1994). Singelyn et al (1991) performed 625 blocks with nerve stimulation in a prospective study; 30 mL of mepivacaine 1% (10 mg/mL) or bupivacaine 0.5% (5 mg/mL) was injected. An adequate block was achieved in 92% of the patients and in another 5% the block was successfully

supplemented. The popliteal artery was punctured in two patients (0.3%). Patient satisfaction was 95%. Popliteal block is considered to be a safe technique (Jan et al 2000). An out-of-plane ultrasound-guided puncture a few centimeters distal to the bifurcation has shown that one injection between the two nerves (tibial nerve, common fibular nerve) leads to a fast, reliable block (Perlas et al 2013, Chapter 12.3.5) so that it is not absolutely necessary to block the two nerves separately in this region.

## 12.3 Distal Block of the Sciatic Nerve ▶

### 12.3.1 Technique

#### Posterior Approach, Continuous Technique According to Meier (Meier 1996)

The sciatic nerve divides, at the latest where it enters the popliteal fossa, into its two main branches, the tibial nerve and the common fibular nerve. The common fascial sheath can no longer be found in the popliteal fossa. For reasons of efficacy, this suggests that the sciatic nerve should be found and anesthetized as far cranially as possible in the popliteal fossa, that is, before it divides—in other words, a distal sciatic nerve block should be performed (▶ Fig. 12.3).

#### Landmarks

Above the popliteal crease, the popliteal fossa is bounded laterally by the tendon of biceps femoris, and medially by the semimembranosus and the tendon of semitendinosus. The needle is inserted at the lateral boundary of the popliteal fossa (corresponding to the inside of the biceps femoris tendon) about 8 to 12 cm above the popliteal crease (▶ Fig. 12.4, ▶ Fig. 12.5, ▶ Fig. 12.6).

#### Position

The patient lies on his or her side with the leg to be anesthetized on top. The lower leg is flexed at the knee; the upper leg is loosely extended (▶ Fig. 12.5).

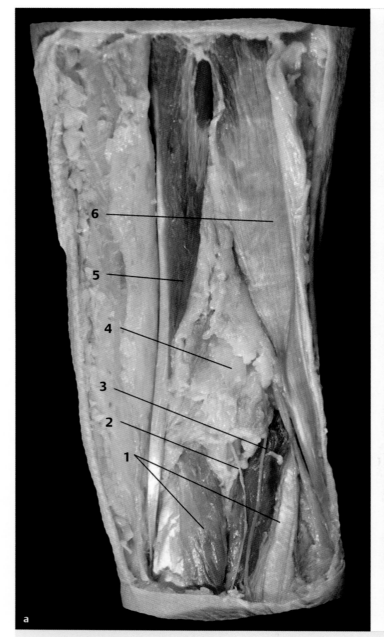

**Fig. 12.3** Popliteal fossa.

**a** Boundaries of a right popliteal fossa: the massive fat body that hides the tibial nerve is easily seen.

1 Inner and outer head of the gastrocnemius muscle
2 Sural nerve
3 Communicating branch of the fibular nerve
4 Fat of the popliteal fossa
5 Semitendinosus muscle
6 Biceps femoris muscle

**b** Right popliteal fossa, view from dorsal. The sciatic nerve, which often divides very proximally into the tibial nerve and common fibular nerve, leaves the common sheath that surrounds the two divisions at the latest on entering the popliteal fossa (about 8–10 cm

above the popliteal crease), and the tibial nerve and common fibular nerves separate here. In order to block both divisions of the sciatic nerve in the region of the popliteal fossa with one injection, this must be performed at least 8 to 10 cm above the popliteal crease. A continuous technique can also be performed here without difficulty.

1 Tibial nerve
2 Semimembranosus muscle
3 Semitendinosus muscle
4 Sciatic nerve
5 Biceps femoris muscle
6 Common fibular nerve

▶ **Variation of position, preferred position.** The patient lies supine, the leg to be anesthetized is lifted and flexed at the hip and knee, also known as the "lithotomy" position, ▶ Fig. 12.7.

## Procedure

The patient is asked to flex the knee. The tendon of the biceps femoris can be readily palpated on the lateral side. The leg is then

extended. A line is drawn about 8 to 12 cm proximal and parallel to the popliteal crease. The intersection with the tendon of the biceps femoris marks the insertion site (▶ Fig. 12.6). The insertion site is medial to the tendon of the biceps femoris and lateral to the popliteal vessels (Meier 1996; ▶ Fig. 12.8).

Following disinfection, infiltration, and prepuncture of the skin at the insertion site, a 6 to 10 cm long 19.5G needle is connected to a nerve stimulator and advanced proximally and slightly

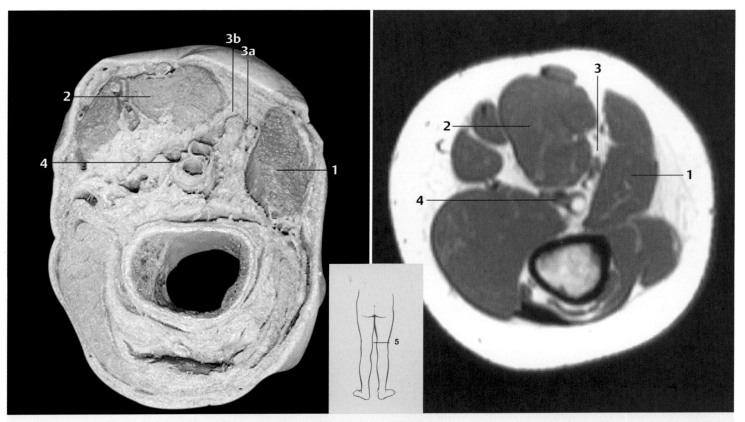

**Fig. 12.4** Cross-section through the right thigh at the level of insertion (here 9 cm above the popliteal crease) for distal sciatic nerve block, and MRI at the same level in prone position. The plane through the right thigh is seen from below.
1 Biceps femoris muscle
2 Semimembranosus/semitendinosus muscle
3 Sciatic nerve
3a Fibular nerve
3b Tibial nerve
4 Popliteal artery
5 Plane (view from caudal)

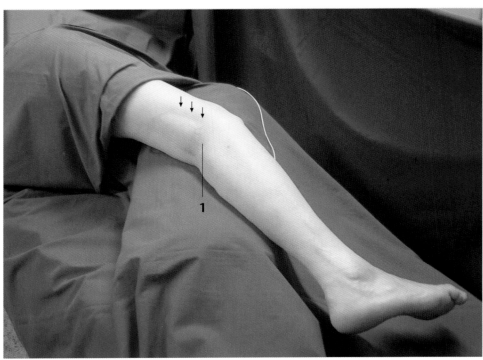

**Fig. 12.5** Distal sciatic nerve block, distal approach in lateral position: there is a posterior and a lateral approach to distal sciatic nerve block. The posterior approach can be performed in the lateral or supine position (see ▶ Fig. 12.7). The tendon of the biceps femoris is used for orientation. A skin groove can often be identified medial to the tendon, and for better orientation the patient can be asked to flex the lower leg against resistance, which makes the tendon more prominent.
1 Popliteal crease

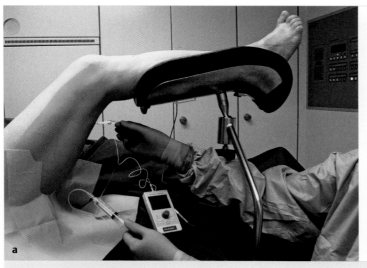
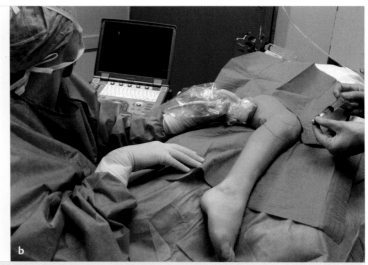

**Fig. 12.6** Distal sciatic nerve block.
**a** Performance in supine position.
**b** In this child with extensor deficits, the lateral position is ideal. However, the supine position is usually preferred.

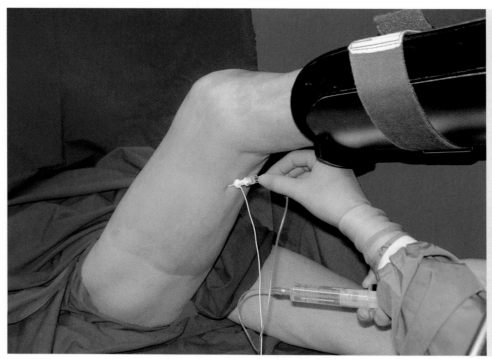

**Fig. 12.7** Posterior distal sciatic nerve block in supine position.

medially at an angle of 30 to 45° to the skin. When the fascia is reached, obvious resistance ("click") can often be felt.

The sciatic nerve or its divisions are reached after 4 to 6 cm. In obese patients, the distance may be greater than 6 cm. Because of the laterally situated insertion site, the common fibular nerve is usually reached first and then the tibial nerve when the needle is advanced deeper and further medially.

### Note

The position of the needle tip is optimal when pronation of the foot with dorsiflexion (fibular division) or a motor response of the tibial nerve (supination of the foot with plantar flexion) can be produced.

Both responses can often be produced by a minimal shift of the needle tip. Then 30 to 40 mL of local anesthetic is injected.

▶ **Supine position.** Alternatively, the distal sciatic nerve block can be performed in supine position (with the leg supported with a positioning aid). The patient then does not need to be turned to their side. In the continuous technique, after the local anesthetic is injected the catheter is advanced proximally by the needle 3 cm beyond its tip.

### Tips and Tricks

- If the tibial nerve is stimulated first, the position of the needle tip should be directed more laterally in order to reach the fibular nerve.
- Vascular puncture is not anticipated with this technique of distal sciatic nerve block (▶ Fig. 12.9).
- The catheter should not be advanced more than 3 cm past the tip of the needle.
- A frequently observed long onset time is possibly caused by fat tissue in the popliteal fossa.

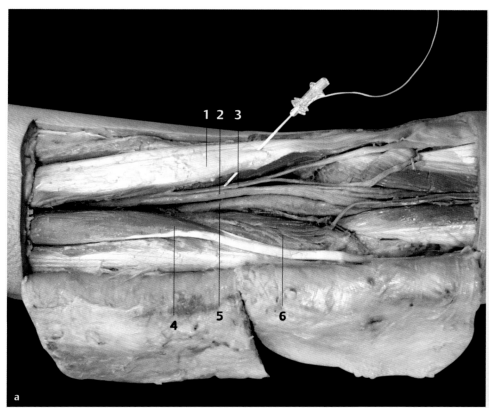

**Fig. 12.8** Right popliteal fossa, posterior view.
1 Biceps femoris muscle
2 Tibial division of the sciatic nerve
3 Fibular division of the sciatic nerve
4 Semitendinosus muscle
5 Popliteal artery
6 Semimembranosus muscle
**a** Posterior distal sciatic nerve block: the insertion site is medial to the tendon of biceps femoris and lateral to the popliteal vessels.
**b** Clinical setting.

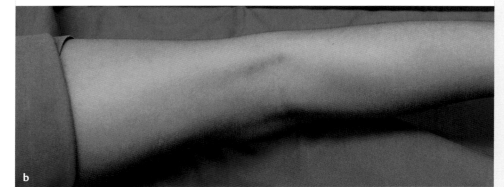

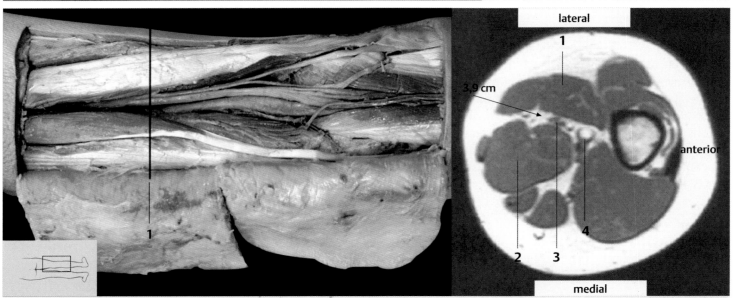

**Fig. 12.9** MRI of right thigh in lateral position, 9 cm above the popliteal crease (seen from below). As the nerve is reached first with the described needle direction, vascular puncture is normally excluded.

Image **a**:
1 Plane for MRI (12 cm above the popliteal crease)

Image **b**:

1 Biceps femoris muscle
2 Semimembranosus/semitendinosus muscle
3 Sciatic nerve
4 Popliteal artery

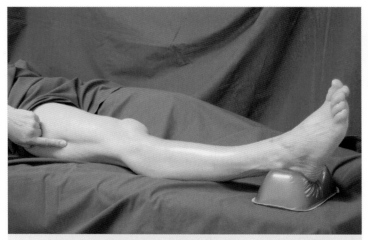

**Fig. 12.10** Distal sciatic nerve block, lateral approach with the patient in supine position. The muscle gap between the vastus lateralis muscle and the biceps femoris muscle is used for orientation. The insertion site is about 12 cm proximal of the popliteal crease.

## Lateral Approach ▶

### Landmarks and Position

Lateral joint line, vastus lateralis, biceps femoris.

Supine position, the leg should be supported at the foot so that the muscles of the thigh can sag freely.

### Procedure

The needle insertion site is at least 8 to 12 cm proximal to the lateral joint line in the gap between the biceps femoris and vastus lateralis (▶ Fig. 12.10).

The angle of the needle in the transverse plane varies with the distance from the lateral femoral epicondyle: the further proximal the insertion site, the lower the angle posteriorly (Neuburger et al 2005); the minimum distance proximal to the joint line should be 8 cm. Distal to this, the sciatic nerve has already separated into the common fibular nerve and tibial nerve and runs without the common connective-tissue sheath (▶ Fig. 12.11).

In addition to posterior needle angle, an angle in proximal direction should be maintained (▶ Fig. 12.12), as this will facilitate advancing a catheter. At a distance of 8 to 12 cm proximal to the lateral joint line, the nerve is reached from in front, so there can be a response from the tibial nerve first, although the common fibular nerve lies more laterally (and somewhat posterior) to the tibial nerve. The skin–nerve distance can be up to 8 cm, sometimes even more, so a needle 10 to 12 cm long should be used (▶ Fig. 12.13).

## 12.3.2 Indications and Contraindications

### Indications for Single-Shot and Continuous Sciatic Nerve Blocks

(sometimes in combination with a saphenous nerve block)
• Anesthesia for operation on the foot or ankle—for example, lateral ligament suture, resection arthroplasty, arthrodesis,

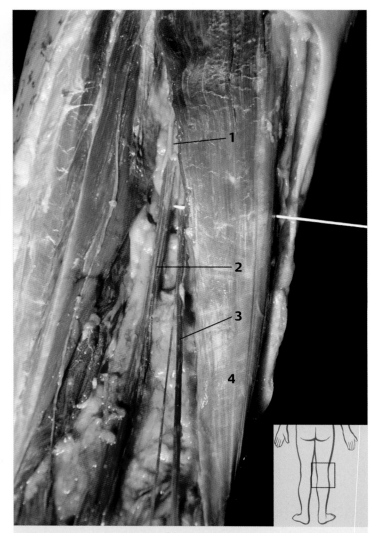

**Fig. 12.11** Lateral distal sciatic nerve block, view from behind, right popliteal fossa.
1 Sciatic nerve
2 Tibial nerve
3 Common fibular nerve
4 Biceps femoris muscle

amputation (▶ Fig. 12.14), free tissue transfer/transplantation with microvascular–vascular attachment to the lower leg/foot region (e.g., latissimus dorsi flap; ▶ Fig. 12.15).
• Anesthesia/pain therapy for fractures distal to the knee.
• Postoperative pain therapy (e.g., ankle and foot region).
• Pain therapy (e.g., diabetic gangrene, CRPS 1).
• Regional sympathetic block (perfusion and wound healing disorders, CRPS 1; ▶ Fig. 12.16 and ▶ Fig. 12.17).

### Contraindications

• General contraindications (see Chapter 20.2).
• Previous peripheral vascular surgery to the legs (relative).

## 12.3.3 Side Effects and Complications

No special complications or side effects are known.

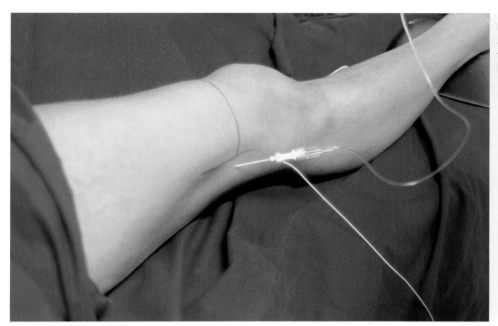

**Fig. 12.12** Lateral distal sciatic nerve block, about 12 cm proximal to the popliteal crease in the gap between the vastus lateralis muscle and biceps femoris muscle.

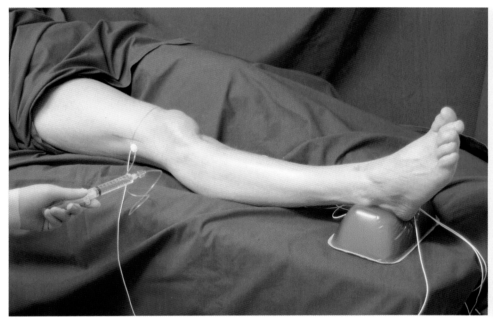

**Fig. 12.13** Lateral distal sciatic nerve block: The needle direction is about 10° in posterior direction and 30° in proximal direction; the nerve is reached after 5 to 8 cm.

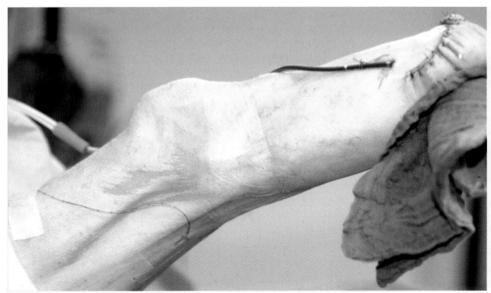

**Fig. 12.14** Distal sciatic nerve block is an ideal alternative to a lumbar epidural catheter for pain therapy and prophylaxis before and after lower leg amputations.

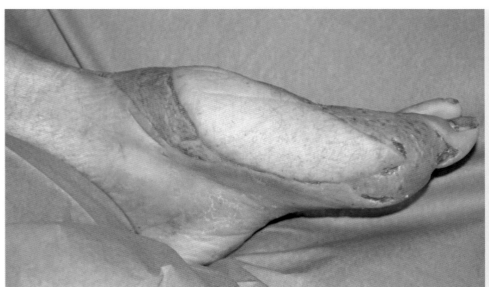

**Fig. 12.15** Distal sciatic nerve block is an ideal alternative to a lumbar epidural catheter for free tissue transfer (e.g., latissimus dorsi flap) in the lower leg or foot.

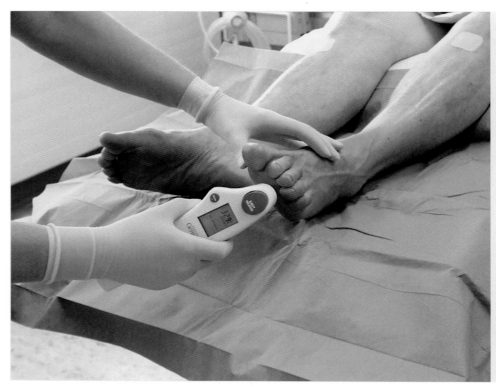

**Fig. 12.16** The sciatic nerve is rich in sympathetic fibers. After injection of the local anesthetic there is a marked sympathetic block with a rise in temperature and vasodilatation, which can be used therapeutically. Continuous sciatic nerve block is an ideal alternative to a continuous lumbar epidural block for various indications.

### Tips and Tricks

- Vascular puncture is not to be expected with the lateral technique and a distal sciatic nerve block.
- In polyneuropathy, peripheral nerve stimulation should be performed with pulse duration of 1.0 ms.
- If the operation is performed with lower leg tourniquet, it is useful to perform supplementary block of the saphenous nerve, the sensory terminal branch of the femoral nerve (Chapter 13.5).
- If there is an indication for sympathetic block, a response from the tibial nerve should be sought.
- If it is not possible to produce a response in the region of the common fibular nerve, the needle should be corrected in a medial direction, for the tibial nerve in lateral direction.

## 12.3.4 Remarks on the Technique

Labat described the sciatic nerve block in the popliteal fossa for the first time in 1924 (Labat 1924). Different variants of popliteal block are employed in clinical practice.

▶ **Postoperative pain therapy.** Operations on the foot can be very painful postoperatively. Opioids are often inadequate for pain therapy (Bonica 1980, 1984). The use of continuous regional techniques for postoperative pain therapy is therefore particularly indicated in painful operations on the ankle and foot.

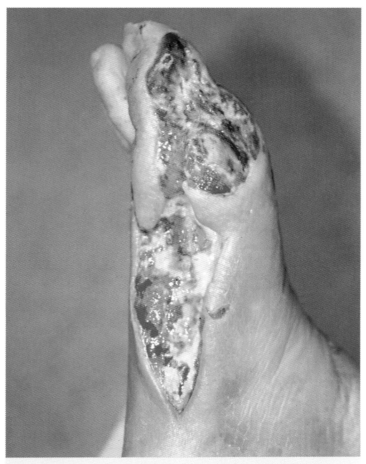

Fig. 12.17 Wound healing disorders due to a poor perfusion can be an indication for a blockade via a distal sciatic nerve catheter.

## Continuous Technique (Catheter Technique)

► **Fascial sheath.** The existence of a fascial sheath around the nerve(s) is an important requirement for the success of a continuous technique (catheter technique). The fascia has been demonstrated in several anatomical studies on dissected specimens (Rorie et al 1980; Vloka et al 1996a, Meier et al 1999a). Radiological examination with contrast reproducibly shows even spread in a space limited by the fascial sheath (Bauereis and Meier 1997). Injection and placement of the catheter within this fascial sheath is therefore recommended.

► **Injection site.** As the selected injection site is quite proximal where the two divisions of the sciatic nerve lie very close together, a double injection technique should be avoided to prevent intraneural injections.

The best response for a successful block is the subject of much discussion. Mach (2000) found no differences in success rates between stimulation of the tibial nerve and common fibular nerve in a study of 112 patients with a posterior popliteal block. As the diameter of the tibial nerve is about twice that of the common fibular nerve, it can be expected that the time required to complete a block of the tibial nerve will be longer.

► **Local anesthetic.** As with all techniques where the local anesthetic is injected into a space bounded by connective tissue or fascia, an adequate volume and adequate concentration of the local anesthetic should be selected. There is a great deal of fat tissue in the popliteal fossa (► Fig. 12.3a), which could be the reason for a relatively long onset time. For distal sciatic nerve blocks 30 to 40 mL of prilocaine 1% or mepivacaine 1% (10 mg/mL), or of ropivacaine 0.5% (5 mg/mL) or 0.75% (7.5 mg/mL), is recommended (Meier 1999b , Meier et al 1999b).

► **Effectiveness of the continuous posterior technique.** Singelyn et al (1997) investigated the course and effectiveness of a continuous posterior sciatic nerve block in 30 patients who had undergone operation on the foot. In 93% of cases, the technique was performed without problems. A motor response was produced at a needle depth of 4 to 5.5 cm. The patients were given 40 mL of mepivacaine 1% (10 mg/mL) with epinephrine and a continuous infusion of bupivacaine 0.25% (2.5 mg/mL). The anesthesia was sufficient in 28 patients (93%). Fewer than 10% of the patients required an opioid in the postoperative period. Singelyn recommends 0.125% (1.25 mg/mL) bupivacaine 7 mL/h for continuous administration and additional patient controlled boluses of 2.5 mL/30 min for 48 to 72 hours if needed (Singelyn 1998).

## Distal Sciatic Nerve Block (Meier 1996)

► **Injection site.** In the continuous technique for distal sciatic nerve block as described by Meier in 1996, the insertion site is relatively far proximal. Because the sciatic nerve (or its two divisions) runs lateral to the popliteal artery, the insertion site is lateral to the tip of the triangle that forms the proximal border of the popliteal fossa and medial to the biceps femoris. The insertion site lateral to the artery was selected in order to avoid inadvertent vascular puncture.

The sciatic nerve is reached at a depth of 5 to 6 cm when the needle is directed cranially at an angle of 30–40° to the skin (Meier et al 1999a). In large thighs, the distance to the sciatic nerve can be greater, particularly with a more tangential needle direction; 10-cm needles are needed for these patients. Advancing the needle at an acute angle to the nerve rather than perpendicular facilitates the insertion of a catheter (Bauereis and Meier 1997; Meier et al 1997, Meier 1999a, 2001).

► **Study.** In a study by Meier et al (1999b) of 303 patients, a distal sciatic nerve catheter was placed for an operation on the foot or ankle and subsequent pain therapy. The patients were given 10 mL of mepivacaine 2% (20 mg/mL) and 20 mL of mepivacaine 1% (10 mg/mL) for anesthesia. The postoperative pain therapy consisted of ropivacaine 0.375% (3.75 mg/mL) or bupivacaine 0.25% (2.5 mg/mL). The catheter remained in situ for an average of 4.5 days (max. 21 days).

> **Note**
>
> No side effects or complications were observed. Patient acceptability of this procedure was extraordinarily high—94% of the patients were satisfied or very satisfied.

► **Lateral approach.** In the lateral approach the patient can remain in supine position. Orientation is simple; it is important that the leg sags freely. The distance to the nerve can be 8 cm or more, depending on needle direction, so a 12-cm needle should be selected.

▶ **Operations in the ankle.** The extent to which distal sciatic nerve block can be employed in conjunction with a saphenous nerve block for anesthesia for operations in the ankle region (ankle fracture, Achilles tendon rupture) depends essentially on whether space will allow lower leg tourniquet.

> **Note**
>
> Lower leg tourniquet should not be less than 6 cm from the head of the fibula. If this distance is maintained, procedures can be performed on the ankle in lower leg exsanguination.

However, in ankle fractures or Achilles tendon rupture, disinfection and draping are usually so far proximal that there is no room for a tourniquet on the lower leg.

It has been reported that a proximal block of the sciatic nerve according to Labat, with its proven anesthetic effect on the posterior femoral cutaneous nerve, has no advantages in relation to the tolerance of a tourniquet. Hence it would follow that surgery in the area of the lower leg/foot with a proximal tourniquet on the thigh would be possible with a combination of femoral nerve/distal sciatic nerve block (Fuzier et al 2005).

The authors' clinical experience, however, shows that the thigh tourniquet is not tolerated without an additional analgesic.

> **Practical Note**
>
> All operations on the foot can be performed with lower leg tourniquet using distal sciatic nerve block in conjunction with saphenous nerve block. For pain therapy and sympathetic block, the distal sciatic block is ideal for the lower leg. The block may be performed on both legs at the same time without problems (▶ Fig. 12.18).

## Summary

Distal techniques of sciatic nerve block are excellent for operations on the lower leg and in the foot region. In combination with a saphenous nerve block (Chapter 13.5), surgery can be performed on a blood-free lower leg. The continuous techniques are suitable for pain therapy and regional sympathetic block. The procedures have few complications and are safe and effective when performed with nerve stimulation.

## 12.3.5 Distal Sciatic Nerve Block Using Ultrasound ▶

Linear transducer (e.g., 7.5–10 MHz)
Needle: 8 to 12 cm

The sciatic nerve has a round to oval, hyperechoic structure in the distal thigh region (about 10 cm proximal to the popliteal crease). It is found anterior (and slightly medial) to the long head of the biceps femoris, which can be identified by its typical, usually triangular shape (Moayeri et al 2010; ▶ Fig. 12.19). The sciatic nerve appears as a "shining moon" above (or slightly medial to) the highest part of the long head of the biceps femoris.

It is embedded here in ample fatty tissue. The start of the division into the common fibular nerve (lateral) and tibial nerve (medial) can often be visualized here (or further distal; ▶ Fig. 12.20). Deeper and somewhat medial to this are the popliteal artery and vein (▶ Fig. 12.19 and ▶ Fig. 12.21). The popliteal vein is lateral to the artery (▶ Fig. 12.19 ▶ ).

### Scanning Technique

The two already separate nerves (tibial nerve, common fibular nerve) can be easily visualized in the region of the popliteal crease, as they are relatively superficial ▶ . The tibial nerve lies medial, the common fibular nerve is lateral and has a diameter about half that of the tibial nerve. From here, the nerves can be followed proximally up to where they join as the sciatic nerve. The sciatic nerve can usually be easily visualized in this region because it is hyperechoic. Here the nerve is posterior and somewhat lateral to the popliteal artery (Tsui and Finucane 2006; ▶ Fig. 12.21). Another identifying feature of the sciatic nerve in this region is the "seesaw sign" (Schafhalter-Zoppoth et al 2004) ▶ .

▶ **Seesaw sign.** On active plantar and dorsiflexion of the foot, the two divisions of the sciatic nerve (tibial and fibular) move in opposite directions ▶ .

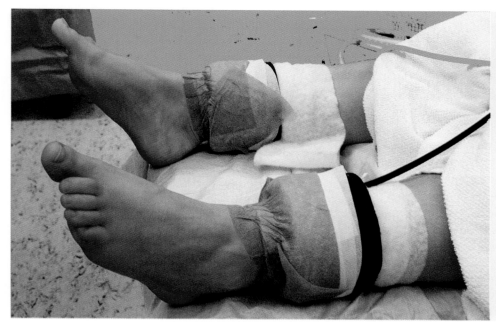

**Fig. 12.18** Bilateral distal sciatic nerve block can be performed in conjunction with a saphenous nerve block for operations on both feet at the same time. A tourniquet can be applied to the leg about four finger breadths above the malleoli and at least 6 cm below the head of the fibula (avoid fibular nerve injury!).

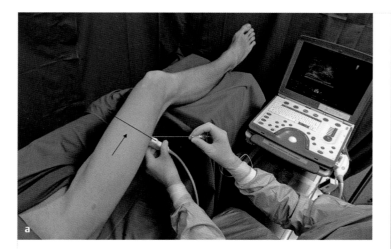
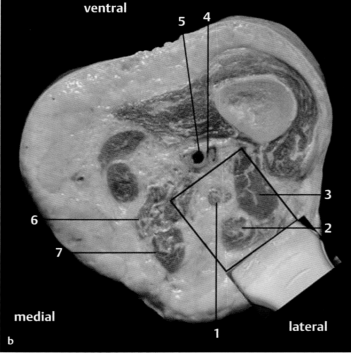
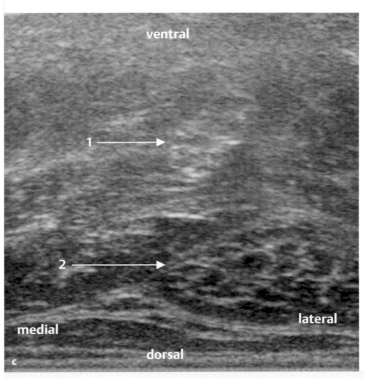
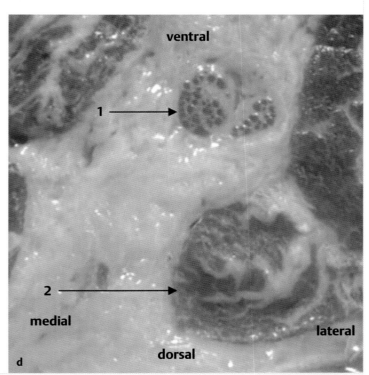

**Fig. 12.19** Plane through the thigh about 10 cm proximal to the knee joint line (→ view toward the plane; note that the bottom in the ultrasound image is near the transducer).
**a** Clinical setting.
**b** Anatomical cross-section.
**c** Corresponding ultrasound image.
**d** Anatomical cross-section corresponding to **c**.

1 Sciatic nerve
2 Long head of the biceps femoris muscle
3 Short head of the biceps femoris muscle
4 Popliteal vein
5 Popliteal artery
6 Semimembranosus muscle
7 Semitendinosus muscle

## Needle Approach

The needle insertion can be made in plane (▶ Fig. 12.22 ▶) or out of plane (▶ Fig. 12.23) in supine, prone, or lateral position. For *needle approach in supine position*, the leg must be positioned high enough (e.g., in a leg holder, ▶ Fig. 12.23) so enough space remains for the transducer. The nerve is always visualized in the short axis. Slight internal rotation of the leg can facilitate visualization.

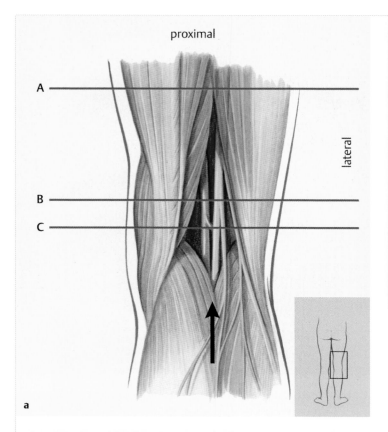

proximal

A

B

C

lateral

a

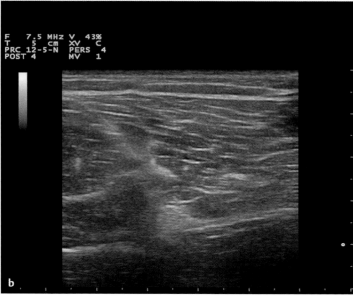

b

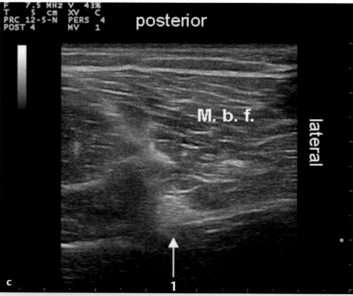

posterior

M. b. f.

lateral

c    1

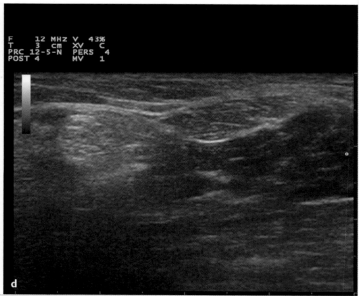

d

**Fig. 12.20 a–g** Sonographic visualization of the bifurcation of the sciatic nerve, from posterior (prone position). In the ultrasound images the top is near the transducer (arrow in a: Perspective as seen on the ultrasound images).
a Anatomical visualization.
b Plane A: penetration depth 5 cm (unlabeled).
c Plane A: penetration depth 5 cm (labeled).
d Plane B: penetration depth 3 cm (unlabeled).
e Plane B: penetration depth 3 cm (labeled).
f Plane C: penetration depth 3 cm (unlabeled).
g Plane C: penetration depth 3 cm (labeled).

1 Sciatic nerve
2 Tibial nerve
3 Common fibular nerve
M.b.f. = biceps femoris muscle

Continued >

▶ **In-plane technique.** In the in-plane technique, the needle insertion is made laterally about 10 cm proximal to the popliteal crease (somewhat proximal to where the sciatic nerve divides). The puncture site can be determined using the depth of the nerve measured by ultrasound, so that the needle direction is approximately parallel to the transducer (▶ Fig. 12.22).

▶ **Out-of-plane technique.** In the out-of-plane technique, the nerve is also visualized in the short axis. The insertion site is around 1 to 1.5 cm distal to the transducer and 0.5 to 1 cm lateral to the nerve. The tip of the needle can be well visualized as a hyperechoic point by tilting the transducer at the end of the needle hub (Girdharry and McQuillan 2004). Small "wobbling"

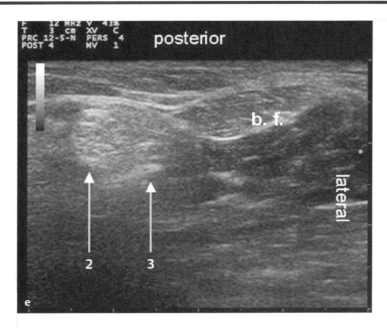

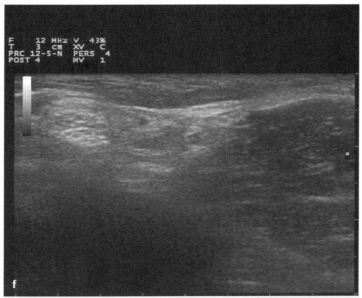

Fig. 12.20 a–g (continued)

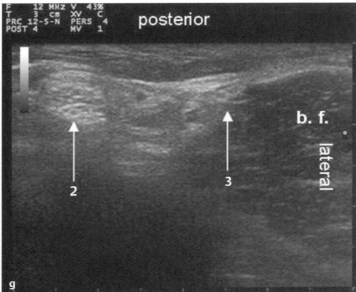

movements of the needle help identify the needle or the tip of the needle (▶ Fig. 12.23 and ▶ Fig. 12.24).

▶ **Spread of local anesthetic.** The local anesthetic should spread in a circle around the nerve like a donut to ensure the success of the block (▶ Fig. 12.21 and ▶ Fig. 12.24). The needle should approach the nerve tangentially to avoid mechanical damage to the nerve (▶ Fig. 12.22).

Many studies have proven a more rapid and better success of the block compared with the technique using nerve stimulation (Perlas et al 2008, Van Geffen et al 2009).

## Catheter Placement

Placing the catheter is sometimes difficult in the lateral in-plane technique ▶.

**Tips and Tricks**

- An out-of-plane approach a few centimeters distal to the bifurcation, in which the tip of the needle is directed between the two nerves (tibial nerve, common fibular nerve) leads to a fast, reliable block (Perlas et al 2013). Visualization is in the short axis. The catheter, advanced 2–3 cm proximally, lies in the immediate vicinity of the sciatic nerve (▶ Fig. 12.24). A comparable technique is described by Buys et al (2010) and Prasad et al (2010). However, both use the in-plane approach in which they look for the tibial nerve and common fibular nerve separately. This has proved to be unnecessary in the out-of-plane technique immediately distal to the bifurcation of the sciatic nerve. In ultrasound, good spread around both nerves can be seen without requiring a correction of the needle and without injuring the epineurium.
- The tibial and common fibular nerves can also be visualized in the long axis. The puncture can then be made in plane (▶ Fig. 12.25).

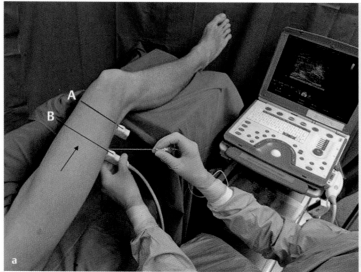

**Fig. 12.21** Finding the sciatic nerve. The popliteal artery anterior and medial to the sciatic nerve. (Note: the bottom of the ultrasound images is near the transducer.)

**a** Clinical setting.

**b** Plane A (popliteal crease): tibial nerve and common fibular nerve are already separated (unlabeled).

**c** As **b** (labeled).

**d** Plane B (about 10 cm proximal to the popliteal crease): tibial nerve and common fibular nerve are still united as the sciatic nerve, but the two divisions can be easily distinguished (unlabeled).

**e** As **d** (labeled).

1 Tibial nerve

2 Common fibular nerve

1 + 2 in **d/e** united as sciatic nerve

*Red*: Popliteal artery

l.h.b.f. = long head of the biceps femoris muscle

Area inside dotted line denotes the spread of local anesthetic

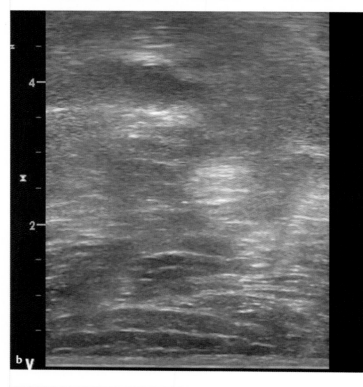

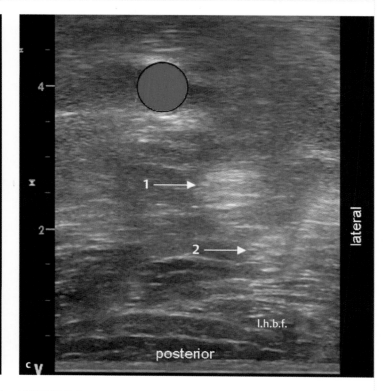

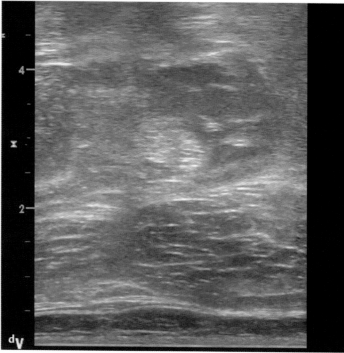

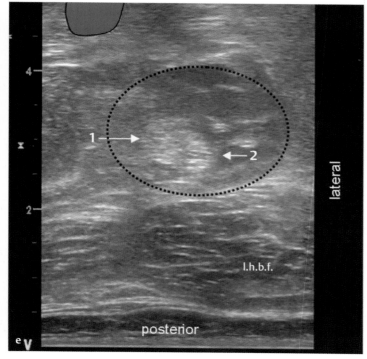

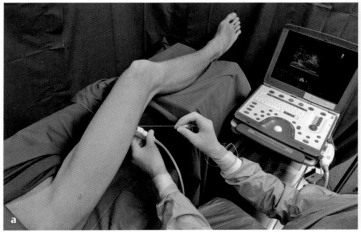

**Fig. 12.22** Distal block of the sciatic nerve (in-plane technique).
(Note: the bottom in the ultrasound image is near the transducer.)
**a** Clinical setting.
**b** Ultrasound image (unlabeled).
**c** Ultrasound image (labeled).
1 Sciatic nerve
l.h.b.f. = Long head of the biceps femoris muscle
Area inside dotted line denotes the spread of local anesthetic (donut sign)
White line = needle

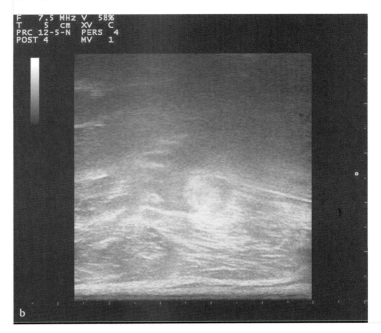

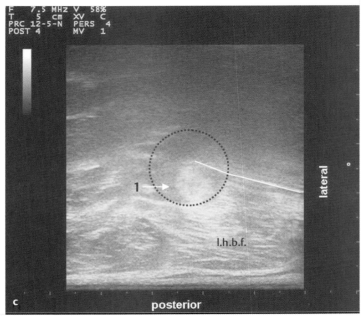

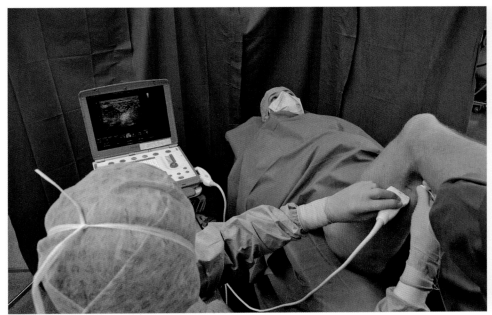

**Fig. 12.23** Distal block of the sciatic nerve in supine position, out of plane.

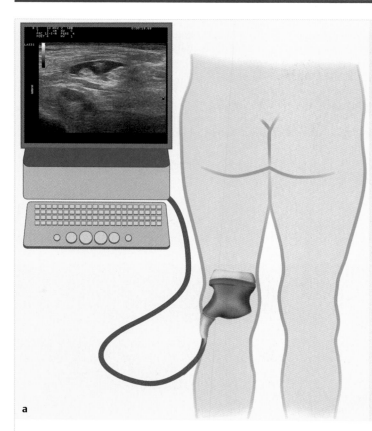

**Fig. 12.24** Puncture at the left slightly distal to the bifurcation of the sciatic nerve (in prone position!).
**a** Clinical setting.
**b** Insertion site after injection of about 10 mL local anesthetic (unlabeled).
**c** Insertion site after injection of about 10 mL local anesthetic (labeled).
**d** Tip of the catheter about 3 to 5 cm proximal to the insertion site on the sciatic nerve (unlabeled).
**e** Tip of the catheter about 3 to 5 cm proximal to the insertion site on the sciatic nerve (labeled).

1 Popliteal vein
2 Common fibular nerve
3 Popliteal artery
4 Tip of the needle
5 Local anesthetic (dotted line)
6 Tibial nerve
7 Tip of the catheter
8 Sciatic nerve

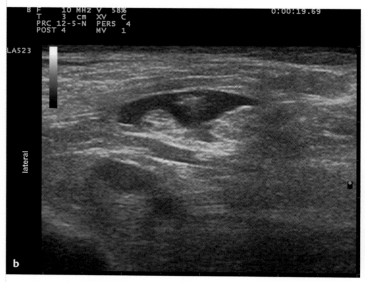

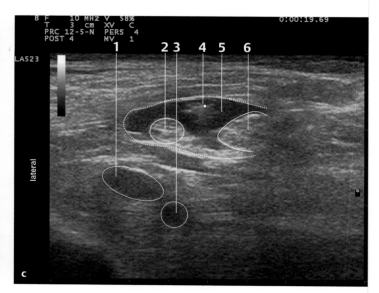

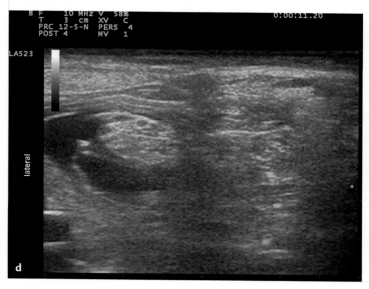

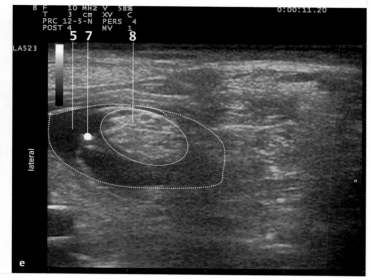

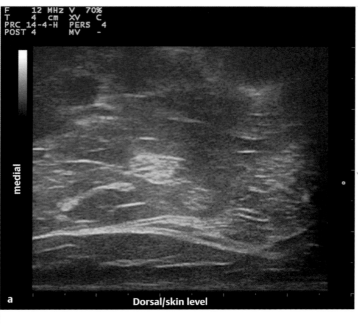
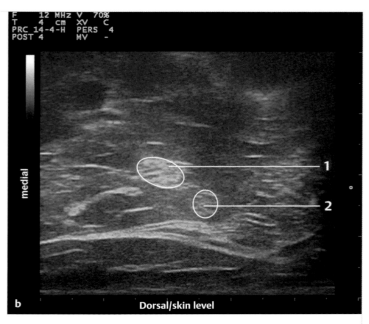
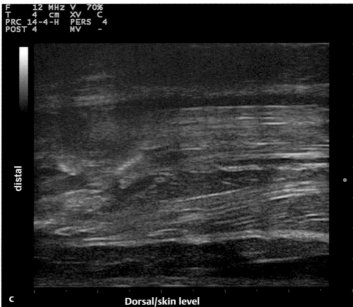
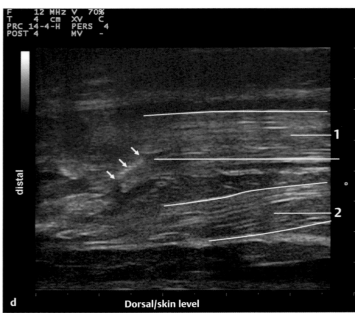

**Fig. 12.25** Visualization of the tibial nerve and the common fibular nerve slightly distal to the bifurcation of the sciatic nerve. (Note: the transducer level is at the bottom of the images.)

a Visualization in the short axis (unlabeled).
b Visualization in the short axis (labeled).
c Visualization in the long axis (unlabeled).
d Visualization in the long axis (labeled).

1 Tibial nerve
2 Common fibular nerve
Arrows: tip of the needle (Sonoplex needle, Pajunk GmbH)

# References

Bailey SL, Parkinson SK, Little WL, Simmerman SR. Sciatic nerve block. A comparison of single versus double injection technique. Reg Anesth 1994; 19: 9–13

Bauereis Ch, Meier G. The continuous distal sciatic nerve block for anaesthesia and postoperative pain management. Intern Monitor Reg Anesth 1997; 9: 96

Bonica JJ. The Management of Pain. Philadelphia: Lea and Febiger;1980: 1205–1209

Bonica JJ. Local anaesthesia and regional blocks. In: Wall PD, Melzack R. Textbook of Pain. Edinburgh: Churchill Livingstone; 1984: 541–557

Buys MJ, Arndt CD, Vagh F, Hoard A, Gerstein N. Ultrasound-guided sciatic nerve block in the popliteal fossa using a lateral approach: onset time comparing separate tibial and common peroneal nerve injections versus injecting proximal to the bifurcation. Anesth Analg 2010; 110: 635–637

Fuzier R, Hoffreumont P, Bringuier-Branchereau S, Capdevila X, Singelyn F. Does the sciatic nerve approach influence thigh tourniquet tolerance during below-knee surgery? Anesth Analg 2005; 100: 1511–1514

Girdharry D, McQuillan P. Popliteal fossa block. Tech Reg Anesth Pain Manage 2004; 8: 164–168

Gligorijevic P. Lower extremity blocks for day surgery. Tech Reg Anesth Pain Manage 2000; 4: 30–37

Jan RA, Kerner M, Provenzano DA et al. Popliteal nerve block and its safety in foot and ankle surgery. Anesth Analg 2000; 59: 371–376

Labat G. Regional Anesthesia: Its Technique and clinical Application. Philadelphia: Saunders; 1924: 45

Mach D. Is the type of motor response an important factor in determining the quality of the sciatic nerve block with a relatively small volume of local anaesthetics. Int Monitor Reg Anesth 2000; 12: 203

Meier G. Der kontinuierliche Ischiadicusblock zur Anästhesie und postoperativen Schmerztherapie. Anaesthesist 1996; 45 S2: 100

Meier G et al. The continuous distal sciatic nerve block for anaesthesia and postoperative pain management. The International Monitor 1997; 9: 96

Meier G. Der distale Ischiadicusblock (DIB) mit Katheter (DIK). In: Büttner J, Meier G, eds. Kontinuierliche periphere Techniken zur Regionalanästhesie und Schmerztherapie—Obere und untere Extremität. Bremen: Uni-Med; 1999a: 140–144

Meier G. Der distale Ischiadicuskatheter (DIK). In: Mehrkens HH, Büttner J, eds. Kontinuierliche periphere Leitungsblockaden. Munich: Arcis; 1999b: 43–46

Meier G, Bauereis Ch, Meier Th et al. Schmerztherapie mit distalen Ischiadicuskathetern—Anatomische Voraussetzungen. Schmerz 1999a; 51: 75

Meier G, Bauereis Ch, Meier Th. Kontinuierliche distale Ischiadicusblockaden zur Schmerztherapie. Schmerz 1999b; S1: 74–75

Meier G. Peripheral nerve block of the lower extremities. [Article in German] Anaesthesist 2001; 50: 536–557, quiz 557, 559

Moayeri N, van Geffen GJ, Bruhn J, Chan VW, Groen GJ. Correlation among ultrasound, cross-sectional anatomy, and histology of the sciatic nerve: a review. Reg Anesth Pain Med 2010; 35: 442–449

Neuburger M, Hendrich E, Lang D et al. Lateral approach to blockade of the sciatic nerve. Biometric data using magnetic resonance imaging. [Article in German] Anaesthesist 2005; 54: 877–883

Perlas A, Brull R, Chan VW, McCartney CJ, Nuica A, Abbas S. Ultrasound guidance improves the success of sciatic nerve block at the popliteal fossa. Reg Anesth Pain Med 2008; 33: 259–265

Perlas A, Wong P, Abdallah F, Hazrati LN, Tse C, Chan V. Ultrasound-guided popliteal block through a common paraneural sheath versus conventional injection: a prospective, randomized, double-blind study. Reg Anesth Pain Med 2013; 38: 218–225

Prasad A, Perlas A, Ramlogan R, Brull R, Chan V. Ultrasound-guided popliteal block distal to sciatic nerve bifurcation shortens onset time: a prospective randomized double-blind study. Reg Anesth Pain Med 2010; 35: 267–271

Rorie DK, Byer DE, Nelson DO, Sittipong R, Johnson KA. Assessment of block of the sciatic nerve in the popliteal fossa. Anesth Analg 1980; 59: 371–376

Schafhalter-Zoppoth I, Younger SJ, Collins AB, Gray AT. The "seesaw" sign: improved sonographic identification of the sciatic nerve. Anesthesiology 2004; 101: 808–809

Singelyn FJ, Gouverneur JM, Gribomont BF. Popliteal sciatic nerve block aided by a nerve stimulator: a reliable technique for foot and ankle surgery. Reg Anesth 1991; 16: 278–281

Singelyn FJ, Aye F, Gouverneur JM. Continuous popliteal sciatic nerve block: an original technique to provide postoperative analgesia after foot surgery. Anesth Analg 1997; 84: 383–386

Singelyn FJ. Continuous femoral and popliteal sciatic nerve blockades. Tech Reg Anesth Pain Manage 1998; 2: 90–95

Tsui BC, Finucane BT. The importance of ultrasound landmarks: a "traceback" approach using the popliteal blood vessels for identification of the sciatic nerve. Reg Anesth Pain Med 2006; 31: 481–482

van Geffen GJ, van den Broek E, Braak GJJ, Giele JL, Gielen MJ, Scheffer GJ. A prospective randomised controlled trial of ultrasound guided versus nerve stimulation guided distal sciatic nerve block at the popliteal fossa. Anaesth Intensive Care 2009; 37: 32–37

Vloka JD, Hadzić A, Kitain E et al. Anatomic considerations for sciatic nerve block in the popliteal fossa through the lateral approach. Reg Anesth 1996a; 21: 414–418

# 13 Peripheral Block (Conduction Block) of Individual Nerves of the Lower Limb

## 13.1 Lateral Cutaneous Nerve of the Thigh ▶

### 13.1.1 Anatomy

The lateral cutaneous nerve of the thigh (L2–L3) is a purely sensory nerve, which crosses the iliacus muscle lateral to the psoas after leaving the lumbar plexus. The nerve lies below the iliac fascia here and emerges through the fascia immediately below and medial to the anterior superior iliac spine, where it divides into anterior and posterior branches that run a few centimeters subcutaneously distal to the anterior superior iliac spine. The anterior branches supply the skin of the lateral thigh down to the knee where they are responsible for innervation of the knee region together with other sensory branches (also known as pre-patellar plexus). The posterior branches innervate the skin of the lateral hip region below the greater trochanter as far as the middle of the thigh (▶ Fig. 13.1, ▶ Fig. 13.2, ▶ Fig. 13.3, ▶ Fig. 13.4).

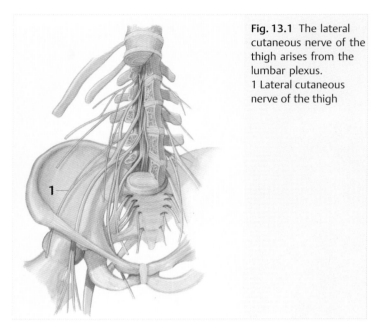

**Fig. 13.1** The lateral cutaneous nerve of the thigh arises from the lumbar plexus.
1 Lateral cutaneous nerve of the thigh

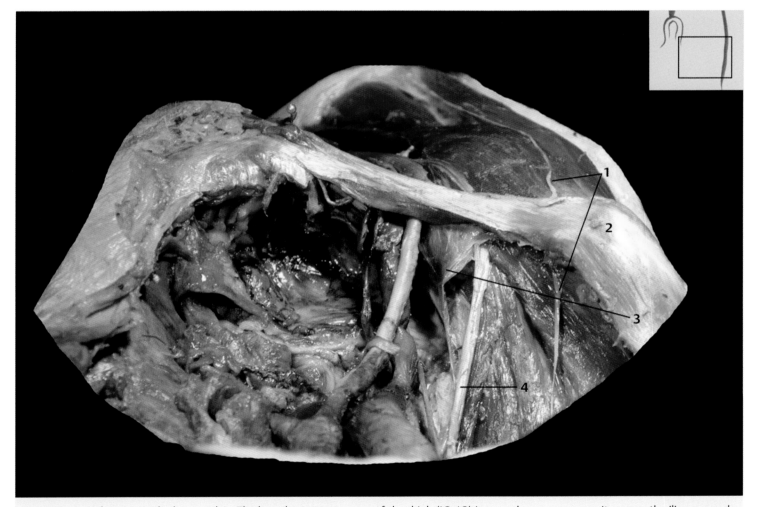

**Fig. 13.2** Cranial view into the lesser pelvis. The lateral cutaneous nerve of the thigh (L2–L3) is a purely sensory nerve. It crosses the iliacus muscle lateral to the psoas muscle after leaving the lumbar plexus. The nerve lies under the iliac fascia and passes through the fascia immediately below and medial to the anterior superior iliac spine and divides into anterior and posterior branches.
1 Lateral cutaneous nerve of the thigh
2 Anterior superior iliac spine
3 Iliac fascia
4 Femoral nerve

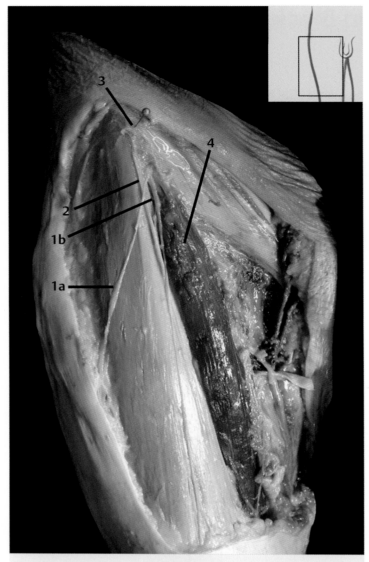

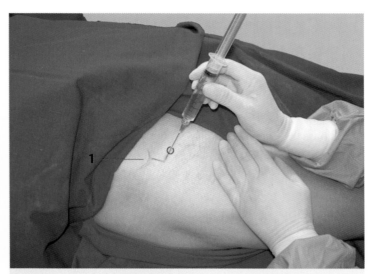

**Fig. 13.4** Right iliac crest. The anterior superior iliac spine on the side to be anesthetized is palpated and the puncture site is located 2 cm distally and 2 cm medially. At the marked site, a 4 to 6 cm long 24 G needle is advanced vertical to the skin. A loss of resistance can be felt when the tip of the needle passes through the fascia. Following negative aspiration, a total of 15 mL of a medium-acting or long-acting local anesthetic is injected, subfascially at first and then in a fan pattern above the fascia after withdrawing the needle. The procedure corresponds to a field block.
1 Anterior superior iliac spine

**Fig. 13.3** Right iliac crest. The lateral cutaneous nerve of the thigh passes through the fascia immediately distal and medial to the anterior superior iliac spine and divides into anterior and posterior branches, which run subcutaneously for a few centimeters distal to the anterior superior iliac spine.
1a Posterior branch of the lateral cutaneous nerve of the thigh
1b Anterior branch of the lateral cutaneous nerve of the thigh
2 Thick fascia lata
3 Anterior superior iliac spine
4 Sartorius muscle

## 13.1.2 Techniques

### Block of the Lateral Cutaneous Nerve of the Thigh (Classical Technique)

#### Landmarks and Position

Anterior superior iliac spine: the insertion site is 2 cm distal and 2 cm medial to the anterior superior iliac spine.

The patient lies supine (▶ Fig. 13.4).

#### Procedure

The anterior superior iliac spine on the side to be anesthetized is palpated and the insertion site is established 2 cm distally and 2 cm medially. Following disinfection, local subcutaneous anesthesia is given. At the marked site, a 24 G needle 4 to 6 cm long is

advanced vertical to the skin (▶ Fig. 13.4). A loss of resistance can be felt when the needle passes through the fascia. Following negative aspiration, a total of 15 mL of a medium-acting or long-acting local anesthetic is injected, subfascially at first and then in a fan pattern above the fascia after withdrawing the needle. The procedure corresponds to a field block (Hallén et al 1991, Cousins and Bridenbaugh 1998, Rosenquist and Lederhaas 1999).

### Block of the Lateral Cutaneous Nerve of the Thigh (Alternative Technique)

#### Procedure

The point 2 cm distal und 2 cm medial to the anterior superior iliac spine is again selected as the insertion site. A 6-cm needle is directed cranially, pierces the fascia lata, and is advanced until a bony resistance indicates that the iliac crest has been reached. Local anesthetic (5 mL) is injected between the fascia lata and the iliac crest. This is repeated twice with 5 mL local anesthetic each time and the needle is directed further medially each time. This produces a depot of 15 mL local anesthetic below the inguinal ligament.

## 13.1.3 Indications, Contraindications, Side Effects

### Indications

- Supplemental analgesia of the lateral side of the thigh in the case of incomplete lumbar plexus block
- Skin graft harvesting on the lateral thigh, muscle biopsy
- Meralgia paresthetica (diagnostic and therapeutic, e.g., after total hip replacement)

## Contraindications and Side Effects

No specific contraindications or clinically important side effects are known.

---

**Tips and Tricks**

- As the anterior parts of the nerve terminate in the prepatellar area, block of the lateral cutaneous nerve of the thigh is usually necessary for extensive (open) operations on the knee (Ellis and Feldman 1996).
- The majority of the local anesthetic must be injected under the fascia.
- The procedure is also possible with peripheral nerve stimulation (PNS; Shannon et al 1995). The pulse duration must be set to 1.0 ms. If the needle is in the correct location, the patient feels tingling paresthesia in the lateral part of the thigh (see below).
- Ultrasound guidance is very suitable for this procedure (Chapter 13.1.5).

---

## 13.1.4 Remarks on the Technique

The course of the nerve is very variable. This refers both to its individual division and to its area of innervation. In 4 to 6% of cases it is believed not to be present at all and can possibly be regarded as a branch of the femoral nerve (Bonniot 1922/23, Hovelacque 1927). Failure of anesthesia after a selective block can thus be explained anatomically. The close relationship between the femoral nerve and the lateral cutaneous nerve of the thigh is emphasized by reports on block effects in the region of the femoral nerve after conduction anesthesia of the lateral cutaneous nerve of the thigh (Sharrock 1980, Lonsdale 1988, Konder et al 1990).

To ensure a higher success rate, Shannon et al (1995) described an alternative PNS technique, which is initially performed transdermally. Morris et al (1999) point out that the paresthesia is reported synchronously with the nerve stimulator pulse and that injection of only 6 mL of local anesthetic leads to successful anesthesia. The possible advantages are a lower volume of local anesthetic and a higher success rate. Shannon reports an increase in the success rate from 85 to 100%. However, Rosenquist regards the procedure as relatively complex. For this reason, PNS is not recommended for routine use (Rosenquist and Lederhaas 1999) and is now replaced by ultrasound guidance.

An isolated block of the lateral cutaneous nerve of the thigh is useful as pain therapy for the treatment of meralgia paresthetica and for anesthesia—for example, for muscle biopsy and superficial operations on the lateral thigh (Jenkner 1983, Bonica 1984, Rybock 1989).

## 13.1.5 Block of the Lateral Cutaneous Nerve of the Thigh Using Ultrasound

Linear transducer: 12 MHz
Penetration depth: 3 to 5 cm
Needle: 5 cm

### Scanning Technique

The lateral cutaneous nerve of the thigh is found in the short axis medial and distal to the anterior superior iliac spine (▶ Fig. 13.5).

The patient lies supine. The lateral cutaneous nerve of the thigh crosses the sartorius muscle from medial to lateral, immediately medial and distal to the anterior superior iliac spine (▶ Fig. 13.6). The course of the lateral cutaneous nerve of the thigh varies greatly; it sometimes crosses within or below the sartorius muscle (▶ Fig. 13.7).

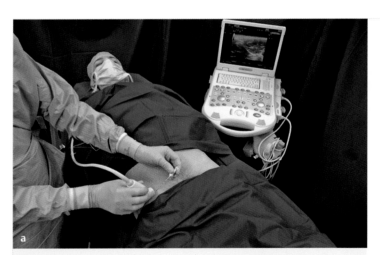
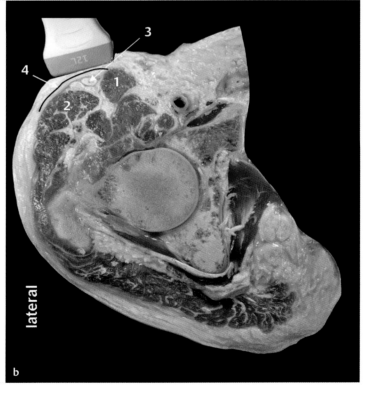

**Fig. 13.5** Visualization of the lateral cutaneous nerve of the thigh using ultrasound (short axis, in-plane puncture). For details see ▶ Fig. 13.6.
**a** Clinical setting.
**b** Anatomical cross-section below the inguinal ligament.
1 Sartorius muscle
2 Tensor fasciae latae
3 Lateral cutaneous nerve of the thigh
4 Fascia lata

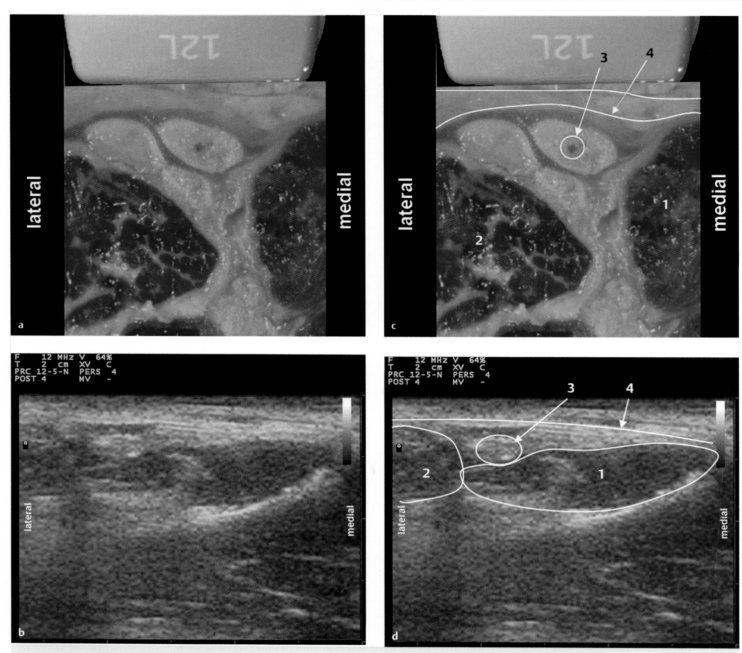

**Fig. 13.6** Visualization of the lateral cutaneous nerve of the thigh using ultrasound.
**a** Anatomical enlargement of ▶ Fig. 13.5. *Note:* The lateral cutaneous nerve of the thigh lies lateral to the sartorius muscle in the triangle between the sartorius and the tensor fasciae latae.
**b** Ultrasound image (short axis) corresponding to **a**.
**c** As **a** (labeled) *Note:* The lateral cutaneous nerve of the thigh lies on the sartorius muscle.
**d** As **b** (labeled).
1 Sartorius muscle
2 Tensor fasciae latae
3 Lateral cutaneous nerve of the thigh
4 Fascia lata

The nerve should not be looked for immediately at the attachment of the sartorius muscle to the superior iliac spine, because it is difficult to distinguish the nerve here in the hyperechoic muscle fascia tissue. Somewhat further medially and distally, the nerve can be visualized as a round hyperechoic structure (diameter 1–3 mm) on, in, or below the sartorius muscle. A few centimeters further distal, it is already lateral to the sartorius in the angle between the sartorius and the tensor fasciae latae muscles (▶ Fig. 13.6).

> **Note**
>
> The best visualization of the lateral cutaneous nerve of the thigh is 1 to 2 cm medial and 4.5 to 5.5 cm distal to the anterior superior iliac spine. The skin–nerve distance here is 0.5 to 0.7 cm (Ng et al 2008).

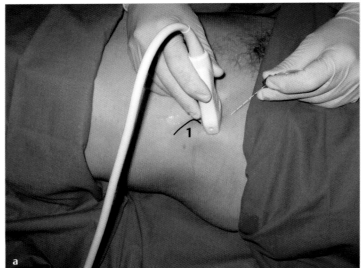

**Fig. 13.7** Visualization of the lateral cutaneous nerve of the thigh using ultrasound (short axis, out-of-plane approach).
**a** Clinical setting.
**b** Visualization of the cutaneous nerve of the thigh in ultrasound (short axis; unlabeled).
*Note:* The lateral cutaneous nerve of the thigh lies below the sartorius muscle.
**c** Visualization of the cutaneous nerve of the thigh in ultrasound (short axis; labeled).
1 Anterior superior iliac spine
2 Lateral cutaneous nerve of the thigh
3 Sartorius muscle
4 Iliac bone

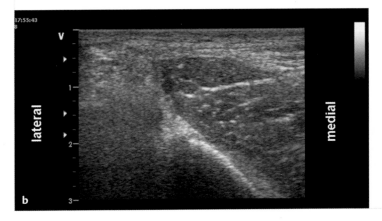

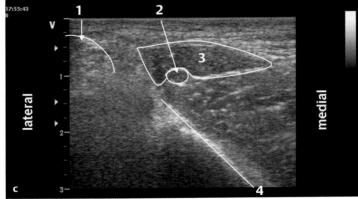

## Needle Approach

The needle insertion can be made in plane (▶ Fig. 13.5; ▶) or out of plane (▶ Fig. 13.7).

▶ **Volume.** Two to 5 mL local anesthetic.

### Tips and Tricks

- The sartorius muscle has a typical triangular to oval shape; it can be followed from distal to proximal with the transducer, 3 to 5 cm before the attachment to the anterior superior iliac spine, the nerve can be found on the muscle. Alternatively, it runs in or below the sartorius. Due to the more hypoechoic structure of the muscle tissue, it can be visualized better in this case.
- The lateral cutaneous nerve of the thigh crosses the sartorius muscle from medial to lateral, so it can also be found lateral to the sartorius further distally.
- If the nerve cannot be visualized, a depot of local anesthetic can be injected between the fascia lata (which appears as a strong hyperechoic band in front of the sartorius) and the sartorius.

# 13.2 Infiltration of the Iliac Crest

## 13.2.1 Indication

Anesthesia and pain therapy for iliac crest bone graft harvesting.

## 13.2.2 Procedure

The area intended for removal of bone chips from the iliac crest is first infiltrated subcutaneously with a medium-acting or long-acting local anesthetic (▶ Fig. 13.8). This is followed by injection as far as the periosteum of the iliac crest. This injection is given as a field block in order to infiltrate the entire harvesting area.

When bone graft harvesting is complete, the surgeon can place a catheter between the subcutaneous fat and the reconstructed musculofascial and periosteal tissue, tunneling the catheter out through the skin (▶ Fig. 13.9).

Pain therapy can commence postoperatively with an intermittent injection of 20 mL of a long-acting local anesthetic. Alternatively, continuous local infiltration of the periosteum through an elastomer pump has proved useful. With this type of system, subcutaneous tunneling of the catheter outside the operation area (▶ Fig. 13.10) is possible.

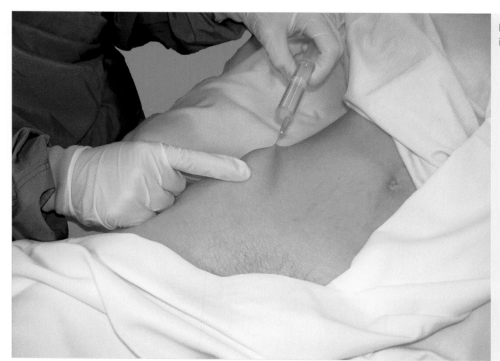

**Fig. 13.8** Infiltration of the right iliac crest; the injection must include the periosteum.

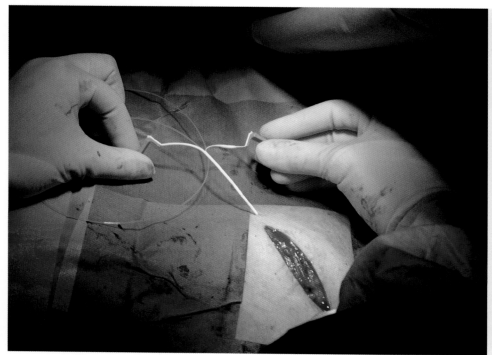

**Fig. 13.9** Inserting a catheter for local pain therapy after harvesting bone chips from the iliac crest.

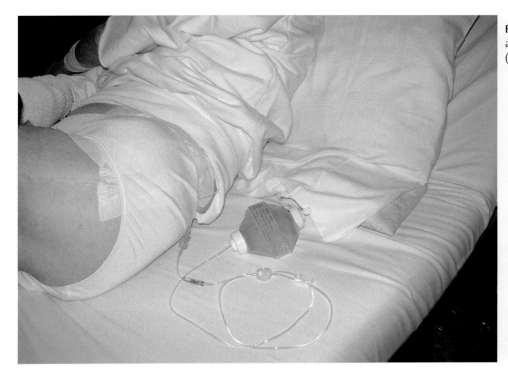

**Fig. 13.10** Continuous administration of local anesthetic by means of an elastomer pump (ropivacaine 2 mg/mL; 5 mL/h).

▶ **Local Anesthetics, dosage.** Anesthesia (single shot): 20 mL of ropivacaine 0.75% (7.5 mg/mL).

Analgesia: 20 mL of ropivacaine 0.375% (3.75 mg/mL) bolus or 5 mL of ropivacaine 0.2% (2 mg/mL) continuously.

---

**Tips and Tricks**

- Bone chip harvesting from the iliac crest is an operation that causes severe postoperative pain. Anesthesia should therefore be provided with a long-acting local anesthetic.
- Continuous administration is very effective. In comparison to results from a placebo group, the continuous application of a local anesthetic at the graft harvesting site at the iliac crest appeared to be effective against pain at that site, even 3 months postoperatively (Blumenthal et al 2005). The elastomer pump system enables insertion outside the operation field and is therefore preferred by some surgeons. There is no increased risk of infection (Hachenberg et al 2010).
- Continuous wound infusion can be an alternative for pain therapy in operations in which regional anesthesia is not generally given (Gottschalk and Gottschalk 2010).
- An alternative is the transversus abdominis plane block, which should be performed only under ultrasound guidance (Chapter 13.3).

---

# 13.3 Transversus Abdominis Plane Block (TAP Block) ▶

## 13.3.1 Anatomy

The abdominal wall is supplied by the anterior branches of spinal nerves T7–T12 (intercostal nerves) and L1–L3 (iliohypogastric nerve [T12/L1], ilioinguinal nerve [L1], genitofemoral nerve [L1/L2], and lateral cutaneous nerve of the thigh [L2/L3]). These nerves lie between the internal oblique and the transversus abdominis muscles and give off cutaneous branches to the

surface during their course (▶ Fig. 13.12). The classical lateral TAP block usually leads only to a block of segments T10–L1. An additional subcostal block (possibly on both sides) is required for a block of segments T6–T9 (Børglum et al 2012). In this region, the transversus abdominis muscle lies directly below the rectus abdominis muscle (Hebbard et al 2010; ▶ Fig. 13.11).

## 13.3.2 Landmarks

The subcostal TAP block is performed immediately below the costal arch in the mid-clavicular line. The transversus abdominis lies directly below the rectus abdominis here. The layer between the two muscles is looked for (▶ Fig. 13.11).

The classical lateral TAP block is performed at the lateral abdominal wall in the middle axillary line between the iliac crest and the 12th rib. The abdominal wall is formed from outside to inside by the following muscles: external oblique, internal oblique, transversus abdominis (▶ Fig. 13.12). Below this is the peritoneal cavity with the corresponding organs (intestines, liver).

## 13.3.3 Indications and Contraindications

### Indications

Pain therapy after:
- Inguinal hernias (Heil et al 2010)
- Open appendectomies (Niraj et al 2009)
- Laparoscopic cholecystectomies (El-Dawlatly et al 2009)
- Bone chip harvesting from the anterior iliac crest (Chiono et al 2010)
- Open retropubic prostatectomies (bilateral; O'Donnell et al 2006)
- Caesarean section (bilateral; Belavy et al 2009)
- Colectomy (bilateral; McDonnell et al 2007)
- Surgical gynecological procedures in the lower abdomen (bilateral; Griffiths et al 2010)

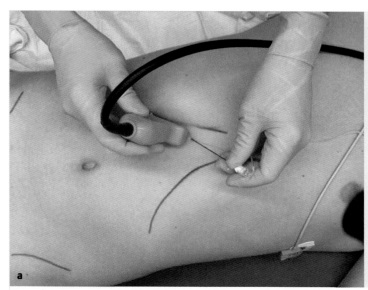

**Fig. 13.11** Subcostal TAP (transversus abdominis plane) block.
**a** Clinical setting.
**b** Ultrasound image (unlabeled).
**c** Ultrasound image (labeled) indicating the needle direction (in plane).
1 Subcutaneous fatty tissue
2 Rectus abdominis muscle
3 Transversus abdominis muscle
4 Peritoneal cavity with intestine

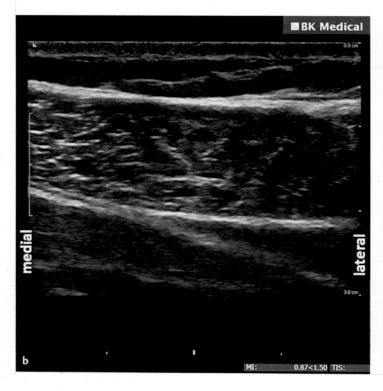

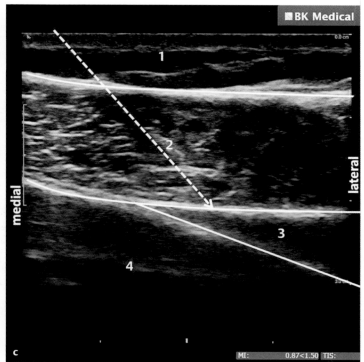

## Contraindications

• Unclear anatomical conditions (e.g., extreme obesity, scars), infections of the abdominal wall, hernias in the puncture region

## Complications

• Perforation of the abdominal wall with injury to organ structures such as intestine or liver
• Femoral nerve block

## 13.3.4 Procedure

The TAP block should be performed only under ultrasound guidance, as otherwise a high rate of failure and complications can be expected.

## Ultrasound-Guided Transversus Abdominis Plane Block ▶

Linear transducer: 6 to 13 MHz
Needle: 6 to 12 cm

## Classical Lateral Transversus Abdominis Plane Block

The abdominal wall is visualized in the axial plane using ultrasound in the middle between the iliac crest and the lower costal arch in the mid-axillary line. The anterior part of the transducer should not extend beyond the anterior axillary line.

Before needle insertion, the following structures (from outside to inside) should be clearly defined (▶ Fig. 13.12):

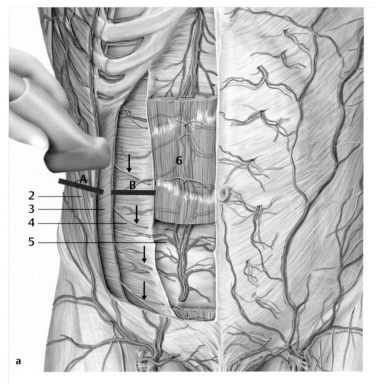

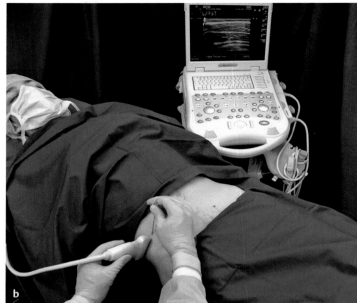

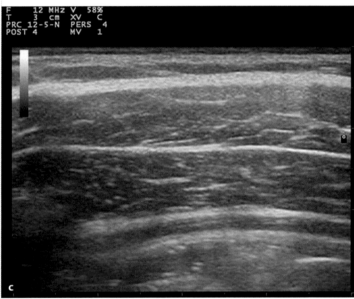

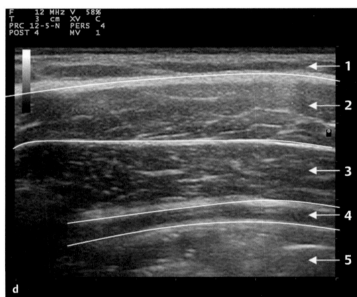

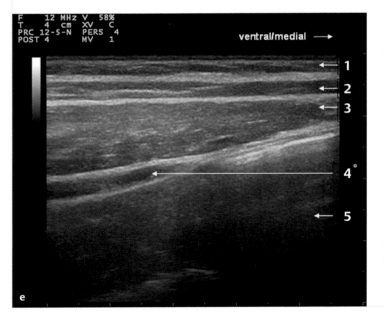

**Fig. 13.12** Classical lateral TAP (transversus abdominis plane) block.
Source: Schünke et al 2011.
a Anatomy.
b Clinical setting.
c Ultrasound image (unlabeled).
d Ultrasound image (labeled).
e Ultrasound image for transducer position B.
1 Subcutaneous fatty tissue
2 External oblique muscle
3 Internal oblique muscle
4 Transversus abdominis muscle
5 Peritoneal cavity with intestine
6 Rectus abdominis muscle
A Transducer position in c and d
B Transducer position in e
↓ Nerve (intercostal nerves T10–12, ilioinguinal nerve)

- Fatty tissue
- External oblique muscle
- Internal oblique muscle
- Transversus abdominis muscle
- Intraperitoneal structures (intestine)

In case of doubt, the transducer can be moved toward the middle of the abdominal wall where the origins of the muscles are visualized and then followed laterally (▶ Fig. 13.12).

After positioning the transducer, the puncture is made in plane; the puncture site should not be too close to the end of the transducer, so that a needle direction which is as tangential as possible can be maintained ▶. The tip of the needle must be in the plane between the internal oblique and transversus abdominis muscles. The tip of the needle should be positioned posterior to the mid-axillary line as otherwise the lateral cutaneous branches of the intercostal nerves, which reach the surface from the layer between the internal oblique and the transversus abdominis muscles at around the mid-axillary line, will not be anesthetized.

The correct position of the needle is checked using 2 to 3 mL of local anesthetic, then the main dose of local anesthetic is injected (▶ Fig. 13.13; ▶).

A catheter can be placed for a continuous technique (▶ Fig. 13.14).

## Subcostal Transversus Abdominis Plane Block

The transducer is positioned subcostally at about the mid-clavicular line at the lower costal arch. The puncture is made in plane from medial to lateral. The local anesthetic is injected in the layer between the rectus abdominis and the transversus abdominis, which lies here directly below the rectus abdominis (▶ Fig. 13.11).

▶ **Local anesthetic, dosage.** Ropivacaine 0.375% (3.75 mg/mL) or mepivacaine 1% (10 mg/mL) at a volume of 20 mL (unilateral) to 40 mL (bilateral). For a complete block of the anterior abdominal wall (4 injections), 60 mL of ropivacaine 0.375% (3.75 mg/mL, 225 mg) have been described (Børglum et al 2012). All dosages apply to adults (> 50 kg).

Caution: Toxic plasma levels of ropivacaine have been measured at a total dose of 3 mg/kg body weight, corresponding to about 200 mg ropivacaine (Griffiths et al 2010; see also Chapter 21.6).

Continuous block: Ropivacaine 0.33% (3.3 mg/mL), 6 to 8 mL/h (max. 12 mL/h).

### Tips and Tricks

- Well suited for postoperative therapy after harvesting bone chips from the iliac crest. Catheter placement is recommended, as the duration of the effect of a single-shot technique is generally not sufficiently long, even if a longer-acting local anesthetic (e.g., ropivacaine) is used.
- The catheter should be tunneled and drained out so that it can be fixated as far as possible from the operation region (▶ Fig. 13.14).
- For bilateral blocks, toxic plasma levels have been measured using a dosage of 3 mg/kg body weight of ropivacaine (corresponds approx. to 40 mL ropivacaine 0.5% (5 mg/mL) at 70 kg; Griffiths et al 2010).
- The block can also be made under general anesthesia.
- In the classical TAP block, a block of the femoral nerve is occasionally observed.
- Skin, muscles, and the parietal peritoneum are anesthetized.
- The visceral peritoneum is not anesthetized (if there is peritonitis, a dull peritoneal pain remains!).

# 13.4 Obturator Nerve Block ▶

## 13.4.1 Anatomy

The obturator nerve (L2–L4) arises from the lumbar plexus and is a nerve with both sensory and motor fibers. It runs on the medial border of the psoas major down through the lesser pelvis, penetrates the parietal pelvic fascia, and is accompanied by the obturator artery and vein. It passes together with them through the obturator foramen and obturator canal to the thigh (▶ Fig. 13.15).

Here the nerve divides into the anterior (superficial) branch, which innervates the anterior adductors and the hip joint and ends in a cutaneous main branch that provides a variable sensory supply to the medial side of the thigh, and the posterior (deep) branch (▶ Fig. 13.16), which is responsible for the posterior adductors and sends a branch to the posterior knee joint.

## 13.4.2 Techniques

### Obturator Nerve Block (Classical Technique)

### Landmarks and Position

The pubic tubercle is the bony landmark for obturator nerve block. The pubic tubercle on the side to be blocked is palpated

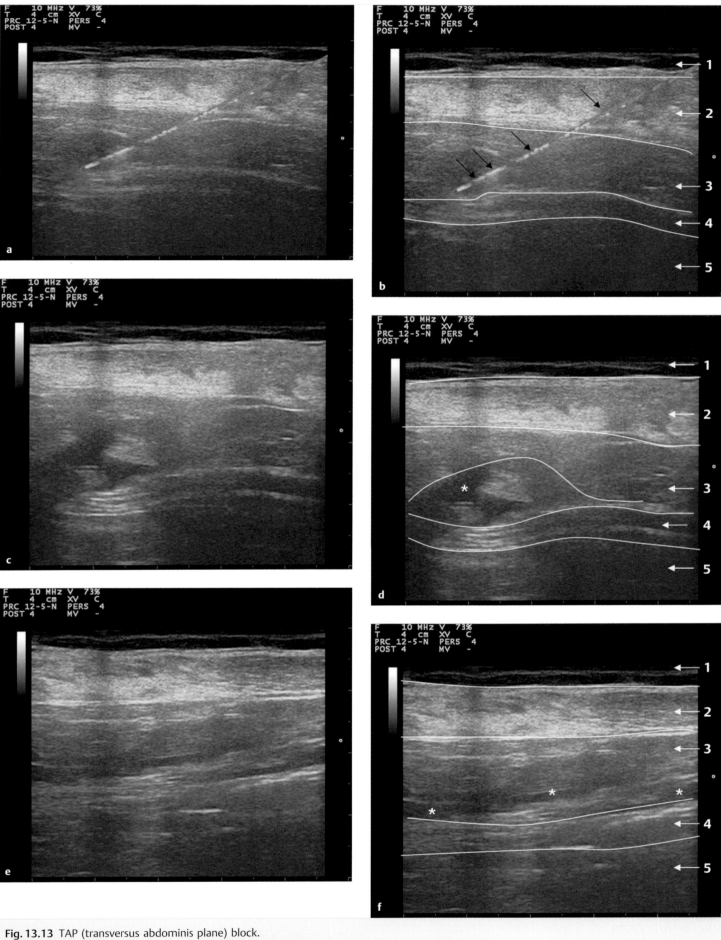

**Fig. 13.13** TAP (transversus abdominis plane) block.
**a** Direction of needle before injection (unlabeled).
**b** Direction of needle before injection (labeled).
**c** After injection of 5 mL local anesthetic (unlabeled).
**d** After injection of 5 mL local anesthetic (labeled).
**e** Spread of local anesthetic after injection of 15 mL (unlabeled).
**f** Spread of local anesthetic after injection of 15 mL (labeled).

1 Subcutaneous fatty tissue
2 External oblique muscle
3 Internal oblique muscle
4 Transversus abdominis muscle
5 Peritoneal cavity with intestine
↓ Needle, * local anesthetic

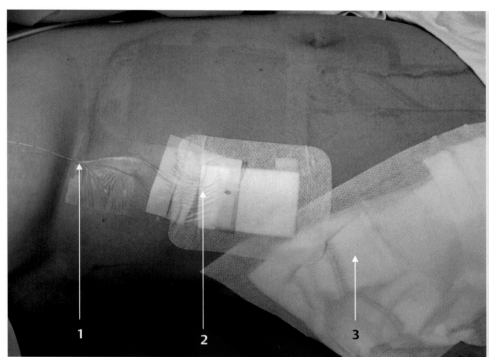

**Fig. 13.14** Continuous TAP block for harvesting bone chips from the iliac crest (note the cranial tunneling of the catheter).
1 Catheter
2 Dressing for catheter
3 Dressing for iliac crest

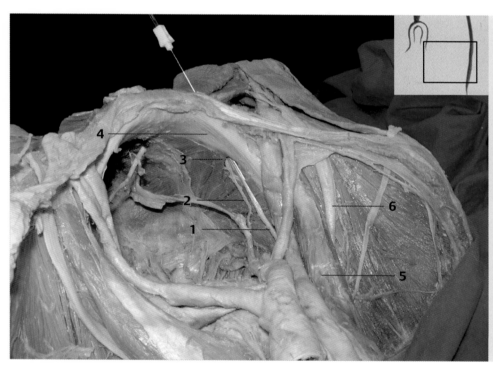

**Fig. 13.15** View from above into the pelvis minor: the obturator nerve leaves the pelvis minor through the obturator canal together with blood vessels. The further course of the nerve is indicated by a needle introduced into the obturator canal from the opposite end.
1 Obturator nerve
2 Blood vessels
3 Obturator canal
4 Pubic bone
5 Psoas major muscle
6 Femoral nerve

and the puncture site is marked 1.5 cm lateral and distal to the pubic tubercle (► Fig. 13.17).

The patient lies supine. The leg is slightly abducted.

## Procedure

An 8-cm needle is inserted perpendicular to the underlying surface at the puncture site and advanced (► Fig. 13.18). After 2 to 5 cm it reaches the horizontal superior ramus of the pubic bone. The distance to the pubic ramus is recorded and the needle is withdrawn somewhat; then the needle is slowly advanced in a more laterocaudal direction (more laterally and only slightly caudally) as far as 2 to 3 cm beyond the previously recorded depth. Here it passes the lower border of the pubic ramus and is close to the obturator canal (► Fig. 13.19 and ► Fig. 13.20).

Following contractions of the adductors and after negative aspiration, 15 mL of a medium-acting or long-acting local anesthetic is injected. Because of the proximity of the obturator artery, there is a risk of accidental intravascular injection (► Fig. 13.21 and ► Fig. 13.22) and a hematoma may develop. If the needle is advanced too far, it can pass through the obturator canal into the lesser pelvis minor, with the risk of injuring internal organs (► Fig. 13.21).

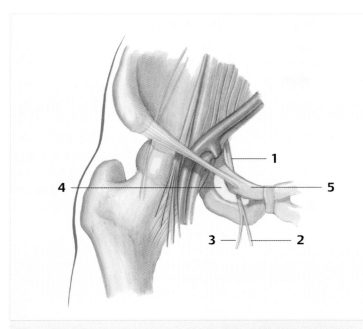

**Fig. 13.16** The obturator nerve comes from the lumbar plexus, passes separately from the other nerves of the lumbar plexus on the inside of the psoas major muscle, and leaves the lesser pelvis through the obturator canal, from where it provides the motor supply to the adductor muscles. The sensory innervation of the obturator nerve is variable: occasionally it is responsible for the sensory supply of medial parts of the knee joint. Whether it can be assigned a sensory area of skin is doubtful; if so, it is on the medial side of the knee. However, there is obvious overlapping with the areas of innervation of other nerves.
1 Obturator nerve
2 Anterior branch (superficial)
3 Posterior branch (deep)
4 Obturator foramen
5 Pubic bone

## Obturator Nerve Block (Alternative Technique)

### Landmarks and Position

Proximal attachment of the tendon of adductor longus, femoral artery, anterior superior iliac spine.

The patient lies supine. The leg on the side to be anesthetized is abducted and externally rotated (▶ Fig. 13.23).

### Procedure

The proximal attachment (origin) of the tendon of adductor longus is palpated. After disinfection and local anesthesia, an 8–12 cm long needle is inserted immediately lateral to or above the tendon attachment (▶ Fig. 13.24). The needle is directed toward the ipsilateral anterior superior iliac spine. The angle of the needle to the long axis of the leg is thus around 45°. The needle is advanced posteriorly in the horizontal plane, or at an angle of about 15 to 20° (▶ Fig. 13.23, ▶ Fig. 13.24, ▶ Fig. 13.25). At a depth of 3 to 8 cm, contractions of the adductors at 0.3 mA/ 0.1 ms indicate the proximity of the anterior branch of the obturator nerve (Bridenbaugh and Wedel 1998, Meier 1999; ▶ Fig. 13.26). Alternatively, the block can be performed under ultrasound guidance (see below).

After negative aspiration, 15 mL of a medium-acting or long-acting local anesthetic is injected. This leads reliably to a complete block of both divisions of the obturator nerve. In ▶ Fig. 13.27, spread toward the obturator canal is visualized using contrast medium. If a continuous technique is performed, the catheter is advanced 3 to 5 cm cranially through the needle after the injection (▶ Fig. 13.28).

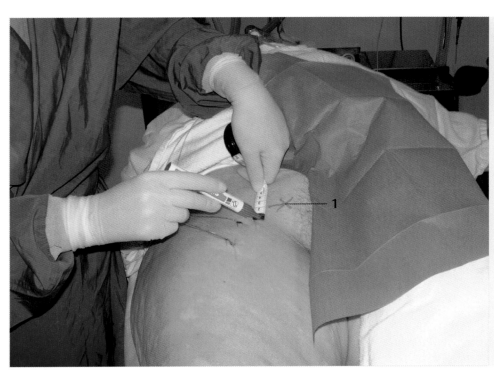

**Fig. 13.17** The pubic tubercle is used for orientation in the classical technique of obturator nerve block. The insertion site is located 1.5 cm lateral and 1.5 cm caudal to the pubic tubercle. Note the femoral nerve and sciatic nerve catheters already in situ.
1 Pubic tubercle

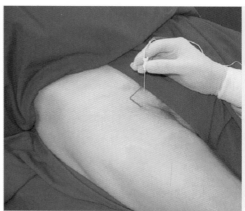

**Fig. 13.18** Obturator nerve block is performed in supine position with the leg slightly abducted. Puncture is performed perpendicular to the underlying surface with an 8-cm insulated needle connected to a nerve stimulator.

# Obturator Nerve Block with Ultrasound

Linear transducer: 7.5 to 10 MHz
Penetration depth: 4 to 8 cm
Needle: 5 to 10 cm

## Scanning Technique

The patient lies supine, the leg to be operated on is extended and slightly abducted in external rotation. The femoral vein is looked for on the medial side in the proximal thigh 2 to 4 cm below the inguinal crease. From here, the transducer is slid medially to find the adductors. Visualization is in the short axis (► Fig. 13.29).

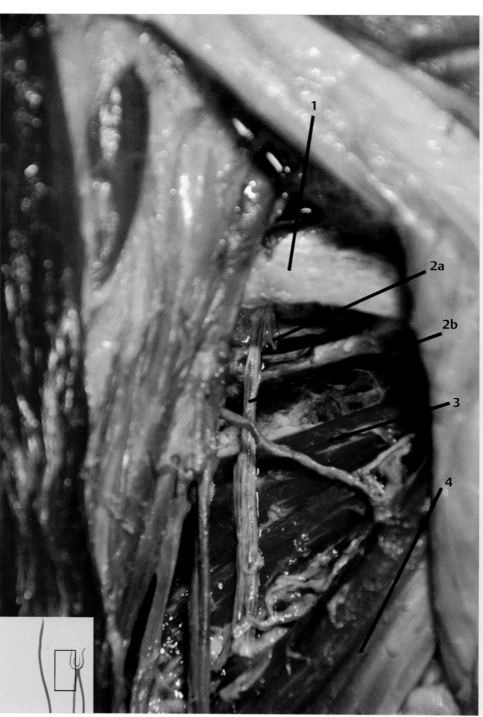

**Fig. 13.19** Right subinguinal region. The obturator nerve leaves the pelvis minor through the obturator canal and immediately divides into its two branches.
1 Superior pubic ramus
2a Posterior branch of the obturator nerve
2b Anterior branch of the obturator nerve
3 Adductor brevis muscle
4 Adductor longus muscle

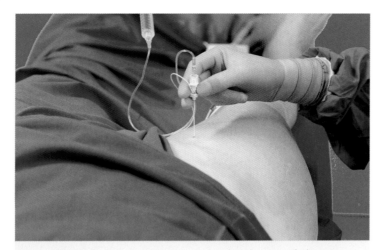

Fig. 13.20 Right leg, cranial view. Classical technique of obturator nerve block. After about 2 to 5 cm, the horizontal superior pubic ramus is reached. Following bone contact, the needle is withdrawn somewhat, the distance to the pubic ramus is recorded, and the needle is again advanced in the laterocaudal direction (more laterally and only slightly caudally) 2 to 3 cm beyond the previously recorded distance. It passes the lower border of the pubic ramus and lies close to the obturator canal. Following contractions of the adductors and negative aspiration, 15 mL of medium-acting or long-acting local anesthetic is injected.

The adductors typically have three layers:
- The upper layer is formed by the pectineus and/or adductor longus (depending on how far distally the transducer is moved).
- The middle layer is formed by the adductor brevis.
- The deepest layer is formed by adductor magnus.

The anterior branch of the obturator nerve is in the layer between the pectineus / adductor longus muscle and the adductor brevis muscle. The posterior branch of the obturator nerve is in the layer between the adductor brevis muscle and the adductor magnus muscle. The septa between the muscles appear hyperechoic (light in comparison with the muscle tissue). Nevertheless, the branches of the obturator nerve can often be found within these septa as flat, oval hyperechoic structures (▶ Fig. 13.30).

The anterior branch is located at a depth of 1 to 2 cm, the posterior branch at 2 to 4 cm below the skin (Soong et al 2007).

## Needle Approach

For a block of both branches of the obturator nerve, the fascia layers between the pectineus / adductor longus and the adductor brevis muscles and between the adductor brevis and the adductor magnus muscles are found. Local anesthetic

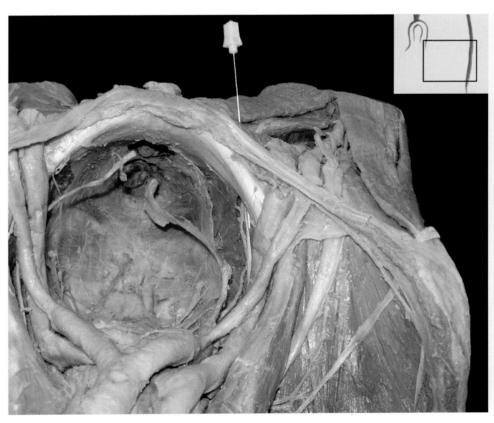

Fig. 13.21 View from above into the lesser pelvis. If the needle is advanced too far, the needle can pass through the obturator canal into the lesser pelvis minor with the risk of injuring internal organs.

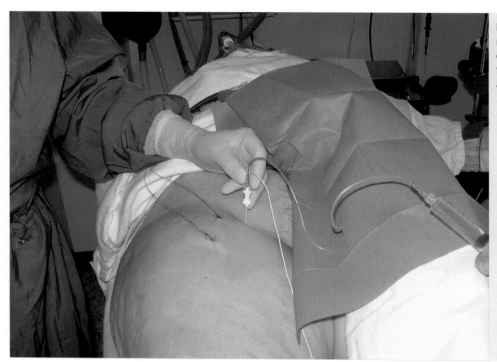

**Fig. 13.22** As the obturator nerve is accompanied by blood vessels when it passes through the obturator canal, vascular puncture with hematoma or intravascular injection of the local anesthetic is possible.

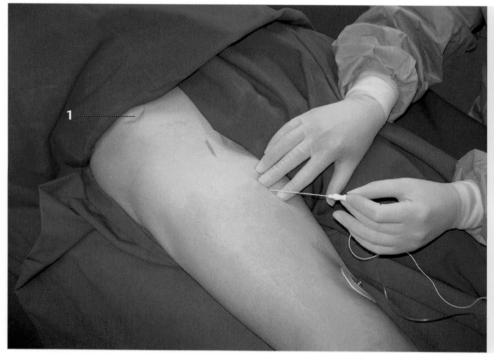

**Fig. 13.23** Alternative technique of obturator nerve block. The proximal attachment (origin) of the adductor longus is palpated. The needle is inserted immediately laterally to the tendon origin with a needle of 8 to 12 cm length. The needle is directed toward the ipsilateral anterior superior iliac spine; the puncture angle to the long axis of the leg is thus about 45°; the needle direction is slightly posterior in the horizontal plane. At a depth of 3 to 8 cm, contractions of the adductors at 0.7 mA/0.1 ms indicate the proximity of the obturator nerve.
1 Anterior superior iliac spine

(5–10 mL) is injected into each of them. This occasionally leads to a better visualization of the nerve (hydrodissection technique).

Similar to the complete block achieved by blocking only of the anterior branch of the obturator nerve described in Chapter 13.4.2, blocking this branch alone is sufficient here as well.

The needle approach can be out of plane (▶ Fig. 13.29) or in plane.

▶ **Volume.** Five to 10 mL local anesthetic per fascia layer, 15 mL for blocking only the anterior branch of the obturator nerve.

## Catheter Placement

A catheter can be placed.

**Tips and Tricks**

- It is useful to use a nerve stimulator (dual-guidance technique).
- Using color Doppler, vessels can be detected in the intermuscular septa that are in the immediate vicinity of nerves (Soong et al 2007).
- The nerves need not be identified directly; the important thing is to inject the local anesthetic into the correct layer or layers.

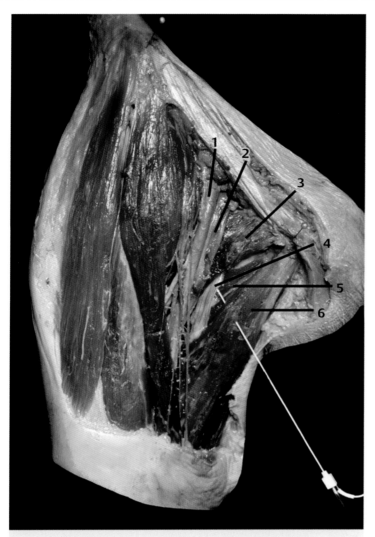

**Fig. 13.24** Alternative technique of obturator nerve block (see
► Fig. 13.23).
1 Femoral artery
2 Femoral vein
3 Pectineus muscle
4 Anterior branch of the obturator nerve
5 Adductor brevis muscle
6 Adductor longus muscle

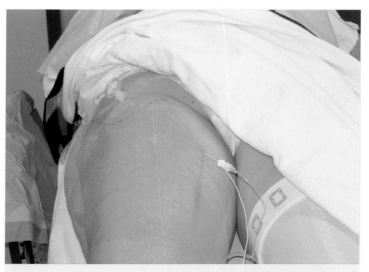

**Fig. 13.25** Needle direction for obturator nerve block (alternative technique).

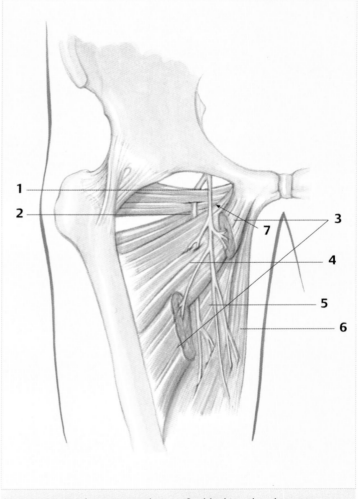

**Fig. 13.26** An alternative technique for blocking the obturator nerve by locating the nerve behind the tendon of adductor longus. The anterior branch is reached and stimulated; after injection of 10 to 15 mL of local anesthetic there should be a complete block of the two divisions of the nerve. The tendon of adductor longus can always be palpated readily when the leg is slightly abducted.
1 Obturator nerve, anterior branch (superficial)
2 Obturator nerve, posterior branch (deep)
3 Adductor longus muscle
4 Adductor brevis muscle
5 Adductor magnus muscle
6 Gracilis muscle
7 Site of needle insertion for the alternative technique

## 13.4.3 Indications and Contraindications

### Indications

- Incomplete lumbar plexus blockade
- Diagnosis and treatment of pain syndromes in the hip and groin (subinguinal) region (Hong et al 1996)
- Adductor spasm (Vloka and Hadzic 1999)
- Transurethral resection of bladder wall tumors (to eliminate the obturator reflex in spinal anesthesia; Augspurger and Donohue 1980)

### Contraindications

- General contraindications (Chapter 20.2)
- Coagulation disorders

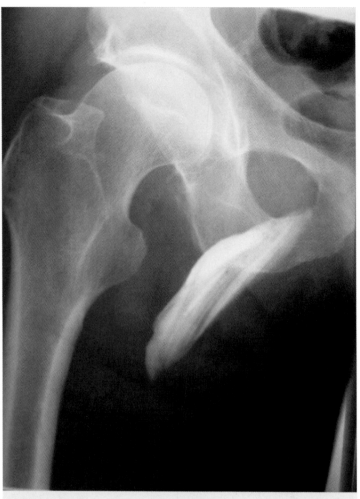

**Fig. 13.27** Spread of contrast after obturator nerve block (alternative technique).

## 13.4.4 Side Effects and Complications

Intravascular injection, hematoma (mainly with the classical technique), nerve injury (Sunderland 1968).

### Tips and Tricks

- In the classical technique, the contact between the needle tip and the superior pubic ramus ensures that the needle has reached the obturator canal and has not perforated adjacent soft tissues such as the bladder or vagina (Bridenbaugh and Wedel 1998; ► Fig. 13.21).
- Successful block can be identified by the reduced adduction force (Platzer 1999).
- It should be ensured that the skin and mucous membranes of the genital region do not come into contact with the disinfectant.
- The modified technique has the advantage that the needle direction does not have to be altered and the usually painful contact with the periosteum is avoided. The complications described in the classical technique (injury of internal organs) can thus also be avoided.
- The modified technique enables catheter placement (Meier 1999).
- When the thigh is abducted (modified technique) the origin of the adductor longus projects obviously under the skin and the muscle gap between adductor longus and sartorius can be readily palpated (Platzer 1999).

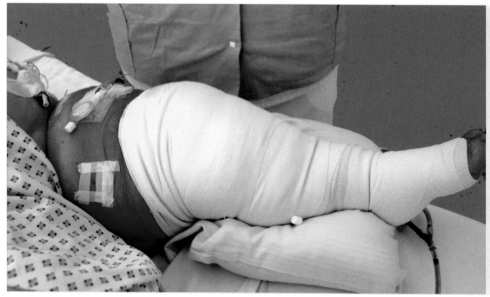

**Fig. 13.28** Obturator nerve catheter at the left (in a short patient, 120 cm tall, and special total knee replacement).

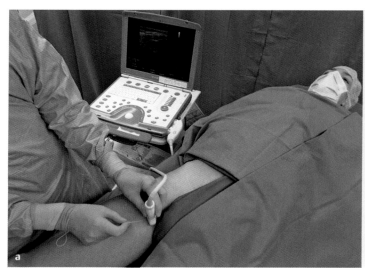

Fig. 13.29 Block of the obturator nerve using ultrasound: anatomical overview. (For details, see ► Fig. 13.30.)
a Clinical setting.
b Anatomical cross-section (unlabeled).
c Anatomical cross-section (labeled).
1 Pectineus / adductor longus muscle
2 Adductor brevis muscle
3 Adductor magnus muscle
4 Intermuscular septum with the anterior branches of the obturator nerve
5 Intermuscular septum with the posterior branches of the obturator nerve
6 Femoral vessels

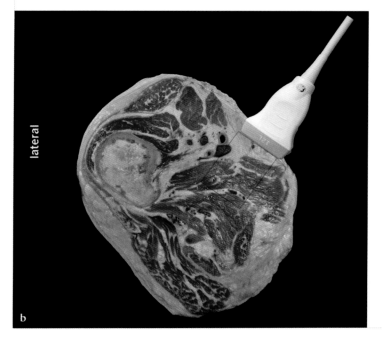

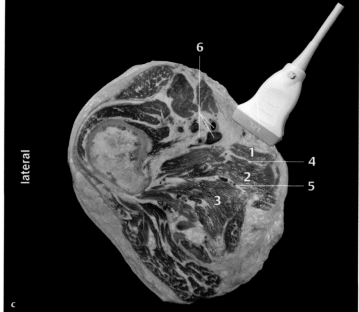

## 13.4.5 Remarks on the Technique

An accessory obturator nerve arises from the roots of L3 and L4 in 30% of patients (Sunderland 1968, Felsenthal 1974). This was described for the first time by Schmitt in 1744 (Bier 1908). The accessory nerve gives branches to the hip and does not pass through the obturator foramen but runs together with the femoral nerve and can thus also be blocked by a femoral nerve block (Cousins and Bridenbaugh 1998). If adductor spasm persists although the obturator nerve has been anesthetized, this can be attributed to the accessory branch of the nerve (Vloka and Hadzic 1999).

To achieve adequate block of the obturator nerve, a volume of 10 to 15 mL of local anesthetic is required (Bonica 1980, Löfström 1980, Hoffmann and Meyer 1980, Auberger and Niesel 1982, Jenkner 1983, Paul et al 1996). Yazaki et al (1985) injected 1% (10 mg/mL) lidocaine at the point of maximum adductor contraction with electrical stimulation until the muscle response disappeared completely. With this procedure, 96% of 78 blocks were successful. This agrees with the results of Parks and Kennedy (1967), who have reported a success rate of over 95%.

► **Supplementary obturator nerve block.** It is often assumed that neuraxial anesthesia leads to elimination of the obturator reflex. This is not the case as the interruption of nerve conduction is blocked proximal to the transurethral electrical stimulus. Particularly in urological operations (e.g., transurethral resection of bladder wall tumors) under spinal anesthesia, a supplementary obturator nerve block can therefore be useful for suppressing an obturator reflex (Augspurger and Donohue 1980, Gasparich et al 1984).

## Selective Block of the Nerve

An important practical indication is selective block of the obturator nerve in incomplete lumbar plexus anesthesia. This applies particularly to the so-called "3-in-1 block" (see Chapter 10).

The sensory supply of the medial side of the thigh is very variable and is therefore unsuitable for monitoring the success of an obturator block (Bergmann 1994, Morris and Lang 1999, Geiger et al 2000). The spread of the zone of analgesia can extend from the medial side of the thigh to the upper tibial third of the lower leg, but in some cases the sensory area of skin can be so small

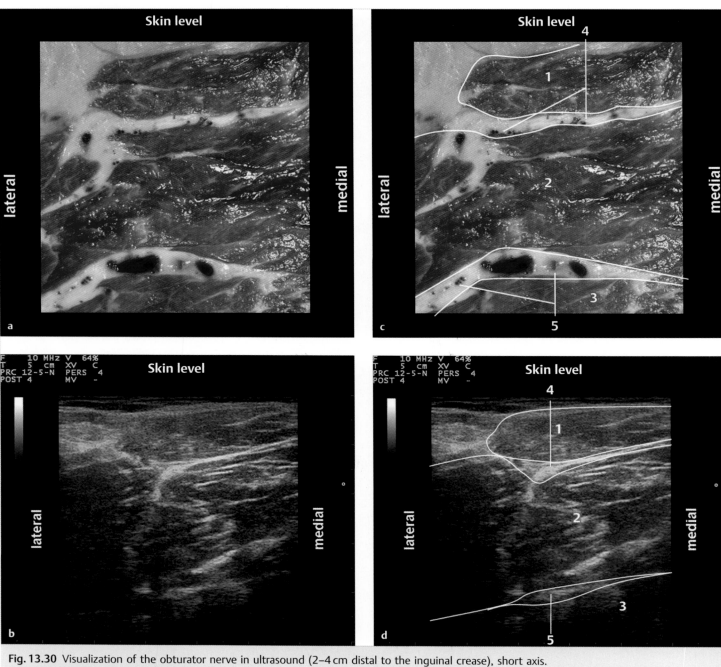

**Fig. 13.30** Visualization of the obturator nerve in ultrasound (2–4 cm distal to the inguinal crease), short axis.
a Anatomical detail of ▶ Fig. 13.29 (unlabeled).
b Corresponding ultrasound image (unlabeled).
c As a (labeled).
d As b (labeled).

1 Pectineus / adductor longus muscle
2 Adductor brevis muscle
3 Adductor magnus muscle
4 Anterior branch of the obturator nerve
5 Posterior branch of the obturator nerve

that cutaneous anesthesia is absent, even though motor block of the adductors indicates an adequate block. However, an insufficient block can lead to pain problems when using a thigh tourniquet, depending on the extent of skin innervation (Vloka and Hadzic 1999). The extent to which the knee joint periosteum is supplied by the obturator nerve is still not completely known.

If a patient complains of pain particularly on the medial side of the knee after an inguinal paravascular block for a knee operation, an insufficient block of the obturator nerve should be suspected (Chapter 10). If selective anesthesia of the nerve is successfully performed in this case, the block serves as both

diagnosis and pain therapy. This also applies for the diagnosis of pain in the hip region (Trainer et al 1986). Anesthesia of the obturator nerve in patients with hemiparesis and adductor spasm can be very effective.

The variant of the technique (see above) is a development described by Wassef (1993), who described it as an "interadductor approach"; this has been performed successfully in quadriplegia and multiple sclerosis for the treatment of adductor spasm. The development leads to simplification of the technical procedure, enables placement of a catheter, and expands the range of indications for the method (Büttner and Meier 1999, Meier and Büttner 2001).

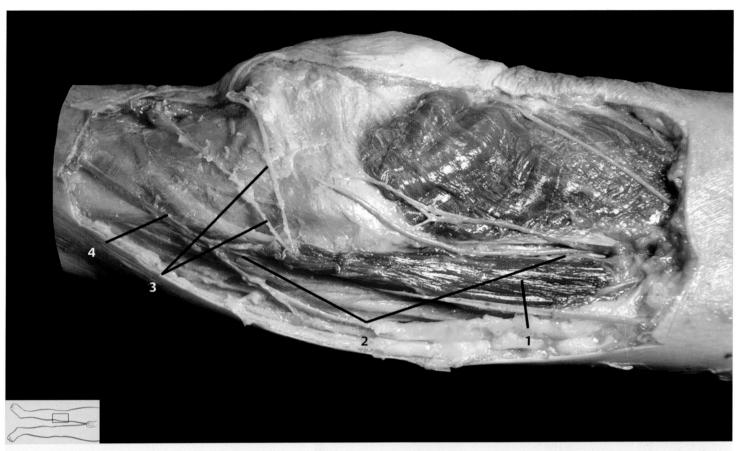

**Fig. 13.31** Right knee, medial view. The saphenous nerve runs under the sartorius muscle, crosses under it, and passes through the fascia lata (knee fascia) behind its tendon at the level of the patella.
1 Sartorius muscle
2 Saphenous nerve
3 Infrapatellar branch of the saphenous nerve
4 Long saphenous vein

# 13.5 Saphenous Nerve Block ▶

## 13.5.1 Anatomy

The saphenous nerve (L2/L4) is a sensory terminal branch of the femoral nerve that travels with the femoral artery and femoral vein in the thigh along with the infrapatellar nerve and a nerve to the vastus medialis muscle. Under the sartorius muscle this complex forms the "subsartorial plexus." While the femoral artery and vein pass further through the adductor hiatus (about at the junction of the middle and the distal thirds of the thigh) in the popliteal fossa, the nerve continues its way separate from the blood vessels and penetrates the vastoadductor membrane together with the descending genicular artery. There it passes behind the sartorius muscle in the subsartorial fat, gives off the infrapatellar branch, and penetrates its tendon and the fascia lata medially at the level of the patella (knee fascia, ▶ Fig. 13.31). As a superficial cutaneous nerve, it divides below the knee (▶ Fig. 13.32 and ▶ Fig. 13.33) and the main branch accompanies the great saphenous vein as far as the medial malleolus or even beyond it (▶ Fig. 13.34).

The saphenous nerve innervates the skin of the inside of the lower leg from the knee to the dorsum of the foot and even reaches as far as the great toe in up to 20% of cases (Morris and Lang 1999).

## 13.5.2 Techniques

### Saphenous Nerve Block (Classical Technique)

#### Landmarks and Position

Tibial tuberosity, medial head of gastrocnemius.

The patient lies supine with the leg extended. A small pad (or pillow) can be placed under the knee (▶ Fig. 13.35).

#### Procedure

The tibial tuberosity is palpated. After disinfecting the skin, a subcutaneous infiltration is performed from the tuberosity toward the medial head of gastrocnemius with a 6-cm 24 G needle and 5 to 10 mL of local anesthetic.
• The technique is simple infiltration anesthesia.
• The main depot should be injected around the great saphenous vein, which runs in the angle between the belly of gastrocnemius and the tibia; this is where the main branch of the saphenous nerve runs (▶ Fig. 13.36).
• Intermittent aspiration tests should be performed to exclude accidental injection into the long saphenous vein.
• The injection can be painful due to periosteal contact by the needle tip, as there is very thin subcutaneous tissue over the tibia.

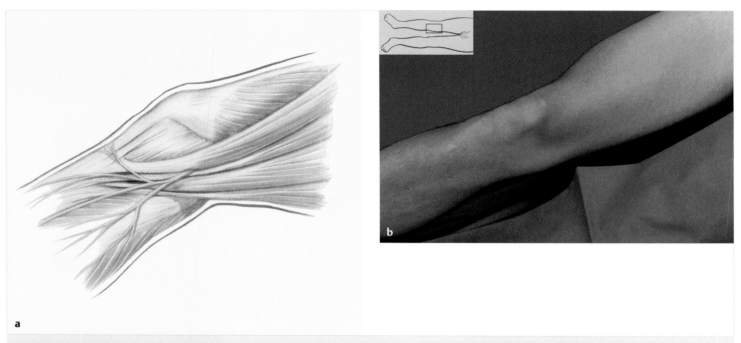

**Fig. 13.32** The saphenous nerve runs under the sartorius muscle, crosses under it, and passes through the fascia lata (knee fascia) behind its tendon at the level of the patella. As a superficial cutaneous nerve, it branches below the knee and accompanies the long saphenous vein as far as the medial malleolus or beyond it.
**a** Anatomy.
**b** Clinical setting.

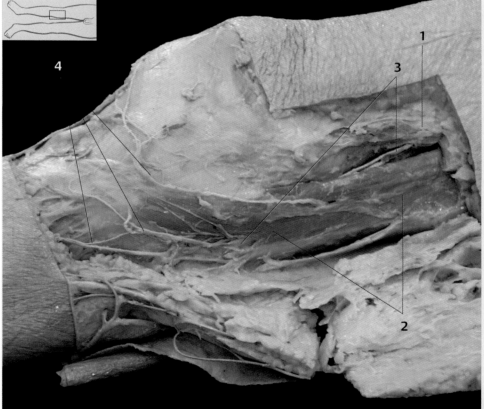

**Fig. 13.33** Anatomical dissection, same view as
▶ Fig. 13.32.
1 Vastus medialis muscle
2 Sartorius muscle
3 Saphenous nerve
4 Infrapatellar branches of the saphenous nerve

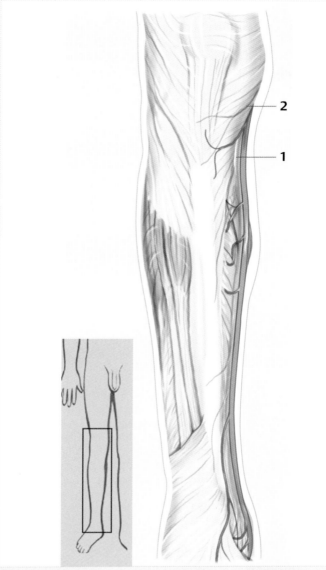

**Fig. 13.34** The main branch of the saphenous nerve runs superficially together with the long saphenous vein on the belly of the gastrocnemius muscle (Platzer 1999).
1 Long saphenous vein with saphenous nerve
2 Infrapatellar branches of the saphenous nerve

## Transsartorial Technique of Saphenous Nerve Block

The transsartorial technique is a compartment block of the saphenous nerve between the sartorius muscle and vastus medialis (intermuscular vastoadductor septum) (Platzer 1999; ► Fig. 13.37).

## Landmarks and Position

Medial side of the thigh, vastus medialis, patella, and sartorius muscle.

The patient lies supine and the leg to be anesthetized is extended.

## Procedure

For anatomical orientation, the patient is asked to extend the leg actively. This causes the sartorius and vastus medialis muscles to contract. The outlines of the two muscles are readily palpable on the medial side of the thigh (► Fig. 13.38). The insertion site is two finger widths proximal to the upper border of the patella in the gap between the sartorius and vastus medialis muscles.

Following disinfection, infiltration anesthesia, and skin prepuncture, a needle is advanced on the medial side of the thigh about three finger widths proximal to the medial knee joint line in the gap between the sartorius and vastus medialis muscles until a loss of resistance after about 2 to 4 cm indicates that the needle tip is in the correct position in the subsartorial fat (► Fig. 13.39, ► Fig. 13.40, ► Fig. 13.41).

Following negative aspiration, 10 mL of a medium-acting to long-acting local anesthetic is injected. For the continuous technique, a catheter is advanced 3 to 5 cm following the injection (► Fig. 13.42). Alternatively, the space can be found through the sartorius muscle; in this case the needle passes through the sartorius until an appropriate loss of resistance is felt after 2 to 4 cm. This is the explanation of the term "transsartorial technique."

• The advantage of this technique is that it is almost pain-free (no periosteal contact) and has a greater success rate than the classical approach (Morris et al 1997).

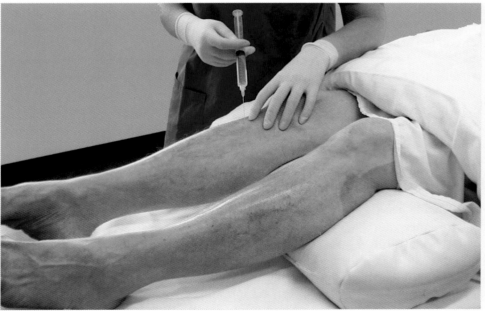

**Fig. 13.35** Technique of the (classical) saphenous nerve block: The tibial tuberosity is palpated. After disinfection, a subcutaneous infiltration is performed from the tuberosity toward the medial head of gastrocnemius with a 6-cm 24 G needle and 5 to 10 mL of local anesthetic.

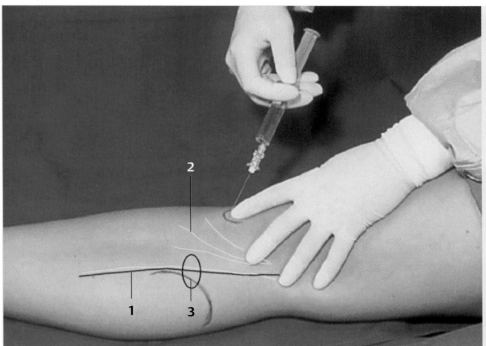

**Fig. 13.36** The main branch of the saphenous nerve passes together with the long saphenous vein superficially along the belly of the gastrocnemius. The depot of local anesthetic must be placed here.
1 Long saphenous vein with saphenous nerve
2 Prepatellar branches of the saphenous nerve
3 Site of the main depot of local anesthetic

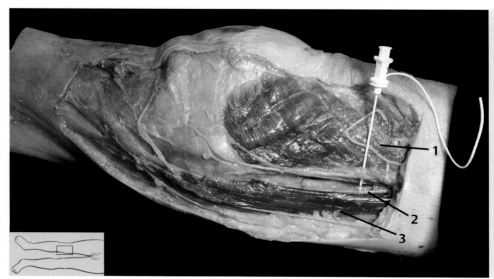

**Fig. 13.37** Right knee, medial view. Transsartorial technique of saphenous nerve block. The transsartorial technique is a compartment block of the saphenous nerve between the sartorius muscle and the intermuscular vastoadductor septum. The space between vastus medialis and sartorius is found about two finger widths above the upper border of the patella. The saphenous nerve runs in this space behind the sartorius muscle.
1 Vastus medialis muscle
2 Saphenous nerve
3 Sartorius muscle

- As this is a "loss-of-resistance" technique, use of a needle with a short bevel is recommended.
- The technique can also be performed with PNS (Comfort et al 1996).
- The technique enables a catheter to be placed (Meier and Büttner 2001; ▶ Fig. 13.42).
- The procedure can be performed and the position of the catheter can be checked using ultrasound (▶ Fig. 13.43; see also Chapter 12.5.1).

## Saphenous Nerve Block with Ultrasound ▶

The saphenous nerve is a sensory branch of the femoral nerve that runs distally in the adductor canal, initially together with the femoral artery and vein. It lies below the sartorius muscle. It is accompanied by a motor branch to the vastus medialis. Approximately at the junction from the middle to the distal third of the thigh, the saphenous nerve passes with the descending genicular artery through the vastoadductor membrane, which

forms the anterior border of the adductor canal. Here it separates from the femoral artery and vein that continue through the adductor hiatus toward the popliteal fossa, while the saphenous nerve continues with the descending genicular artery in close proximity to the sartorius muscle to the medial side of the knee joint. The course of the saphenous nerve varies greatly.

## Ultrasound-Guided Saphenous Nerve Block in the Mid-Thigh (Subsartorial Plexus Block, Adductor Canal Block)

Linear transducer: 6 to 13 MHz
Penetration depth: 5 to 8 cm
Needle: 7 to 10 cm

In the middle of the thigh (about 12–15 cm proximal to the popliteal crease) the femoral artery is sought from medial in the triangle between the sartorius and the vastus medialis muscles in the short axis (▶ Fig. 13.44). The sartorius muscle usually has the

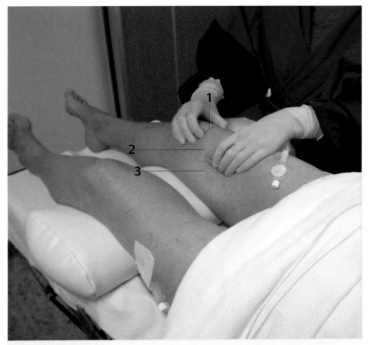

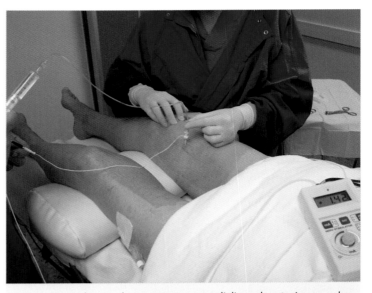

**Fig. 13.39** In the gap between vastus medialis and sartorius muscles the needle is advanced some three finger widths proximal to the medial knee joint line behind the sartorius muscle until a loss of resistance after about 2 to 4 cm indicates that the tip of the needle is in the correct position in the subsartorial fat. Following negative aspiration, 10 mL of a medium-acting to long-acting local anesthetic is injected.

**Fig. 13.38** Transsartorial technique of saphenous nerve block. The transsartorial technique is a compartment block of the saphenous nerve between the sartorius muscle and the intermuscular vasto-adductor septum. The space between vastus medialis and sartorius is found about two finger widths above the upper border of the patella. The saphenous nerve runs in this space behind the sartorius muscle.
1 Upper border of the patella
2 Vastus medialis muscle
3 Sartorius muscle

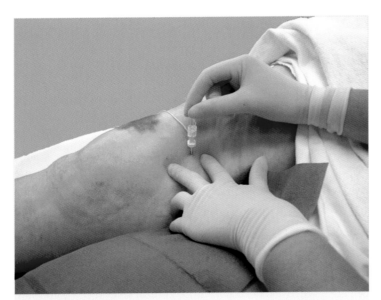

**Fig. 13.40** Right-handed persons can stand on the patient's left side to perform a block of the right leg.

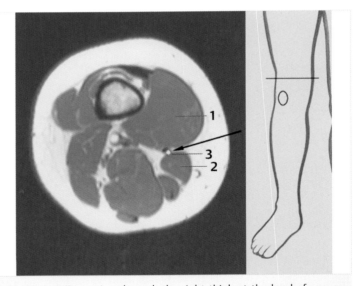

**Fig. 13.41** MRI section through the right thigh at the level of transsartorial saphenous nerve block, caudal view. The arrow indicates an alternative needle direction to the previous images.
1 Vastus medialis muscle
2 Sartorius muscle
3 Saphenous nerve

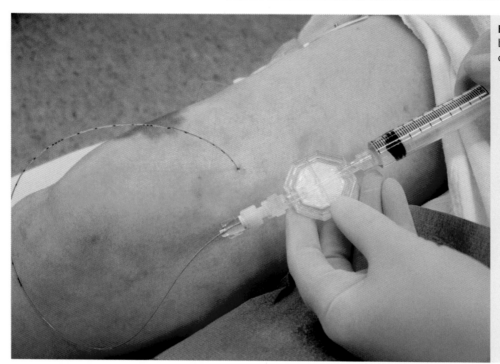

Fig. 13.42 The transsartorial technique can also be performed as a continuous technique with a catheter.

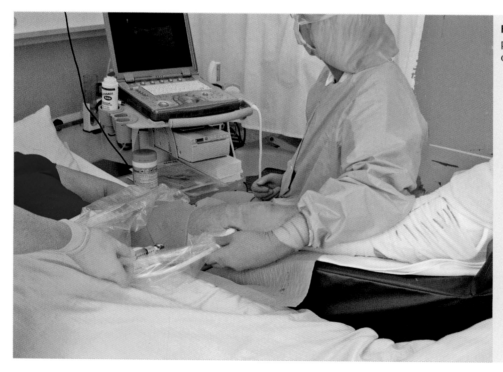

Fig. 13.43 Check of catheter position for postoperative analgesia after an ankle prosthesis operation.

typical shape of a flat isosceles triangle with its base facing the skin or a flat oval shape. The saphenous nerve lies here in the immediate vicinity of the femoral artery in a space filled with fatty tissue (▶ Fig. 13.44). Sometimes the motor branch to the vastus medialis, which runs along with saphenous nerve here, can also be visualized. The nerve closer to the artery is always the saphenous nerve.

The nerve is found here in plane from anterior direction (Manickam et al 2009, Tsui and Özelsel 2009). An out-of-plane needle insertion with the same visualization of the structures is also possible. A depot of 8 to 10 mL of anesthetic is sufficient. If the saphenous nerve cannot be visualized, a circular depot (8–10 mL) can be injected around the artery. A catheter can be placed. Motor impairment due to the secondary block of

individual motor branches that supply the vastus medialis is conceivable, but is likely to have little clinical relevance (Manickam et al 2009).

## Ultrasound-Guided Transsartorial Saphenous Nerve Block in the Distal Thigh

Linear transducer: 6 to 13 MHz
Penetration depth: 3 to 5 cm
Needle: 5 to 7 cm

The saphenous nerve leaves the adductor canal together with a branch of the femoral artery (femoral genicular artery) in the distal third of the thigh and thus is no longer in the vicinity of the

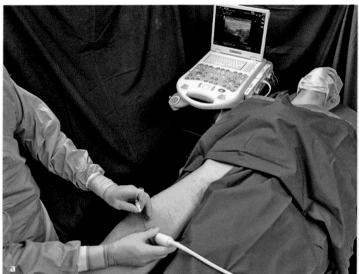

**Fig. 13.44** Saphenous nerve block of the mid-thigh.
**a** Clinical setting.
**b** Anatomical cross-section of the mid-thigh with acoustic window.
**c** Anatomical detail of **b**.
**d** Ultrasound image corresponding to **c**.
**e** As d, labeled.
→ View toward the plane
1 Vastus medialis muscle
2 Sartorius muscle
3 Subcutaneous fatty tissue
4 Femoral artery
5 Saphenous nerve
6 Motor branches of the femoral nerve to the vastus medialis muscle
   (not visualized here in ultrasound)
V Vein (collapsed in specimen)
C Needle (SonoPlex Pajunk GmbH)

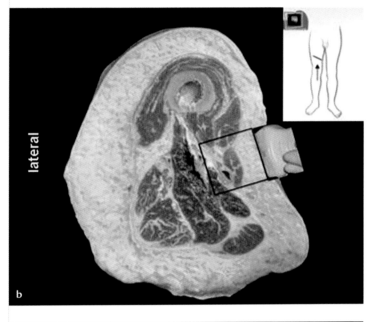

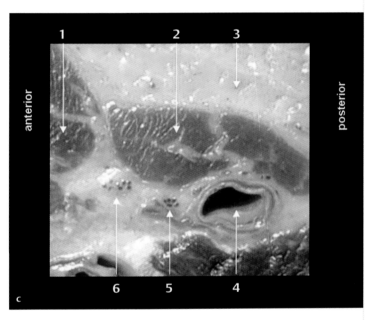

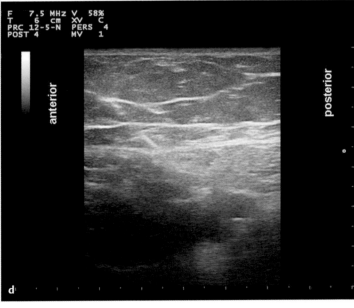

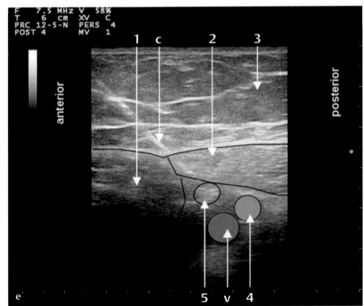

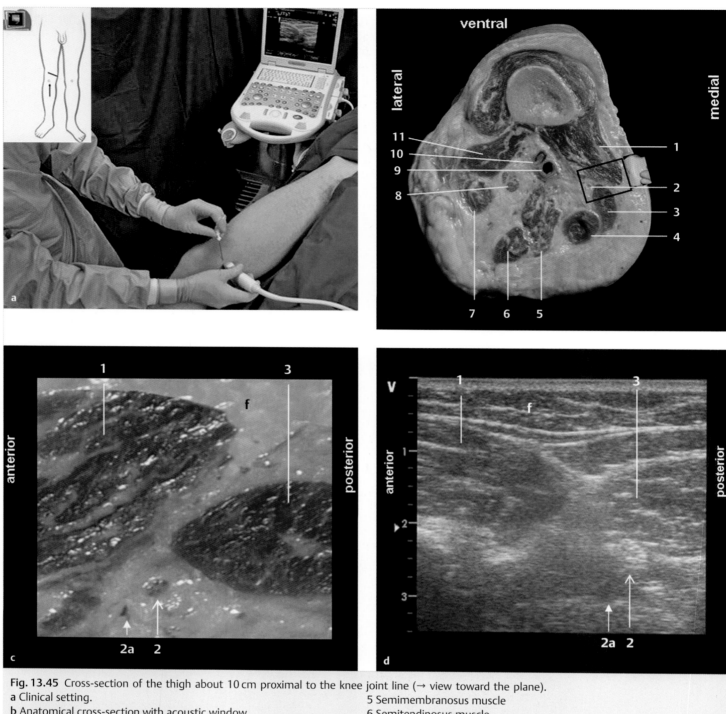

**Fig. 13.45** Cross-section of the thigh about 10 cm proximal to the knee joint line (→ view toward the plane).
a Clinical setting.
b Anatomical cross-section with acoustic window.
c Detail of b.
d Ultrasound image corresponding to c.
1 Vastus medialis muscle
2 Saphenous nerve
2a Descending genicular artery
3 Sartorius muscle
4 Gracilis muscle
5 Semimembranosus muscle
6 Semitendinosus muscle
7 Long head of the biceps femoris muscle
8 Sciatic nerve
9 Femoral artery
10 Femoral vein
11 Short head of the biceps femoris muscle
f Subcutaneous fatty tissue

femoral artery. It first continues in the vicinity of the sartorius muscle. It can be found about 2.5 cm proximal to the upper border of the patella (about 10 cm proximal to the knee joint line; Horn et al 2009), before giving off the infrapatellar branch. It is visualized in the short axis (► Fig. 13.45); needle insertion is generally made in plane (► Fig. 13.46) but an out-of-plane approach is possible. The nerve can often be visualized here as a hyperechoic structure in the space between the sartorius and vastus medialis muscles (► Fig. 13.45 and ► Fig. 13.46). The depot is then injected in the immediate vicinity of the nerve.

The descending genicular artery runs in the immediate vicinity of the saphenous nerve. It appears as a pulsating, hypoechoic point and can also be visualized using color Doppler and used for orientation. A volume of 8 to 10 mL of local anesthetic is sufficient for a block; a catheter can be placed.

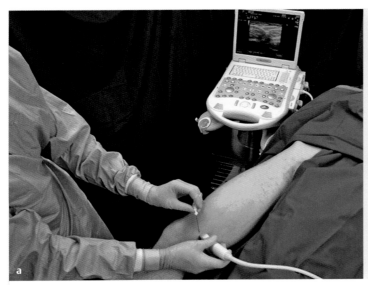

**Fig. 13.46** Cross-section of the thigh ca. 10 cm proximal to the knee joint line. (→ View toward the plane from distal.)
a Clinical setting.
b Ultrasound image (labeled).
c Anatomical cross-section.
1 Vastus medialis muscle
2 Saphenous nerve
2a Descending genicular artery
3 Sartorius muscle
The dashed line indicates the course of the needle in the in-plane technique.

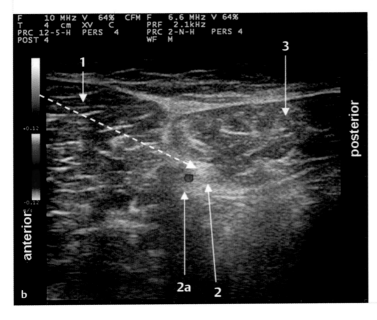

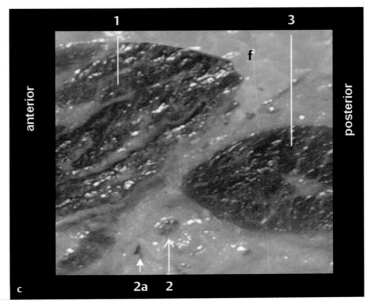

## 13.5.3 Indications and Contraindications

### Indications

- Supplement for incomplete lumbar plexus block (in the distal innervation region of the femoral nerve).
- Combination with distal sciatic block (Chapter 12.3) or popliteal block (lower leg tourniquet, operations in the region of the medial lower leg, varicose vein surgery).
- Operations and pain therapy in the region of the medial lower leg (e.g., muscle biopsy, skin graft harvesting; ▶ Fig. 13.47).

### Contraindications

No special contraindications. Relative contraindication: marked varicosity.

## 13.5.4 Side Effects and Complications

There are no reported special side effects or complications.

## 13.5.5 Remarks on the Technique

The transsartorial technique was described in 1993 by van der Wal as a "loss-of-resistance" (LOR) method (van der Wal et al 1993). In 1997, Morris et al reported a 100% success rate with transsartorial saphenous nerve block in 80 patients (Morris et al 1997). The block was performed with 10 mL lidocaine 1.5% (15 mg/mL) with epinephrine 1:200,000 and the onset of effect was within 5 minutes.

For the patient, the transsartorial technique offers the advantage of an almost pain-free procedure, as the periosteum of the tibia is not touched by the needle. A comparison of the different techniques of saphenous nerve block has shown that this technique is not only the most effective, but also has the lowest failure rate (Benzon et al 2005). Saphenous nerve block below the knee (classical technique) has the relatively common disadvantage of resulting in an inadequate block. According to Morris, the classical technique of saphenous nerve block has a success rate of only 39% (Morris and Lang 1999).

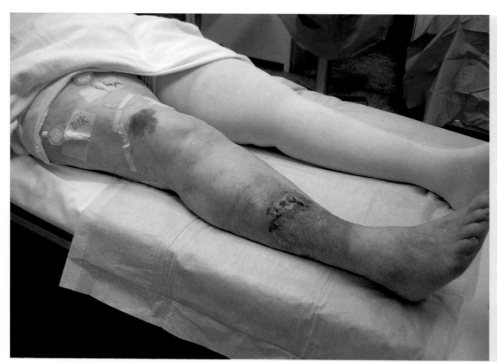

**Fig. 13.47** Patient with an extremely painful soft-tissue disease of the lower leg. A distal sciatic catheter alone did not provide adequate relief; in conjunction with the transsartorial catheter, complete freedom from pain was achieved.

► **Subsartorial technique with PNS.** Mansour reported on subsartorial block of the saphenous nerve in 1993. In comparison with the transsartorial technique, the subsartorial technique described by Mansour is difficult to perform with regard to the given landmarks and position of the patient (Bouaziz et al 1999). However, an interesting observation made by Mansour was the combination with peripheral nerve stimulation. Here he made use of the fact that the sensory saphenous nerve runs together with a motor branch from the femoral nerve that innervates the vastus medialis muscle. The motor nerve to the vastus medialis can be found by nerve stimulation. Contractions of vastus medialis indicate the correct position of the needle tip, and injection of 5 to 10 mL of local anesthetic will block the two nerves.

Then 5 to 10 mL of local anesthetic is injected (see femoral nerve block, multi-injection technique). In a pilot study, the success rate was 80% (Bouaziz et al 1999).

► **Stimulation of the saphenous nerve.** Another possibility for verifying that the needle is in the correct position is stimulation of the sensory saphenous nerve; a pulse duration of 1.0 ms should be selected. If the tip of the needle is in the correct position, the patient reports tingling paresthesia in the innervation area of the saphenous nerve.

> **Practical Note**
>
> For clinical practice, a combination of the LOR method (van der Wal) with PNS (contractions of the vastus medialis muscle) as described by Mansour is optimal for saphenous nerve block. This allows the advantages of both methods to be used (Meier and Büttner 2001).

PNS can be used for diagnostic block of the saphenous nerve, for example, in saphenous neuralgia. If the sensory saphenous nerve is sought exclusively, a pulse duration of 1.0 ms and cooperation of the patient are required (Defalque and McDanal 1994).

► **Continuous saphenous nerve block.** The transsartorial technique was originally described as a single-shot technique. So far, no study has been published of a continuous technique of transsartorial saphenous nerve block. However, catheter placement is easy to perform with the transsartorial approach (Büttner and Meier 1999). The catheter is advanced 3 cm into the subsartorial space.

This possibility expands the indications for saphenous nerve block beyond supplementary block in the case of incomplete lumbar plexus anesthesia or combined anesthesia in foot block. A catheter technique can usefully be employed, for example, in neuralgic disorders or inadequate wound healing or for plastic surgery (skin grafting, ulcers, burns, etc.).

The relevance of the saphenous nerve in pain therapy is possibly underestimated. Patients report postoperative pain on the medial side of the ankle after surgical treatment of complex fractures of the ankle and after ankle prostheses, even with a well-functioning sciatic nerve block, which can be treated with a saphenous nerve block. A continuous saphenous nerve block in the adductor canal is a valuable adjunct for postoperative analgesia after major knee surgery (Lund et al 2011, Andersen et al 2013), reducing the fall risk associated with a femoral nerve block (Kwofie et al 2013).

## 13.6 Fibular Nerve Block

(Synonym in anatomical nomenclature: peroneal nerve block.)

### 13.6.1 Anatomy

The common fibular nerve (L4–L5 and S1–S2) has both sensory and motor nerve fibers and is the smaller of the two terminal branches of the sciatic nerve. It runs initially between the tendon of the biceps femoris and the lateral head of gastrocnemius, then passes distal to the head of the fibula around the neck and subsequently lies on the bone immediately under the fascia (► Fig. 13.48 and ► Fig. 13.49). From there it penetrates the

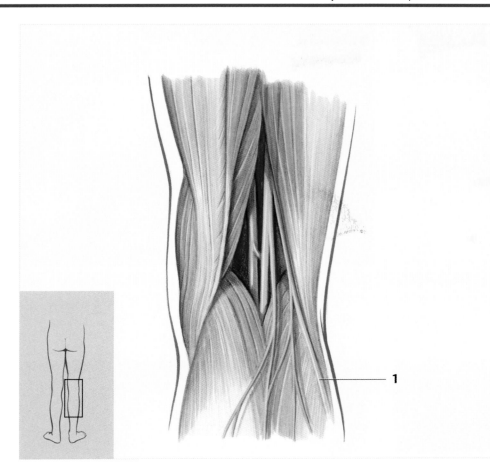

Fig. 13.48 Right popliteal fossa. The common fibular nerve (L4–L5 and S1–S2) has both sensory and motor nerve fibers and is the smaller of the two terminal branches of the sciatic nerve. It runs initially between the tendon of the biceps femoris muscle and the lateral head of the gastrocnemius muscle, then passes around the head of the fibula and subsequently lies on the bone immediately under the fascia. The common fibular nerve provides the sensory supply to the knee, the skin of the lateral lower leg, the ankle, and the heel. It provides motor innervation to the muscles of the anterolateral lower leg and is responsible for dorsiflexion and pronation (eversion) of the foot.
1 Common fibular nerve

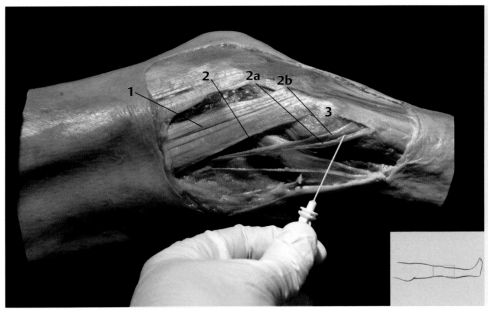

Fig. 13.49 Right knee, lateral view. The common fibular nerve runs initially between the tendon of the biceps femoris muscle and the lateral head of the gastrocnemius muscle, then passes around the head of the fibula and subsequently lies on the bone immediately under the fascia. Note the division of the common fibular nerve into its two terminal branches before entering the fibular compartment.
1 Biceps femoris muscle
2 Common fibular nerve
2a Superficial fibular nerve
2b Deep fibular nerve
3 Head of fibula

posterior intermuscular septum of the leg to the fibular compartment and divides into its terminal branches.

The common fibular nerve is the sensory supply to parts of the knee, the skin of the lateral lower leg, the ankle, and the heel. It provides motor innervation to the muscles of the anterolateral lower leg and is responsible for dorsiflexion and pronation of the foot (▸ Fig. 13.50).

## 13.6.2 Techniques

### Fibular Nerve Block (Posterior Technique)

#### Landmarks and Position

The leg to be anesthetized is bent slightly and the head of the fibula is marked. The patient lies supine.

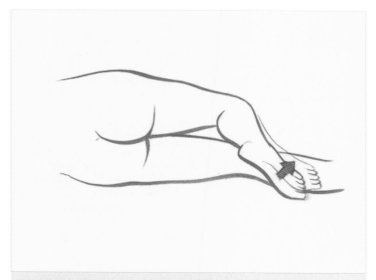

Fig. 13.50 The response to stimulation of the common fibular nerve consists of dorsiflexion and pronation of the foot.

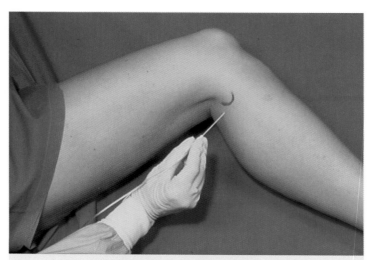

Fig. 13.51 The common fibular nerve is found immediately distal and posterior to the head of the fibula. To do this, the leg is bent slightly.

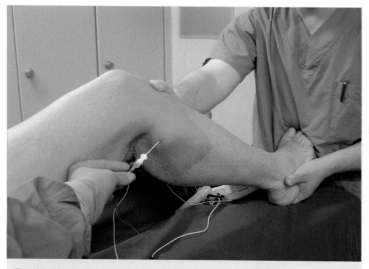

Fig. 13.52 An assistant to hold the leg can be helpful.

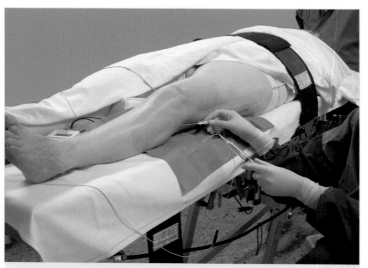

Fig. 13.53 The common fibular nerve can also be blocked with the leg extended. Here, too, the nerve is found just distal and posterior to the head of the fibula.

## Procedure

The head of the fibula is palpated. Following disinfection and subcutaneous or intracutaneous anesthesia, the puncture is made 2 cm caudal and posterior to the head of the fibula, vertically to the skin (▶ Fig. 13.51 and ▶ Fig. 13.52). The short 24 G or 22 G needle is advanced cautiously until it is felt to penetrate the fascia or the motor response of the common fibular nerve (dorsiflexion of the foot) becomes visible. This is followed by injection of 2 to 5 mL of local anesthetic. Paresthesia does not occur.

## Fibular Nerve Block (Lateral Technique)

### Landmarks and Position

The patient lies supine with the legs extended (or flexed slightly; ▶ Fig. 13.53).

## Procedure

Following skin disinfection, a fine needle is inserted about 2 cm distal and posterior to the head of the fibula (▶ Fig. 13.53). The needle is advanced around 1 cm in a mediocaudal direction until a response is produced and a depot of local anesthetic is placed in the space behind the head of the fibula (Hoerster 1988). The block can also be performed using ultrasound (▶ Fig. 13.54).

## 13.6.3 Indications and Contraindication

### Indications

- Incomplete anesthesia after proximal block of the sciatic nerve
- Diagnostic block
- Pain therapy

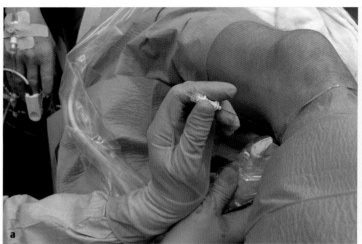

**Fig. 13.54** Selective block of the fibular nerve using ultrasound.
**a** Clinical setting.
**b** Ultrasound image (unlabeled).
**c** Ultrasound image (labeled).
1 Fibula
2 Common fibular nerve

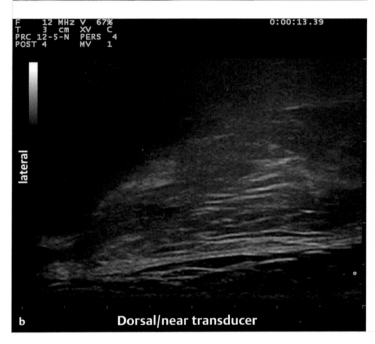

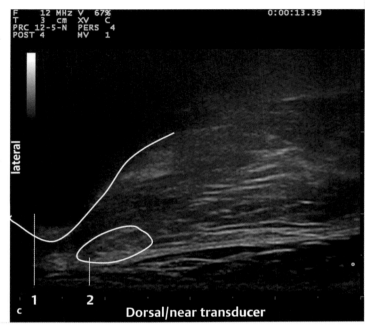

## Contraindication

Relative: nerve lesion (previous documentation required).

## 13.6.4 Side Effects and Complications

Neuropathy (intraneural injection and pressure injury due to excessive volume of local anesthetic must be avoided).

> **Tips and Tricks**
>
> - As the nerve reacts very sensitively to paresthesia—in the literature there are reports of persistent dysesthesia—PNS or ultrasound is recommended.
> - Successful block leads to paresis of the dorsiflexors ("foot drop").

## 13.6.5 Remarks on the Technique

The fibular nerve can in principle be blocked over its entire course through the popliteal fossa as far as distal to the head of the fibula. In their anatomical investigations, Snyder et al (1989) constantly found the nerve to be 0.5 cm (to 1 cm) medial to the most prominent (posterior) part of the head of the fibula and medial to the tendon of the biceps femoris. A number of variations for blocking the common fibular nerve at the knee have been described. An injection of 5 to 10 mL of local anesthetic is adequate for anesthesia. It should be noted that anesthesia of the outside of the lower leg and the dorsum of the foot can be obtained, but the lateral border of the foot is supplied by the sural nerve and this nerve may have to be blocked additionally. The techniques can be subdivided into blocks in the region of the popliteal fossa (see under "knee block"; Adriani 1951, Lecron 1990), the head of the fibula (Adriani 1951, Hoerster 1988, Sparks and Higeleo 1989), and distal to the head of the fibula in the fibular extensor compartment (Zinke 1985). The two methods described are easily learned and are considered to be safe (Niesel 1994).

Fibular neuritis and fibular paresis have been described as a complication of fibular nerve block (Hoerster 1988). In fibular paresis, pressure injury due to positioning or a lesion resulting from a tourniquet (Chapter 20.1) must be considered (Moore et al 1994, Stöhr 1996). The most elegant and often the best technique for practical purposes consists of blocking the common fibular nerve in the proximal part of the popliteal fossa together with the tibial nerve (see under "knee block," distal sciatic nerve block).

# References

Adriani J. Local and regional anesthesia for minor surgery. Surg Clin North Am 1951; 31: 1507–1529

Andersen HL, Gyrn J, Møller L, Christensen B, Zaric D. Continuous saphenous nerve block as supplement to single-dose local infiltration analgesia for postoperative pain management after total knee arthroplasty. Reg Anesth Pain Med 2013; 38: 106–111

Auberger HG, Niesel HC. Praktische Lokalanästhesie. 4th ed. Stuttgart: Thieme; 1982: 11–127

Augspurger RR, Donohue RE. Prevention of obturator nerve stimulation during transurethral surgery. J Urol 1980; 123: 170–172

Belavy D, Cowlishaw PJ, Howes M, Phillips F. Ultrasound-guided transversus abdominis plane block for analgesia after Caesarean delivery. Br J Anaesth 2009; 103: 726–730

Benzon HT, Sharma S, Calimaran A. Comparison of the different approaches to saphenous nerve block. Anesthesiology 2005; 102: 633–638

Bergmann RA. Compendium of Human Anatomic Variations. Munich: Urban & Schwarzenberg; 1994: 143–147

Bier A. Über einen neuen Weg Lokalanästhesie an den Gliedmaßen zu erzeugen. Arch Klin Chir 1908; 86: 1007–1016

Blumenthal S, Dullenkopf A, Rentsch K, Borgeat A. Continuous infusion of ropivacaine for pain relief after iliac crest bone grafting for shoulder surgery. Anesthesiology 2005; 102: 392–397

Bonica JJ. The Management of Pain. Philadelphia: Lea & Febiger; 1980: 1205–1209

Bonica JJ. Local anaesthesia and regional blocks. In: Wall PD, Melzack R, eds. Textbook of Pain. Edinburgh: Churchill Livingstone; 1984: 541–557

Bonniot A. Anatomie du Plexus Lombaire chez l'Homme [Thesis]. Lyon: Université de Lyon; 1922/23

Børglum J, Jensen K, Christensen AF et al. Distribution patterns, dermatomal anesthesia, and ropivacaine serum concentrations after bilateral dual transversus abdominis plane block. Reg Anesth Pain Med 2012; 37: 294–301

Bouaziz H, Narchi P, Zetlaoui PJ et al. Lateral approach to the sciatic nerve at the popliteal fossa combined with saphenous nerve block. Tech Reg Anesth Pain Manage 1999; 3: 19–22

Bridenbaugh PhO, Wedel DJ. The lower extremity. In: Cousins MJ, Bridenbaugh PhO, eds. Neural Blockade in Clinical Anesthesia and Management of Pain. 3rd ed. Philadelphia: Lippincott-Raven; 1998: 373–409

Büttner J, Meier G. Kontinuierliche periphere Techniken zur Regionalanästhesie und Schmerztherapie—Obere und untere Extremität. Bremen: Uni-Med; 1999

Chiono J, Bernard N, Bringuier S et al. The ultrasound-guided transversus abdominis plane block for anterior iliac crest bone graft postoperative pain relief: a prospective descriptive study. Reg Anesth Pain Med 2010; 35: 520–524

Comfort VK, Lang SA, Yip RW. Saphenous nerve anaesthesia—a nerve stimulator technique. Can J Anaesth 1996; 43: 852–857

Cousins MJ, Bridenbaugh PhO. Neural Blockade. In: Cousins MJ, Bridenbaugh PhO, eds. Neural Blockade in Clinical Anesthesia and Management of Pain. 3rd ed. Philadelphia: Lippincott-Raven; 1998: 378–388

Defalque RJ, McDanal JT. Proximal saphenous neuralgia after coronary bypass. Reg Anesth 1994; (A)9: 90

El-Dawlatly AA, Turkistani A, Kettner SC et al. Ultrasound-guided transversus abdominis plane block: description of a new technique and comparison with conventional systemic analgesia during laparoscopic cholecystectomy. Br J Anaesth 2009; 102: 763–767

Ellis H, Feldman S. Anatomy for Anaesthetists. 7th ed. Cambridge: Blackwell Science; 1996

Felsenthal G. Nerve blocks in the lower extremities: anatomic considerations. Arch Phys Med Rehabil 1974; 55: 504–507

Gasparich JP, Mason JT, Berger RE. Use of nerve stimulator for simple and accurate obturator nerve block before transurethral resection. J Urol 1984; 132: 291–293

Geiger M, Wild M, Bartl A et al. 3-in-1 block: reality or fantasy? Int Monitor Reg Anesth 2000; (A)12: 74

Gottschalk A, Gottschalk A. Continuous wound infusion of local anesthetics: importance in postoperative pain therapy. [Article in German] Anaesthesist 2010; 59: 1076–1082

Griffiths JD, Barron FA, Grant S, Bjorksten AR, Hebbard P, Royse CF. Plasma ropivacaine concentrations after ultrasound-guided transversus abdominis plane block. Br J Anaesth 2010; 105: 853–856

Hachenberg T, Sentürk M, Jannasch O, Lippert H. Postoperative wound infections. Pathophysiology, risk factors and preventive concepts. [Article in German] Anaesthesist 2010; 59: 851–868

Hallén J, Rawal N, Harrtvig P. Pharmacocinetic and pharmacodynamic studies of 11C-lidocaine following intravenous regional anaesthesia (IVRA) using positron emission tomography. Acta Anaesthesiol Scand 1991; 35: 214

Hebbard PD, Barrington MJ, Vasey C. Ultrasound-guided continuous oblique subcostal transversus abdominis plane blockade: description of anatomy and clinical technique. Reg Anesth Pain Med 2010; 35: 436–441

Heil JW, Ilfeld BM, Loland VJ, Sandhu NS, Mariano ER. Ultrasound-guided transversus abdominis plane catheters and ambulatory perineural infusions for outpatient inguinal hernia repair. Reg Anesth Pain Med 2010; 35: 556–558

Hoerster W. Blockaden im Bereich des Fußgelenkes. In: Astra Chemicals GmbH, ed. Regionalanästhesie. Stuttgart: Gustav Fischer; 1988:133–139

Hoffmann P, Meyer O. Der Obturatoriusreflex und seine Ausschaltung durch gezielte Blockade. Reg Anaesth 1980; 3: 55–56

Hong Y, O'Grady T, Lopresti D, Carlsson C. Diagnostic obturator nerve block for inguinal and back pain: a recovered opinion. Pain 1996; 67: 507–509

Horn JL, Pitsch T, Salinas F, Benninger B. Anatomic basis to the ultrasound-guided approach for saphenous nerve blockade. Reg Anesth Pain Med 2009; 34: 486–489

Hovelacque A. Anatomie des Nerfs Craniens et Rachidiens du Système Grand Sympathique chez l'Homme. Paris: Doin; 1927: 534–638

Jenkner FL. Nervenblockaden. 4th ed. Vienna: Springer; 1983: 65–75

Konder H, Moysich F, Mattusch W. Akzidentelle motorische Blockade des N. cutaneus femoris lateralis. Region Anästh 1990; 13: 122–123

Kwofie MK, Shastri UD, Gadsden JC et al. The effects of ultrasound-guided adductor canal block versus femoral nerve block on quadriceps strength and fall risk: a blinded, randomized trial of volunteers. Reg Anesth Pain Med 2013; 38: 321–325

Lecron L. Anesthésie du membre inférieur. In: Lecron L. Anesthésie loco-regionale. 2nd ed. Paris: Arnette; 1990: 327–348

Löfström B. Blockaden der peripheren Nerven des Beines. In: Eriksson E, ed. Atlas der Lokalanästhesie. 2nd ed. Berlin: Springer; 1980: 101–115

Lonsdale M. 3-in-1 block: confirmation of Winnie's anatomical hypothesis. Anesth Analg 1988; 67: 601–602

Lund J, Jenstrup MT, Jaeger P, Sørensen AM, Dahl JB. Continuous adductor-canal-blockade for adjuvant post-operative analgesia after major knee surgery: preliminary results. Acta Anaesthesiol Scand 2011; 55: 14–19

Manickam B, Perlas A, Duggan E, Brull R, Chan VW, Ramlogan R. Feasibility and efficacy of ultrasound-guided block of the saphenous nerve in the adductor canal. Reg Anesth Pain Med 2009; 34: 578–580

Mansour NY. Reevaluating the sciatic nerve block: another landmark for consideration. Reg Anesth 1993; 18: 322–323

McDonnell JG, O'Donnell B, Curley G, Heffernan A, Power C, Laffey JG. The analgesic efficacy of transversus abdominis plane block after abdominal surgery: a prospective randomized controlled trial. Anesth Analg 2007; 104: 193–197

Meier G. Technik der kontinuierlichen anterioren Ischiadicusblockade (KAI). In: Büttner J, Meier G, ed. Kontinuierliche periphere Techniken zur Regionalanästhesie und Schmerztherapie—Obere und untere Extremität. Bremen: Uni-Med; 1999: 132–137

Meier G, Büttner J. Regionalanästhesie—Kompendium der peripheren Blockaden. Munich: Arcis; 2001

Moore DC, Mulroy MF, Thompson GE. Peripheral nerve damage and regional anaesthesia. [Editorial] Br J Anaesth 1994; 73: 435–436

Morris GF, Lang SA, Dust WN, Van der Wal M. The parasacral sciatic nerve block. Reg Anesth 1997; 22: 223–228

Morris GF, Lang SA. Innovations in lower extremity blockade. Tech Reg Anesth Pain Manage 1999; 3: 9–18

Ng I, Vaghadia H, Choi PT, Helmy N. Ultrasound imaging accurately identifies the lateral femoral cutaneous nerve. Anesth Analg 2008; 107: 1070–1074

Niesel HCh, ed. Regionalanästhesie, Lokalanästhesie, Regionale Schmerztherapie. Stuttgart: Thieme; 1994

Niraj G, Searle A, Mathews M et al. Analgesic efficacy of ultrasound-guided transversus abdominis plane block in patients undergoing open appendicectomy. Br J Anaesth 2009; 103: 601–605

O'Donnell BD, McDonnell JG, McShane AJ. The transversus abdominis plane (TAP) block in open retropubic prostatectomy. Reg Anesth Pain Med 2006; 31: 91

Parks CR, Kennedy WF, Jr. Obturator nerve block: a simplified approach. Anesthesiology 1967; 28: 775–778

Paul W, Wiesner D, Drechsler HJ. Postoperative pain after total knee replacement: obturator nerve block may be needed additionally to sciatic and high volume femoral nerve block. Internat Monitor 1996: (A)31–32

Platzer W. Color Atlas of Human Anatomy. 7th ed. Vol 1: Locomotor System. Stuttgart: Thieme; 2014

Rosenquist RW, Lederhaas G. Femoral and lateral femoral cutaneous nerve block. Tech Reg Anesth Pain Manage 1999; 3: 33–38

Rybock JD. Diagnostic and therapeutic nerve blocks. In: Tollison CD, ed. Handbook of Chronic Pain management. Baltimore: Williams and Wilkins; 1989: 115–224

Schünke M, Schulte E, Schumacher U. Prometheus. LernAtlas der Anatomie. Allgemeine Anatomie und Bewegungssystem. Illustrationen von M. Voll und K. Wesker. 3rd ed. Stuttgart: Thieme; 2011: 206

Shannon J, Lang SA, Yip RW, Gerard M. Lateral femoral cutaneous nerve block revisited. A nerve stimulator technique. Reg Anesth 1995; 20: 100–104

Sharrock NE. Inadvertent "3-in-1 block" following injection of the lateral cutaneous nerve of the thigh. Anesth Analg 1980; 59: 887–888

Snyder MD, DeBoard JW, Beger TH, Gibbons JJ. Anatomy of the common peroneal nerve at the knee: A cadaver study. Reg Anesth 1989; (S)14: 38

Soong J, Schafhalter-Zoppoth I, Gray AT. Sonographic imaging of the obturator nerve for regional block. Reg Anesth Pain Med 2007; 32: 146–151

Sparks CJ, Higeleo T. Foot surgery in Vanuatu: results of combined tibial, common peroneal and saphenous nerve blocks in fifty-six adults. Anaesth Intensive Care 1989; 17: 336–339

Stöhr M. Iatrogene Nervenläsionen: Injektionen, Operation, Lagerung, Strahlentherapie. 2nd ed. Stuttgart: Thieme; 1996

Sunderland S. Obturator nerve. In: Sunderland S, ed. Nerves and Nerve Injuries. Edinburgh: Livingstone; 1968: 1096–1109

Trainer N, Bowser BL, Dahm L. Obturator nerve block for painful hip in adult cerebral palsy. Arch Phys Med Rehabil 1986; 67: 829–830

Tsui BCH, Özelsel T. Ultrasound-guided transsartorial perifemoral artery approach for saphenous nerve block. Reg Anesth Pain Med 2009; 34: 177–178, author reply 178

van der Wal M, Lang SA, Yip RW. Transsartorial approach for saphenous nerve block. Can J Anaesth 1993; 40: 542–546

Vloka JD, Hadzic A. Obturator and genitofemoral nerve blocks. Tech Reg Anesth Pain Manage 1999; 3: 28–32

Wassef MR. Interadductor approach to obturator nerve blockade for spastic conditions of adductor thigh muscles. Reg Anesth 1993; 18: 13–17

Yazaki T, Ishikawa H, Kanoh S, Koiso K. Accurate obturator nerve block in transurethral surgery. Urology 1985; 26: 588–589

Zinke R. Die perivasale Anästhetikuminfiltration als einfache Methode zur peripheren Sympathikusblockade bei Schmerzzu ständen der Extremitäten. Z Ärztl Fortbild 1985; 79: 77

# 14 Peripheral Nerve Blocks at the Ankle

## 14.1 Anatomy

The foot is supplied by five nerves. Four of them are derived from the sciatic nerve (tibial nerve, superficial fibular nerve, deep fibular nerve, and sural nerve). The sural nerve is a joint terminal branch with sensory nerve fibers from the fibular nerve and the tibial nerve. The fifth nerve, the saphenous nerve, is the sensory terminal branch of the femoral nerve from the lumbar plexus (Chapter 8).

Three of the five nerves run in the subcutaneous fat directly above the deep fascia of the leg: the saphenous, sural, and superficial fibular nerves. These are anesthetized by subcutaneous infiltration. The remaining two nerves—the tibial nerve and the deep fibular nerve—run below the deep fascia of the leg in the ankle region and are anesthetized by selective subfascial injections (▶ Fig. 14.1; Platzer 2009).

> **Note**
>
> Each of the five nerves in the ankle can be blocked separately. The success rate is very high.

### 14.1.1 Tibial Nerve

The tibial nerve (L4–L5 to S1–S3) is the larger of the two branches of the sciatic nerve and in the distal segment of the lower leg it becomes superficial medial to the Achilles tendon. It lies behind and lateral to the posterior tibial artery and between the tendons of flexor digitorum longus and tibialis posterior and the flexor hallucis longus muscles, covered by the flexor retinaculum (▶ Fig. 14.1, ▶ Fig. 14.2, ▶ Fig. 14.3, ▶ Fig. 14.4). The tibial nerve always runs close to the posterior tibial vessels. The tibial nerve gives off medial calcaneal branches on the inside of the heel and then divides behind the medial malleolus into the medial plantar nerve and the lateral plantar nerve. These two nerves run downward, toward the sole of the foot, covered by abductor hallucis, and provide the sensory innervation of the sole. The tibial nerve is the motor supply of the flexor muscles (plantar flexion) and the sensory supply of the anterior and medial regions of the sole.

### 14.1.2 Saphenous Nerve

The saphenous nerve is the sensory terminal branch of the femoral nerve. It passes through the deep fascia of the leg in the region of the pes anserinus at the medial knee joint line and runs distally very close to the long saphenous vein on the medial side of the tibia subcutaneously, reaches the ankle region anterior to the medial malleolus, and continues as far as the great toe, giving off branches on the medial border of the foot (▶ Fig. 14.1, ▶ Fig. 14.2, ▶ Fig. 14.3, ▶ Fig. 14.5). The sensory innervation of the medial region of the heel, the medial malleolus, and the medial border of the foot, sometimes as far as the great toe, is provided by the saphenous nerve.

### 14.1.3 Sural Nerve

The sural nerve is a cutaneous nerve that is a branch of the tibial nerve, which unites with the fibular communicating branch of

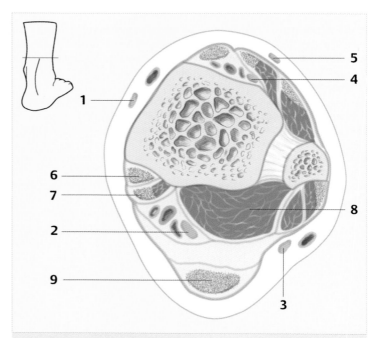

Fig. 14.1 Section through the lower leg at the level of the malleoli. Three of the five nerves supplying the foot run in the subcutaneous fat directly over the deep fascia of the leg: the saphenous, sural, and superficial fibular nerves. These are anesthetized by subcutaneous infiltration. The remaining two nerves—the tibial and the deep fibular nerves—run under the deep fascia of the leg in the ankle region and are anesthetized by direct blockade. While the former three nerves are essentially responsible for the sensory supply of the skin, the tibial and the deep fibular nerves are important for the sensory (and motor) innervation of more deeply situated structures.
1 Saphenous nerve
2 Tibial nerve
3 Sural nerve
4 Deep fibular nerve
5 Superficial fibular nerve
6 Tendon of tibialis posterior muscle
7 Tendon of flexor digitorum longus muscle
8 Flexor hallucis longus muscle
9 Calcaneal tendon (Achilles tendon)

the lateral sural cutaneous nerve (from the common fibular nerve). The nerves usually unite in the middle third of the lower leg. In the further course it passes through the fascia. The sural nerve (which is also called the external saphenous nerve) then runs in the subcutaneous layer and passes downward together with the short saphenous vein on the deep fascia of the leg behind the lateral malleolus to the outer edge of the foot (▶ Fig. 14.6 and ▶ Fig. 14.7). It is the sensory supply of the lateral heel region and lateral malleolus and, as the lateral dorsal cutaneous nerve, it innervates the lateral border of the foot as far as the small toe.

### 14.1.4 Superficial Fibular Nerve

The superficial fibular nerve comes from the common fibular nerve and branches off in the fibular compartment or even sooner. It passes cutaneously, either as a trunk or already divided into its two terminal branches, between the middle and distal third of the lower leg lateral to the anterior edge of the tibia. Lying directly on the deep fascia of the leg, it passes distally and

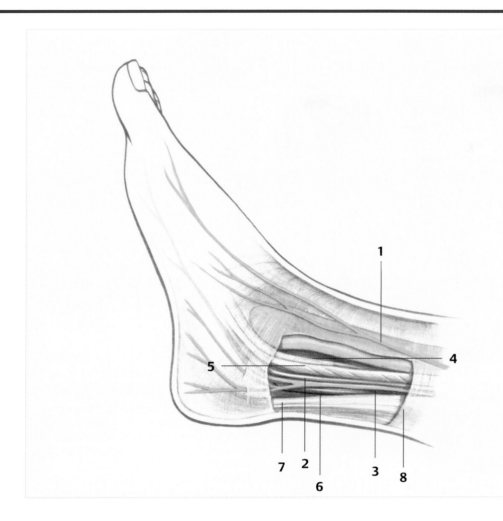

**Fig. 14.2** Right foot, medial view.
1 Saphenous nerve
2 Tibial artery
3 Tibial nerve
4 Tendon of tibialis posterior muscle
5 Tendon of flexor digitorum longus muscle
6 Tendon of flexor hallucis longus muscle
7 Calcaneal tendon (Achilles tendon)
8 Deep fascia of the leg

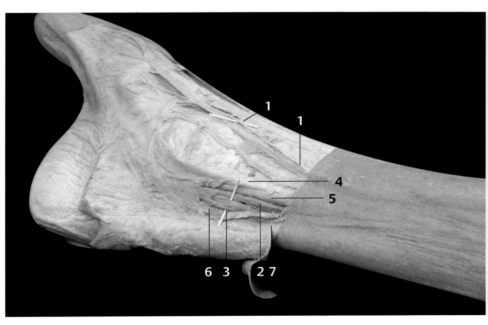

**Fig. 14.3** Right foot, medial view. The tibial nerve (L4–L5 to S1–S3) reaches the surface in the distal segment of the lower leg medial to the Achilles tendon. It lies behind the posterior tibial artery and between the tendons of flexor digitorum longus and tibialis posterior and flexor hallucis longus, covered by the flexor retinaculum (▶ Fig. 14.1).
1 Saphenous nerve
2 Tibial artery
3 Tibial nerve
4 Tendon of tibialis posterior
5 Tendon of flexor digitorum longus
6 Tendon of flexor hallucis longus
7 Calcaneal tendon (Achilles tendon)

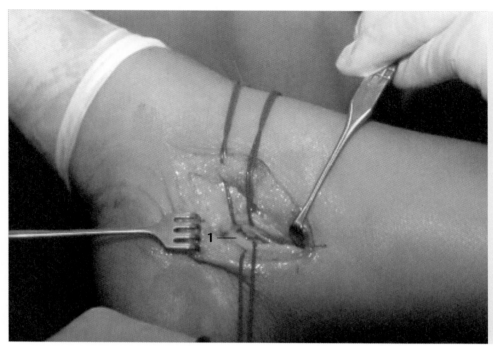

**Fig. 14.4** Right foot, medial view. Surgical exposure of the tibial nerve.
1 Tibial nerve

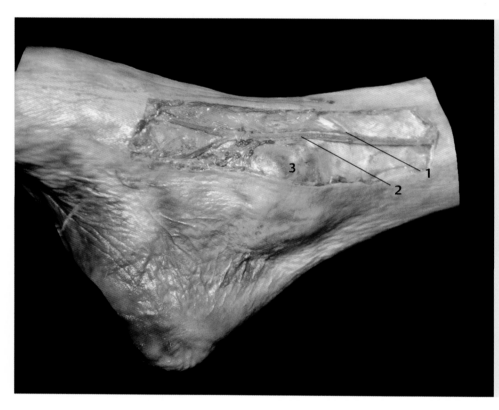

**Fig. 14.5** Right foot, medial view. The main branch of the saphenous nerve runs together with the long saphenous vein on the inside of the lower leg as far as the ankle; occasionally it can extend as far as the great toe.
1 Saphenous nerve
2 Long saphenous vein
3 Medial malleolus

branches above ankle level in a broad fan shape over the entire dorsum of the foot, for which it is the sensory supply with its terminal branches, namely the medial and intermediate cutaneous dorsal nerves (► Fig. 14.6, ► Fig. 14.7, ► Fig. 14.8, ► Fig. 14.9). The superficial fibular nerve is also called the musculocutaneous nerve of the leg (Bridenbaugh and Wedel 1998).

## 14.1.5 Deep Fibular Nerve

The deep fibular nerve passes downward on the anterior surface of the interosseous membrane of the leg deep to the extensor digitorum longus muscle. It is always lateral to the anterior tibial artery between the tibialis anterior and the extensor digitorum

longus and extensor hallucis longus muscles that are located laterally.

It then continues along the dorsum of the foot, covered by the superior and inferior extensor retinaculum. There it innervates the short toe extensors and the skin on the lateral side of the great toe and the medial side of the second toe—that is, the first interdigital space. During its course in the lower leg, the tibial artery is, at first, medial to the nerve. However, further distally the nerve crosses above the artery, which then lies lateral to it. At the level of the extensor retinaculum the nerve and artery are crossed by the tendon of extensor hallucis longus coming from the medial side. At the front of the ankle joint, the anterior tibial artery is therefore lateral to the deep fibular nerve, while the

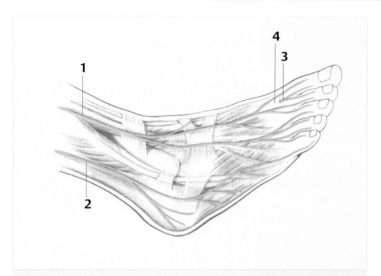

Fig. 14.6 Right foot, lateral view. Note the subfascial position of the deep fibular nerve until its emergence peripherally.
1 Superficial fibular nerve
2 Sural nerve
3 Deep fibular nerve
4 Fascia

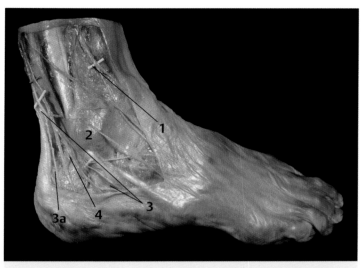

Fig. 14.7 Right lower leg and foot, lateral view. A block of the sural nerve can be made by continuing the subcutaneous depot, as described for the block of the superficial fibular nerve, to the Achilles tendon (dissected by Miriam Petrac).
1 Superficial fibular nerve (yellow marker)
2 Lateral malleolus
3 Sural nerve and its continuation in the lateral dorsal cutaneous nerve (yellow marker)
3a Lateral calcaneal branch of sural nerve
4 Small saphenous vein (blue marker)

tendon of extensor hallucis longus is medial to the nerve (▶ Fig. 14.6, ▶ Fig. 14.8, ▶ Fig. 14.10).

## 14.1.6 Sensory Innervation of the Foot

(▶ Fig. 14.11)

# 14.2 Saphenous Nerve, Sural Nerve, and Superficial Fibular Nerve Block

▶ **Position and landmarks.** Anterior border of the tibia, medial and lateral malleolus, Achilles tendon.

The patient lies supine.

▶ **Procedure.** Following disinfection of the lower leg and foot on the side to be anesthetized, conduction anesthesia is performed with a 6 cm long 24 G needle.

## 14.2.1 Saphenous Nerve Block

### Landmarks and Procedure

Starting from the anterior border of the tibia, 10 mL of a medium-acting or long-acting local anesthetic is injected subcutaneously four finger widths above the medial malleolus to the Achilles tendon (▶ Fig. 14.12).

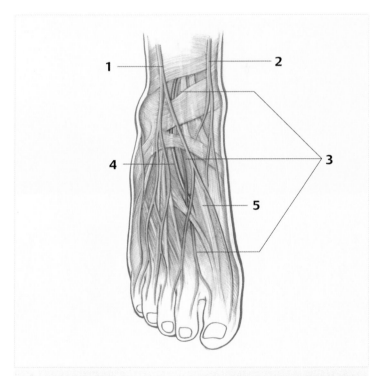

Fig. 14.8 Right foot. Note the subfascial position of the deep fibular nerve: it continues along the dorsum of the foot covered by the inferior and superior extensor retinaculum. At the ankle joint, the anterior tibial artery is lateral to the deep fibular nerve, while the tendon of extensor hallucis longus runs medial to the nerve. The sensory terminal branches innervate the skin on the lateral side of the great toe and the medial side of the second toe.
1 Superficial fibular nerve
2 Saphenous nerve
3 Deep fibular nerve
4 Dorsalis pedis artery
5 Tendon of extensor hallucis longus muscle

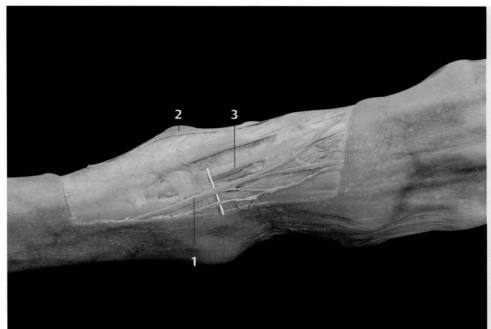

**Fig. 14.9** Right foot.
1 Superficial fibular nerve
2 Saphenous nerve
3 Tendon of extensor hallucis longus muscle

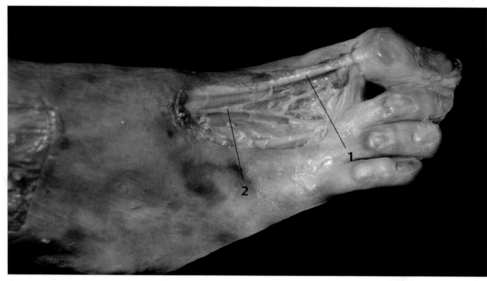

**Fig. 14.10** Right foot, anterolateral view.
1 Tendon of extensor hallucis longus muscle
2 Deep fibular nerve with divisions into its sensory terminal branches for innervation of the first interdigital space

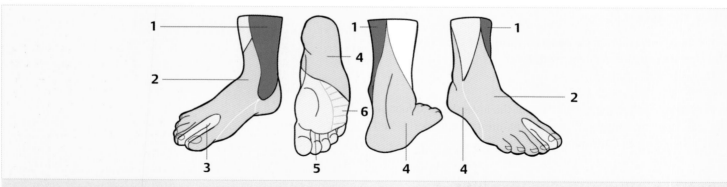

**Fig. 14.11** Sensory supply of the foot. The foot is supplied by five nerves. Four of these originate from the sciatic nerve (tibial nerve, superficial fibular nerve, deep fibular nerve, and sural nerve). The sural nerve is a common terminal branch with sensory nerve fibers from the fibular nerve and the tibial nerve. The fifth nerve, the saphenous nerve, is the sensory terminal branch of the femoral nerve from the lumbar plexus (Chapter 8).
1 Saphenous nerve
2 Superficial fibular nerve
3 Deep fibular nerve
4 Sural nerve
5 Medial plantar nerve
6 Lateral plantar nerve (tibial nerve)
Blue: Terminal branch of the femoral nerve (lumbar plexus)
Yellow: Terminal branches of the sciatic nerve (sacral plexus)

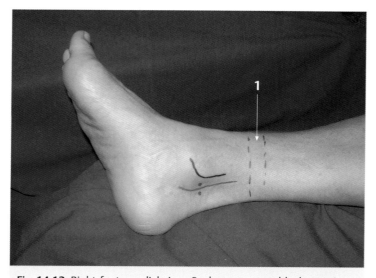

**Fig. 14.12** Right foot, medial view. Saphenous nerve block: starting from the anterior border of the tibia, 10 mL of a medium-acting or long-acting local anesthetic is injected subcutaneously four finger widths above the medial malleolus as far as the Achilles tendon.
1 Subcutaneous injection to block saphenous nerve

## 14.2.2 Superficial Fibular Nerve Block and Sural Nerve Block

### Landmarks and Procedure

Three to four finger widths above the lateral malleolus, a subcutaneous skin depot is created with 5 to 10 mL of local anesthetic (e.g., prilocaine 1%) on the lateral side of the lower leg; the depot should continue backward as far as the Achilles tendon to block the sural nerve (▶ Fig. 14.13 and ▶ Fig. 14.14).

### Alternative Method for Selective Block of the Sural Nerve

The sural nerve can also be blocked by subcutaneous infiltration between the Achilles tendon and the lateral malleolus with 5 to 10 mL of local anesthetic (▶ Fig. 14.15).

The sural nerve is a purely sensory nerve formed from fibers from the tibial and common fibular nerves. It innervates the lateral malleolus and the lateral border of the foot.

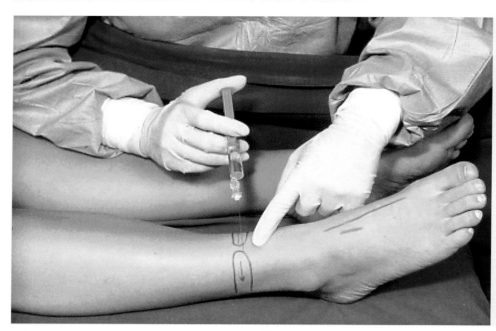

**Fig. 14.13** Superficial fibular nerve and sural nerve block: 5 to 10 mL of local anesthetic is injected to create a subcutaneous skin depot between the anterior border of the tibia about three to four finger widths above the lateral malleolus. Following the superficial fibular nerve block, injection of local anesthetic can be continued further laterally toward the Achilles tendon.

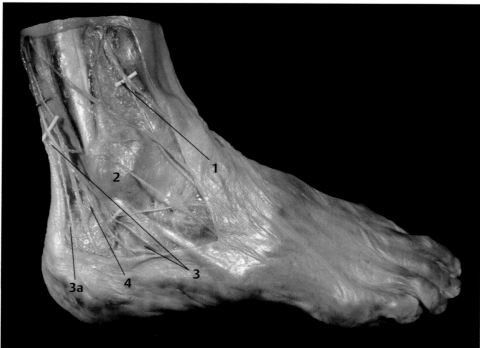

**Fig. 14.14** Right lower leg and foot, lateral view. A block of the sural nerve can be performed by laterally continuing the subcutaneous depot, as described for common fibular nerve block, as far as the Achilles tendon (dissected by Miriam Petrac).
1 Superficial fibular nerve (yellow marker)
2 Lateral malleolus
3 Sural nerve and its continuation in the lateral dorsal cutaneous nerve (yellow marker)
3a Lateral calcaneal branch of the sural nerve
4 Short saphenous vein (blue marker)

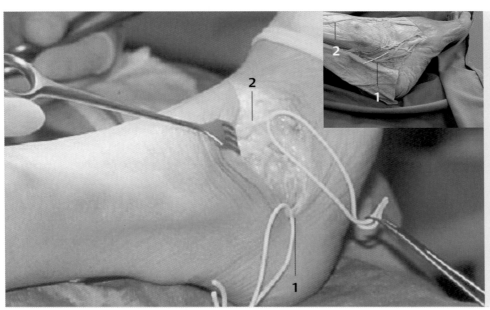

Fig. 14.15 Right foot, lateral view. The sural nerve can also be blocked selectively by a subcutaneous injection of about 5 mL of local anesthetic behind the lateral malleolus.
1 Sural nerve (here exposed surgically)
2 Superficial fibular nerve

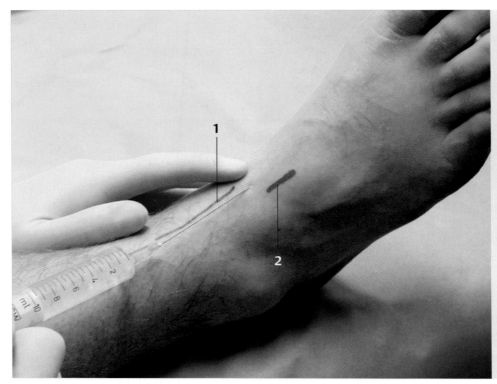

Fig. 14.16 The needle insertion site for the deep fibular nerve block is on the dorsum of the foot immediately between the tendon of extensor hallucis longus (medial) and the dorsalis pedis artery (lateral). The needle is advanced deeply between the artery and tendon under the fascia, the extensor retinaculum, and after negative aspiration about 3 mL of local anesthetic (e.g., mepivacaine 1% [10 mg/mL] or ropivacaine 0.75% [7.5 mg/mL]) is injected. The needle is then withdrawn, and after negative aspiration about 3 mL of local anesthetic is again injected.
1 Tendon of extensor hallucis longus muscle
2 Dorsalis pedis artery

## 14.3 Deep Fibular Nerve Block

### 14.3.1 Landmarks

Tendon of extensor hallucis longus, dorsalis pedis artery.

### 14.3.2 Procedure

The insertion site is on the dorsum of the foot immediately between the tendon of extensor hallucis longus (medial) and the dorsalis pedis artery (lateral). The needle is advanced between the artery and tendon deep under the fascia, the extensor retinaculum.

After negative aspiration, about 3 mL of local anesthetic is injected (▶ Fig. 14.16). The needle is then withdrawn and, after negative aspiration, about 3 mL of local anesthetic (e.g., prilocaine 1% [10 mg/mL] or ropivacaine 0.75% [7.5 mg/mL]) is injected again.

- Orientation is sometimes difficult if the pulse is not palpable. Use of a small Doppler probe or ultrasound can be helpful.
- The tendon of extensor hallucis longus is readily palpable on dorsiflexion of the foot. The artery is always lateral to this tendon.
- A selective block is useful only in the case of pain or operations on the medial side of the great toe and/or lateral side of the second toe (e.g., ingrown toenail).

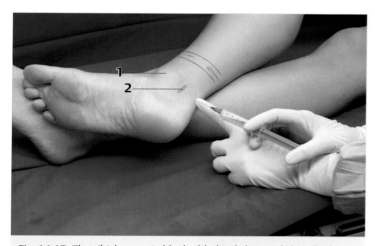

**Fig. 14.17** The tibial nerve is blocked behind the medial malleolus. Somewhat lateral to the posterior tibial artery or immediately medial to the Achilles tendon at the level of the cranial segment of the medial malleolus, a 5 to 8 cm needle is introduced and advanced as far as the posterior border of the tibia (motor response with PNS: plantar flexion of the toes). After reaching the posterior border of the tibia, the needle is withdrawn about 1 cm and 10 mL of a medium-acting or long-acting local anesthetic is injected.
1 Medial malleolus
2 Posterior tibial artery

## 14.4 (Posterior) Tibial Nerve Block ▶

### 14.4.1 Landmarks and Position

Medial malleolus, Achilles tendon.

The patient remains supine, and the lower leg is crossed on the tibia of the other leg (▶ Fig. 14.17).

### 14.4.2 Procedure

The nerve is blocked behind the medial malleolus. After disinfection, the skin is infiltrated somewhat lateral to the posterior tibial artery (i.e., between the Achilles tendon and posterior tibial artery) or—if this is not palpable—immediately medial to the

Achilles tendon at the level of the cranial section of the medial malleolus. A 24 G needle 5 to 8 cm long is introduced at this point vertically to the skin and is advanced cautiously and with intermittent aspiration as far as the posterior border of the tibia (motor response on PNS: plantar flexion of the toes; ▶ Fig. 14.17 and ▶ Fig. 14.18). Paresthesia is not deliberately sought but is relatively frequent. After reaching the posterior border of the tibia, the needle is withdrawn about 1 cm. Following negative aspiration, 10 mL of a medium-acting or long-acting local anesthetic is injected. The analgesia extends to the sole of the foot (with the exception of the heel) and the medial border of the foot. No particular complications are expected. There have been isolated reports of dysesthesia after this block (Schurman 1976).

### Tips and Tricks

- Paresthesia should not be sought. However, if paresthesia (plantar) is produced, the patient must be prepared for this unpleasant sensation so that the patient and therapist are not endangered by a sudden withdrawal movement.
- Anesthesia can be performed very well with PNS (response: plantar flexion of the toes; Frédéric and Bouchon 1996).
- An additional injection below the fascia on the contralateral side (medial) of the artery ensures the success of the block, even when the course of the tibial nerve is variable relative to the artery, particularly when a nerve stimulator is not used or no paresthesia is produced.
- Performing the block under ultrasound guidance allows good visualization of the relevant anatomical structures (▶ Fig. 14.19). Proximity to the nerve can be sought specifically. The lower leg is placed on the tibia of the other leg (see above) or a positioning aid is used (see distal sciatic nerve block) for positioning and to facilitate performing the block.

## 14.5 Ankle Block

Complete block of the foot can be obtained by joint block of all five nerves supplying the foot—the so-called ankle block.

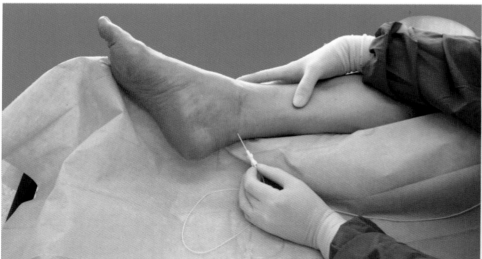

**Fig. 14.18** Block of the tibial nerve can also be performed with the nerve stimulator. The response consists of plantar flexion of the toes.

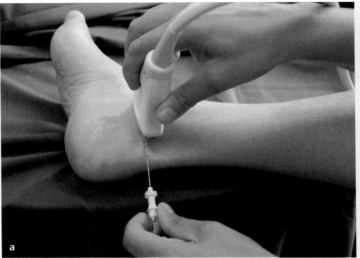

**Fig. 14.19** Puncture of the posterior tibial nerve using ultrasound.
**a** Clinical setting.
**b** Ultrasound image (unlabeled).
**c** As **b**, labeled.
1 Medial malleolus
2 Posterior tibial artery
3 Tibial nerve

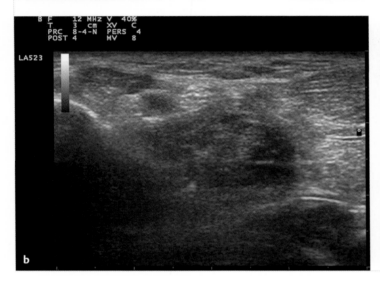

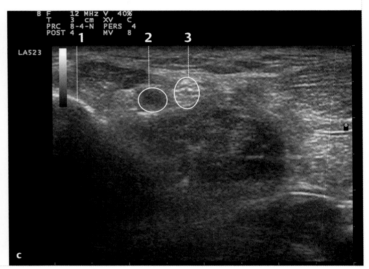

### Tips and Tricks

- The saphenous, superficial fibular, and sural nerves can be blocked relatively easily at the upper level of the ankle joint by subcutaneous infiltration anesthesia. If the procedure starts with these subcutaneous blocks, penetration of the skin in the subsequent blocks is painless. The order is important for minimizing pain when performing an ankle block.
- A complete circular depot should be avoided so as not to endanger blood perfusion of the foot. Subcutaneous infiltration depots can instead be made at different levels.
- The tibial and deep fibular nerves must be sought selectively.
- Epinephrine-free local anesthetics should be used.
- Depending on experience and the anatomical situation, performing an ankle block takes between 5 and 15 minutes; the effect commences after 15 minutes and is complete after 30 minutes. If areas of the foot remain sensitive, these gaps can also be filled by peripheral (subcutaneous) infiltration.
- The pressure of a tourniquet over the subcutaneous infiltration depot is tolerated for up to 2 hours. The actual pain caused by a tourniquet is an ischemic pain and is thus dependent on the ischemic muscle mass that is produced by the tourniquet; for this reason, a tourniquet sited further peripherally (e.g., two to three finger widths above the malleoli) is always tolerated better.

# 14.6 Indications, Contraindications, Complications, Side Effects

## 14.6.1 Indications

- Incomplete lumbosacral plexus anesthesia
- Operations on the foot (e.g., hallux valgus, foot gangrene)
- Pain therapy
- Diagnostic blocks

## 14.6.2 Contraindications

- General contraindications (see Chapter 20.2)
- Nerve lesions (relative; previous documentation required)

## 14.6.3 Side Effects and Complications

No special complications or side effects are known.

# 14.7 Remarks on the Combination Block (Ankle Block)

Combination of the individual blocks described is traditionally called ankle block and is described in many textbooks. It is an easily performed technique with a low rate of complications and a high rate of success (Kay 1999; Malloy 1999).

For operations in the ankle region, it must always be ensured that the block is performed above the actual ankle region. In these cases it should be considered whether a popliteal block or distal sciatic block (Chapter 12.3) could be a helpful alternative.

A complete ankle block—despite its relative safety—is technically rather complex for the novice as it involves two individual blocks in addition to the superficial ring blocks, namely block of the posterior tibial nerve and the deep fibular nerve. Because of the variable anastomoses and the large range of anatomical variation, blocking all the nerves requires either a good technique or injection of rather large volumes of anesthetic. In 100 blocks of the areas of distribution of the sural nerve and saphenous nerve, McCutcheon (1965) reported that only 60% and 84%, respectively, correlated with the information in anatomical textbooks. He obtained a success rate for blockade of the tibial nerve of only 88%. Others, however, have reported very high success rates of 95% (Kofoed 1982) and 100% (Schurman 1976).

Sharrock and Mineo (1988) found low blood levels of local anesthetic after ankle block, so it may be assumed that the volumes required for successful anesthesia are well tolerated. The combination of two ankle blocks in one patient is therefore regarded as justifiable (Concepcion 1999). Nevertheless, the maximum dosages of the individual local anesthetics should not be exceeded.

Ankle block can also be performed for operations with a lower leg tourniquet. In a prospective study, Delgado-Martinez et al (2001) investigated whether block of individual nerves is then adequate. On the basis of their results, they recommend that a complete ankle block (i.e., anesthesia of all five nerves) can be used. If a tourniquet is required, it can be applied just above the ankle. Different levels of pressure in the cuff have been reported (Frédéric and Bouchon 1996). A study in volunteers found that pressures of 225 mmHg (± 46 mmHg) with a narrow cuff and 284 mmHg (± 42 mmHg) with a wide cuff can be regarded as safe and effective (Biehl et al 1993). Other authors regard it as sufficient to measure the individually required pressure with Doppler or a stethoscope (Diamond et al 1985, Pauers and Carocci 1994).

In an electrophysiological study of the use of a tourniquet above the ankle, no increased risk to the nerves was found (Chu et al 1981). In a retrospective study of 3,027 patients who had a tourniquet during operation with a cuff pressure of 325 mmHg, a post-tourniquet syndrome was found in three patients (Derner and Buckholz 1995). As it is obviously dependent on the cuff pressure, the incidence of 0.1% in this study should be even lower at a recommended pressure of 250 mmHg or less.

Ankle block is regarded as a safe anesthesia procedure. Complications have been described only rarely. Isolated cases of persistent paresthesia have been reported in a few studies, but these symptoms subsided spontaneously after 4 to 6 weeks (Sharrock et al 1986, Sharrock and Mineo 1988). In a study of 1,295 patients who had an ankle block, four complications were recorded (three vasovagal reactions, one supraventricular tachycardia), while neuritis, hematoma, or infection was not found in any patient (Myerson et al 1992). In a prospective study of 284 patients, no postanesthetic neuralgia or other complications was reported (Kofoed 1982). In other studies, also, no complications were reported (Sarrafian et al 1983, Wassef 1991, Needoff et al 1995).

## 14.8 Summary

So-called ankle block is a safe anesthetic procedure with few complications for operations on the foot. The technique is eminently suitable for selective block of individual nerves for diagnosis or to complete regional anesthesia. However, it should be ensured that the patient receives as few painful punctures as possible during the procedure. Complete anesthesia of the foot also can be achieved with one injection in a distal sciatic block or popliteal block (see Chapter 12).

## 14.9 Blocks at the Toes

### 14.9.1 Anatomy

The sensory nerves supplying the foot are terminal branches of the sciatic nerve. The medial border of the foot is occasionally supplied as far as the great toe by the terminal branch of the femoral nerve, the saphenous nerve. The tibial and deep fibular nerves supply the more deeply located structures (bone, joints, muscles); the tibial nerve also supplies the sole of the foot and the deep fibular nerve supplies the skin on the lateral side of the great toe and the medial side of the second toe. The other nerves run subcutaneously and innervate the skin of the medial (saphenous nerve) and lateral side (sural nerve) of the foot and also the dorsum of the foot and toes (superficial fibular nerve).

### 14.9.2 Block Anesthesia of the Toes (Oberst Anesthesia)

Digital block anesthesia according to Oberst is a widely used, reliable method that is employed especially for blockade in the fingers. However, the method is also employed for anesthesia in the toes.

### Landmarks and Position

Dorsal side of the toe, patient in supine position.

### Procedure

The toe is punctured subcutaneously with a fine needle at the middle and on both sides of the proximal phalanx from above, tangentially to the bone; the plantar side should almost be reached. By supporting the plantar side of the toe with one's own finger, it is possible to check how far the needle has reached in the plantar direction. On each side, 0.5 to 1 mL of a 1% (10 mg/mL) medium-acting local anesthetic is injected (▶ Fig. 14.20).

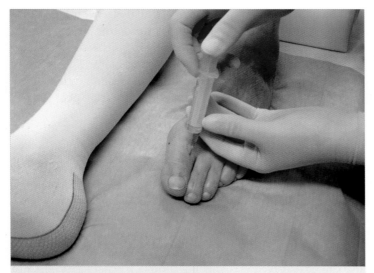

**Fig. 14.20** Oberst block anesthesia of the toes. A fine needle is inserted subcutaneously at the middle and on both sides of the proximal phalanx from above, tangentially to the bone; the plantar side should almost be reached. By supporting the plantar side of the toe with one's own finger, it is possible to check how far the needle has reached in the plantar direction. On each side, 0.5 to 1 mL of 1% (10 mg/mL) medium-acting local anesthetic is injected.

### Tips and Tricks

- The injection should be given slowly as the pressure produced by the injection volume may be perceived as very unpleasant by the patient.
- Oberst block anesthesia can be recommended for the great toe but is less suitable for the other toes because of their tough tissue.
- A gentle alternative is interdigital block in the distal or proximal toe region or in the metatarsal region.

## Remarks on the Technique

In principle there is a risk of block-related gangrene, so only epinephrine-free solutions should be used. No more than 8 mL to a maximum of 10 mL of local anesthetic per toe should be infiltrated. These peripheral block techniques are indicated particularly in the outpatient area and in at-risk patients in whom minor operations on the toes or forefoot must be performed (e.g., nail removal, corrective operations for fractures or hammer toe, toe amputations, or other operations in the area of the phalanges).

Because of the risk of gangrene, the digital block techniques are relatively contraindicated in patients with peripheral perfusion disorders, including Raynaud syndrome, and should be performed only after thorough consideration of the advantages and disadvantages and alternatives (e.g., distal sciatic nerve block, Chapter 12.3). In these cases a tourniquet should not be applied for more than 15 minutes, and the maximum dose of local anesthetic per toe is reported to be 8 mL (Adriani 1984).

## References

Adriani J. Labat Regional Anesthesia. Techniques and Clinical Applications. 4th ed. St. Louis: Green; 1984: 373–384

Biehl WC, III, Morgan JM, Wagner FW, Jr, Gabriel RA. The safety of the Esmarch tourniquet. Foot Ankle 1993; 14: 278–283

Bridenbaugh PhO, Wedel DJ. The lower extremity. In: Cousins MJ, Bridenbaugh PhO, eds. Neural Blockade Clinic Anesthesia and Management of Pain. 3rd ed. Philadelphia: Lippincott-Raven; 1998: 373–409

Chu J, Fox I, Jassen M. Pneumatic ankle tourniquet: clinical and electrophysiologic study. Arch Phys Med Rehabil 1981; 62: 570–575

Concepcion M. Ankle block. Tech Reg Anesth Pain Manage 1999; 3: 241–246

Delgado-Martínez AD, Marchal JM, Molina M, Palma A. Forefoot surgery with ankle tourniquet: complete or selective ankle block? Reg Anesth Pain Med 2001; 26: 184–186(letter)

Derner R, Buckholz J. Surgical hemostasis by pneumatic ankle tourniquet during 3027 podiatric operations. J Foot Ankle Surg 1995; 34: 236–246

Diamond EL, Sherman M, Lenet M. A quantitative method of determining the pneumatic ankle tourniquet setting. J Foot Surg 1985; 24: 330–334

Frédéric A, Bouchon Y. Analgesia in surgery of the foot. Apropos of 1373 patients [Article in French] Cah Anesthesiol 1996; 44: 115–118

Kay J. Ankle block. Tech Reg Anesth Pain Med 1999; 3: 3–8

Kofoed H. Peripheral nerve blocks at the knee and ankle in operations for common foot disorders. Clin Orthop Relat Res 1982: 97–101

Malloy RE. Ankle block. In: Benson B, Malloy RE, Strichartz G, eds. Essentials of Pain Medicine and Regional Anesthesia. Philadelphia: Churchill Livingstone; 1999: 437

McCutcheon R. Regional anaesthesia for the foot. Can Anaesth Soc J 1965; 12: 465–474

Myerson MS, Ruland CM, Allon SM. Regional anesthesia for foot and ankle surgery. Foot Ankle 1992; 13: 282–288

Needoff M, Radford P, Costigan P. Local anesthesia for postoperative pain relief after foot surgery: a prospective clinical trial. Foot Ankle Int 1995; 16: 11–13

Pauers RS, Carocci MA. Low pressure pneumatic tourniquets: effectiveness at minimum recommended inflation pressures. J Foot Ankle Surg 1994; 33: 605–609

Platzer W. Color Atlas of Human Anatomy. 7th ed. Vol 1: Locomotor System. Stuttgart: Thieme; 2014

Sarrafian SK, Ibrahim IN, Breihan JH. Ankle-foot peripheral nerve block for mid and forefoot surgery. Foot Ankle 1983; 4: 86–90

Schurman DJ. Ankle-block anesthesia for foot surgery. Anesthesiology 1976; 44: 348–352

Sharrock NE, Waller JF, Fierro LE. Midtarsal block for surgery of the forefoot. Br J Anaesth 1986; 58: 37–40

Sharrock NE, Mineo R. Venous lidocaine and bupivacaine levels following midtarsal ankle block. Reg Anesth 1988; 13(S): 75

Wassef MR. Posterior tibial nerve block. A new approach using the bony landmark of the sustentaculum tali. Anaesthesia 1991; 46: 841–844

# Part 4

**Peripheral Regional Anesthesia in Pediatrics**

# 15 General Overview

Interest in regional anesthesia procedures in pediatric anesthesia has increased significantly in recent years. Due in part to the spread of ultrasonography, peripheral regional anesthesia is increasingly performed in children. In principle, all peripheral regional procedures that are known in adult anesthesia are possible in pediatric patients. But the smaller the child, the higher are the requirements for handling, the material used, and knowledge of the specific physiological, anatomical, and pharmacological characteristics of these patients.

▶ **Local anesthetic toxicity.** In children up to the age of 6 months, there is an increased risk of toxic complications after administration of local anesthetics (Berde 1992). Local anesthetics of the amide type are weak bases and are bound mainly to proteins in plasma. There is more than 90% binding of bupivacaine, ropivacaine, and levobupivacaine to alpha 1-acid glycoprotein and albumin in the serum. The free, unbound fraction of the local anesthetic is responsible for the pharmacological, but also for the toxic effects on the heart and central nervous system. In children under 6 months, plasma concentrations of the above-mentioned proteins are still low, so that higher levels of free local anesthetic may result in the serum.

Amino amide local anesthetics are metabolized by the hepatic cytochrome P450 system. But enzyme activity in children reaches the levels of adult patients only after the age of 1 year.

Due to the immaturity of the P450 system in infants, there is limited clearance of local anesthetics of the amide type with the risk of accumulation. In addition, due to their higher total body water, newborns and infants have a larger distribution volume and a longer elimination half-life than children and adults (Suresh and Wheeler 2002).

▶ **Dosage.** Continuous peripheral regional anesthesia offers great advantages in terms of effective postoperative pain management. Nevertheless, elevated plasma levels with dangerous accumulation of local anesthetics can occur due to the mechanisms described here.

▶ **Short duration of action.** Owing to the smaller diameter and the still incomplete myelination of the nerve fibers in children up to toddler age, lower local anesthetic concentrations than required for adults are sufficient for a successful block. However, the duration of the regional anesthesia is shorter than in adults due to higher cardiac output and the associated rapid systemic absorption.

---

**Caution**

The plasma concentrations of the local anesthetics that can lead to toxic reactions are largely unknown in children. For this reason especially in children, the recommended local anesthetic dosage limits should not be exceeded (▶ Table 15.1). The maximum quantity of local anesthetic must be calculated based on the body weight of children, and only that amount should be drawn up into a syringe to prevent accidental overdose.

---

▶ **Main indication: postoperative analgesia.** The main indication for the use of regional anesthesia in children is postoperative analgesia. These procedures are therefore usually performed after induction of general anesthesia until about the age of 10 years. The use of peripheral regional anesthesia in children after general anesthesia is widely accepted and is even recommended (Dalens 2006, Taenzer et al 2014).

---

**Note**

Without sedation or general anesthesia, children usually tolerate regional anesthesia inadequately or not at all. A movement at the "wrong time" can have devastating effects and provoke a faulty puncture or even a nerve lesion. On the other hand nerve blocks under sedation or general anesthesia involve the risk of undetected complications. Signs of puncture-induced nerve injury or intravascular injection are missing.

---

▶ **But how safe is regional anesthesia in children?** In a study of 24,409 conventional regional anesthesias, Giaufré et al (1996) found a complication rate of < 1‰. Complications occurred only in neuraxial procedures. None of the complications resulted in permanent damage. In the new edition of this study from the year 2010, the French working group examined 31,132 regional anesthesias and published a slightly higher complication rate of 1.2‰ (Ecoffey et al 2010). Complications occurred significantly more often in neuraxial procedures than peripheral procedures. The age of the children also played a role in the incidence of complications. According to the present study, complications occurred four times more often in children under 6 months than in the age group over 6 months. This study also reported no complications that led to permanent damage.

▶ **What can still be improved?** Can direct sonographic visualization of the peripheral nervous structures and the adjacent

---

**Table 15.1** Maximum recommended doses of local anesthetics for peripheral regional anesthesia (modified according to Berde 1992 and Ross et al 2000)

| Local anesthetic | "Single shot" (mg/kg) | Continuous, any age over 6 months (mg/kg/h) | Continuous, infants < 6 months (mg/kg/h) |
|---|---|---|---|
| Ropivacaine | 3–3.5 | 0.4 | 0.2 |
| Bupivacaine | 2.5–3 | 0.4 | 0.2 |

In infants younger than 6 months, the maximum local anesthetic dose should be reduced by 50% to account for the lower plasma protein binding capacity.

anatomical structures increase the safety and success rate of blocks in children? An advantage of ultrasound-guided regional anesthesia compared to conventional nerve stimulator-guided regional anesthesia has not been yet been demonstrated and it remains to be seen whether such an advantage will ever be proven. Up to now, complications during ultrasound-guided regional procedures have been described only in adults (see below). Similar studies do not yet exist for children, but it is likely that complications will occur and be described in ultrasound-guided regional anesthesia in children as well. The complications in adults described in this chapter can certainly be transferred to the *pediatric* area.

▶ **Advantages.** What are the arguments now for the use of *ultrasound-guided regional anesthesia* in pediatric anesthesia?

• In some regional anesthesia procedures, a relatively high failure rate was described using conventional techniques. Weintraud et al (2008) found a success rate of only 61% after landmark-based ilioinguinal block. In contrast, success rates of 96% after ultrasound-guided block are described in literature (Willschke et al 2005).

• Especially in children there is often very little space between the block site and adjacent vulnerable structures. For this reason, the use of ultrasound provides an advantage, especially in abdominal wall blocks (intra-abdominal organs) and in supraclavicular blocks of the brachial plexus (pleura). The adjacent structures can be visualized by ultrasound and complications can be avoided using an appropriate technique.

> **Note**
>
> In ultrasound scanning, not only the nerves to be blocked can be visualized, but also the anatomical structures that must be avoided with the needle as well.

• Sonography makes regional anesthesia possible in infants and young children even if anatomical landmarks are not found and nerve stimulator-guided regional anesthesia is thus difficult to perform.

• "The local anesthetic makes the block!" During the entire block, the injection and the spread of the local anesthetic can and must be observed. In case of insufficient spread the needle is repositioned and the local anesthetic can be injected optimally around the nerve structures.

• The amount of local anesthetic required for a successful block can be reduced in children by using ultrasound (Willschke et al 2006, Oberndorfer et al 2007). This makes it possible to reduce the risk of toxic local anesthetic complications.

▶ **Sonography machine.** In addition to relevant experience in pediatric anesthesia and performing regional anesthesia procedures in children, especially in infants and young children, there are also special demands on the sonography machine. In pediatric regional anesthesia, a high-resolution ultrasound system with a high-frequency linear transducer (at least 12 MHz) is necessary because the nerve courses are often superficial. Since the space available for placing the transducer is sometimes very limited, especially in infants and young children, transducers with a small contact area are used.

▶ **Ultrasonography and nerve stimulation.** Due to the use of regional anesthesia procedures on the anesthetized child, it is advisable to use ultrasound and nerve stimulation in parallel—dual guidance. The advantage of this approach lies in the additional information gained by nerve stimulation that may be very helpful in poor sonographic conditions or unclear sonoanatomical situations. Sometimes a successful block is not possible without dual guidance.

Many of the common childhood surgical procedures are covered by the peripheral blocks described below, making it a good basis for an anesthetist who regularly treats children.

# 15.1 Needle-Transducer Alignment

▶ **Out of plane.** The regional anesthesia needle is inserted at the long side of the transducer (see ▶ Fig. 16.6 and ▶ Fig. 17.3). At best, only the needle tip or the needle shaft can be visualized. The position of the needle tip can be indirectly visualized through small test injections (0.5–1 mL).

▶ **In plane.** The needle is inserted at the narrow side of the transducer (see ▶ Fig. 16.3 and ▶ Fig. 18.7). The needle is inserted within the scanning plane. This makes it possible to visualize the needle over its entire length.

# 15.2 Ultrasound Axes

▶ **Short axis.** The nerve or nerve plexus is visualized by ultrasound in the cross-section. This transducer position is the typical axis for ultrasound-guided regional anesthesia.

▶ **Long axis.** The target structure is displayed in longitudinal section.

# References

Berde CB. Convulsions associated with pediatric regional anesthesia. Anesth Analg 1992; 75: 164–166

Dalens B. Some current controversies in paediatric regional anaesthesia. Curr Opin Anaesthesiol 2006; 19: 301–308

Ecoffey C, Lacroix F, Giaufré E, Orliaguet G, Courrèges P; Association des Anesthésistes Réanimateurs Pédiatriques d'Expression Française (ADARPEF). Epidemiology and morbidity of regional anesthesia in children: a follow-up one-year prospective survey of the French-Language Society of Paediatric Anaesthesiologists (ADARPEF). Paediatr Anaesth 2010; 20: 1061–1069

Giaufré E, Dalens B, Gombert A. Epidemiology and morbidity of regional anesthesia in children: a one-year prospective survey of the French-Language Society of Pediatric Anesthesiologists. Anesth Analg 1996; 83: 904–912

Oberndorfer U, Marhofer P, Bösenberg A et al. Ultrasonographic guidance for sciatic and femoral nerve blocks in children. Br J Anaesth 2007; 98: 797–801

Ross AK, Eck JB, Tobias JD. Pediatric regional anesthesia: beyond the caudal. Anesth Analg 2000; 91: 16–26

Suresh S, Wheeler M. Practical pediatric regional anesthesia. Anesthesiol Clin North Am 2002; 20: 83–113

Taenzer AH, Walker BJ, Bosenberg AT et al. Asleep versus awake: does it matter?: Pediatric regional block complications by patient state: a report from the Pediatric Regional Anesthesia Network. Reg Anesth Pain Med 2014; 39: 279–283

Weintraud M, Marhofer P, Bösenberg A et al. Ilioinguinal/iliohypogastric blocks in children: where do we administer the local anesthetic without direct visualization? Anesth Analg 2008; 106: 89–93

Willschke H, Marhofer P, Bösenberg A et al. Ultrasonography for ilioinguinal/iliohypogastric nerve blocks in children. Br J Anaesth 2005; 95: 226–230

Willschke H, Bösenberg A, Marhofer P et al. Ultrasonographic-guided ilioinguinal/iliohypogastric nerve block in pediatric anesthesia: what is the optimal volume? Anesth Analg 2006; 102: 1680–1684

# 16 Upper Limb

## 16.1 Supraclavicular Block of the Brachial Plexus

### 16.1.1 Anatomy

The three trunks of the brachial plexus run distally from where they exit the interscalene groove toward the first rib (▶ Fig. 2.3). The upper trunk arises from roots of C5 and C6, the middle trunk is formed from the C7 nerve root, and the lower trunk consists of the roots of C8 and T1 (▶ Fig. 2.1). The brachial plexus crosses the first rib lateral to the subclavian artery. The pleural dome is in the immediate vicinity of the supraclavicular brachial plexus (▶ Fig. 2.11). It extends clearly beyond the first rib.

In the clavicular region, each trunk splits into an anterior and a posterior division and these form the cords. All posterior divisions unite to form the posterior cord (C5–C8, T1). The anterior divisions of the upper and middle trunks form the lateral cord (C5–C7) and the medial cord arises from the anterior divisions of the lower trunk (C8, T1; ▶ Fig. 2.1).

### 16.1.2 Sonoanatomy

A linear transducer is placed directly supraclavicular, parallel to the clavicle, and is directed toward the thorax in the coronal plane (▶ Fig. 16.1). The subclavian artery is visualized in the short axis. The supraclavicular brachial plexus is usually found lateral to the subclavian artery and appears as a (grapelike) cluster of round, hypoechoic structures with a hyperechoic border (▶ Fig. 16.2). As the subclavian artery is usually examined from a slightly oblique direction, it is not seen as round, hypoechoic structure, but shows blurring at the edges. The vessel can be safely identified based on the visible pulsations or by using color Doppler.

The first rib is found in the ultrasound image below, that is, distal to the plexus from the transducer, which thus provides a degree of protection against accidental pleural puncture, as the

pleura is in close proximity to the subclavian artery and the brachial plexus. The pleura should always be visualized.

### 16.1.3 Technique of Supraclavicular Brachial Plexus Block

**Landmarks**

Clavicle, the subclavian artery, and first rib in ultrasound visualization.

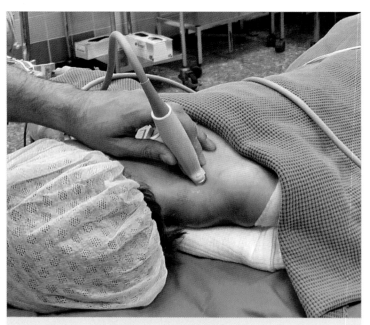

**Fig. 16.1** The transducer position of the sonographic visualization of the right supraclavicular brachial plexus in a 3½-year-old child. The linear transducer is placed directly parallel and cranial to the clavicle and shows the plexus in the short axis. For optimal transducer position, the head is turned slightly to the contralateral side and the shoulders are padded with a towel roll to achieve sufficient hyperextension of the head.

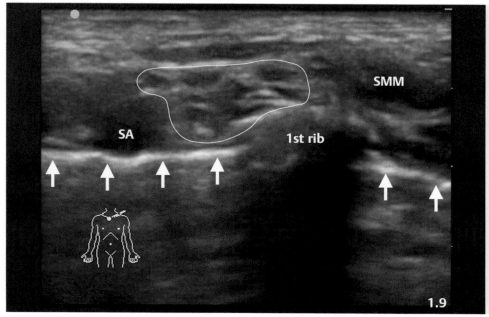

**Fig. 16.2** Sonographic visualization of the left supraclavicular brachial plexus in a 5-year-old child in the short axis. The brachial plexus (white outline) is located lateral to the subclavian artery (SA) and cranial to the first rib. The artery is examined obliquely, so that it shows significant blurring at the edges. The pleura (arrows) is located in the immediate proximity of the brachial plexus. SMM Scalenus medius muscle.

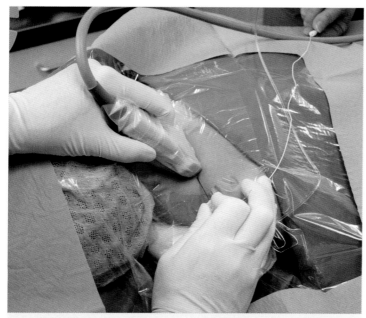

**Fig. 16.3** Ultrasound-guided single-shot block of the right supra-clavicular brachial plexus in a 5-year-old child. The plexus is displayed in the short axis; the needle-transducer alignment is in plane. The shoulder girdle is padded with a towel roll. The head is hyperextended and rotated to the contralateral side.

## Position

The child lies supine, the ipsilateral arm is adducted, and the head is turned slightly to the contralateral side. Due to the limited space in the supraclavicular region, particularly in small children, the shoulder girdle should be padded with a towel roll so that there is a sufficient hyperextension of the neck.

## Procedure

The clavicle is palpated and the transducer is placed parallel and directly cranial to the clavicle (▶ Fig. 16.1). The brachial plexus is sought lateral to the subclavian artery in the short axis. Subsequently, the pleura is identified (▶ Fig. 16.2). Then the region is disinfected, draped, and the transducer is covered with a sterile sleeve. The transducer is placed again at the previously determined position. After a stab incision with a lancet, the regional anesthesia needle is inserted for an in-plane technique on the narrow side of the transducer and the needle is advanced under repeated aspiration from lateral to medial to the plexus (▶ Fig. 16.3).

> **Practical Note**
>
> An in-plane technique should always be used for a single-shot method. Even for a catheter method, in-plane needle guidance should be preferred; however, an out-of-plane technique is possible in exceptions. It is advisable to place a local anesthetic depot between the brachial plexus and first rib. Another depot can be injected above the plexus. Throughout the whole block process, the pleura must be visualized and kept in view.

If a continuous technique is planned, the catheter is then advanced 1 to 3 cm beyond the end of the needle.

## Local Anesthetic, Dosage

▶ **Single-shot block.** Administer 0.4 to 1 mL/kg body weight of a long-acting local anesthetic (e.g., ropivacaine 0.2 to 0.5% [2–5 mg/mL]), maximum 20 mL.

> **Caution**
>
> The maximum permissible local anesthetic dose per kilogram body weight must be observed!

▶ **Continuous block.** Maximum dosage for infants, toddlers, and children older than 6 months is 0.4 mg/kg body weight per hour of ropivacaine.

## 16.1.4 Indications and Contraindications

### Indications

All interventions in the area of the entire arm, especially the upper arm ("spinal anesthesia of the arm"; Tsui and Suresh 2010).

### Contraindications

General contraindications (Chapter 20.2).

Owing to the risk of pneumothorax, no bilateral block should be conducted and no block at all if there is contralateral pneumothorax. This technique should also not be used in children with severe respiratory failure or contralateral paresis of the diaphragm or vocal cords.

## 16.1.5 Complications, Side Effects, Method-Specific Problems

### Complications

The Horner syndrome and accidental puncture of the subclavian artery after conventional, landmark-based, supraclavicular block (Pande et al 2000).

The following complications have been reported only in adult patients up to now:

- Ipsilateral phrenic nerve block with paresis of the diaphragm. Transient neurological deficit in the ipsilateral hand after ultrasound-guided block (Perlas et al 2009).
- Horner syndrome after ultrasound-guided block (Renes et al 2009).
- Permanent damage to the radial nerve after ultrasound-guided block (Reiss et al 2010).
- Symptomatic pneumothorax after ultrasound-guided block (Bhatia et al 2010).
- Respiratory failure after landmark-based block due to simultaneous block of the recurrent laryngeal nerve in a patient with contralateral vocal cord paresis after previous thyroidectomy (Solanki et al 2011).

## Method-Specific Problems

Due to the immediate proximity of the pleural dome to the supraclavicular brachial plexus, this technique has an increased risk of pneumothorax compared with other regional anesthetic approaches to the plexus. Even ultrasound guidance does not eliminate this risk completely.

> **Practical Note**
>
> In children, for the single-shot as well as the continuous technique, preference should be given to in-plane needle direction to guarantee the best possible control of the needle and the needle tip. An out-of-plane technique for catheter placement is possible in principle, but should remain reserved for exceptional cases owing to the difficult placement of the needle tip.

### 16.1.6 Remarks on the Technique

In the supraclavicular region, the suprascapular artery runs above the brachial plexus. In the ultrasound image the artery can be visualized above the plexus close to the transducer head. To avoid an accidental puncture of this vessel, the plexus should be found in an area where the artery is not visualized in the ultrasound plane.

Because the supraclavicular brachial plexus runs very superficially, it may be useful to tunnel an inserted catheter subcutaneously. Otherwise there is a risk of retrograde flow of local anesthetic into the penetration canal of the catheter and it will not adequately reach the parts of the plexus.

Due to the risk of pneumothorax, the supraclavicular approach is not a routine technique in children (Hillmann and Döffert 2009). The indication should be very carefully weighed and pneumothorax should be excluded after each supraclavicular block. In order to minimize the radiation exposure of the children, a thorax ultrasound may be performed (Lichtenstein 2009; see Chapter 1).

## 16.2 Axillary Block of the Brachial Plexus

### 16.2.1 Anatomy

The anatomy is described in Chapter 6.

### Sonoanatomy

A linear transducer is placed slightly distal to the point where the pectoralis major muscle crosses the short head of the biceps brachii muscle (► Fig. 16.4). The axillary artery is visualized in the short axis.

> **Caution**
>
> Accompanying axillary veins may be compressed even by only slight pressure of the transducer; hence the pressure of the transducer should be regularly reduced to visualize the veins.

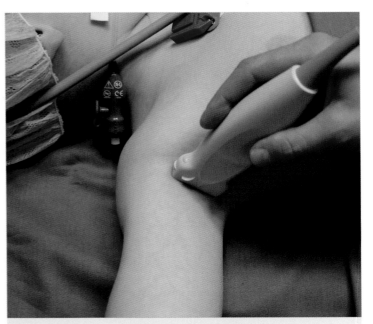

**Fig. 16.4** Transducer position for the sonographic visualization of the right axillary brachial plexus in a 5-year-old child. The linear transducer is placed at the intersection of the pectoralis major muscle and the short head of the biceps brachii muscle. The axillary artery and the brachial plexus are visualized in the short axis.

The nerves of the brachial plexus are distributed around the axillary artery and are usually hyperechoic with a hypoechoic fascicular ("honeycomb-like") internal structure (► Fig. 16.5). In children, however, the nerves may occasionally have a round hypoechoic structure with a hyperechoic border and be the size of the axillary artery.

The position of the individual nerves around the artery is highly variable. Usually the median nerve is found between the axillary artery and the biceps brachii muscle. The ulnar nerve lies in the ultrasound image above the artery, near the transducer and partially adjacent to the medial nerve, so the two nerves can hardly be distinguished from each other. The individual nerves can be clearly distinguished only if they are followed distally.

In rare cases, the ulnar nerve may be lateral to the axillary vein and is therefore difficult to locate and block. Usually, the radial nerve can be visualized in the ultrasound image somewhat below the axillary artery or further from the transducer head.

> **Caution**
>
> The posterior enhancement of the artery should not be confused with the radial nerve.

The musculocutaneous nerve can almost always be visualized very well in the double fascia between the biceps brachii and the coracobrachialis muscles as a lenticular structure with a hyperechoic border (► Fig. 16.5).

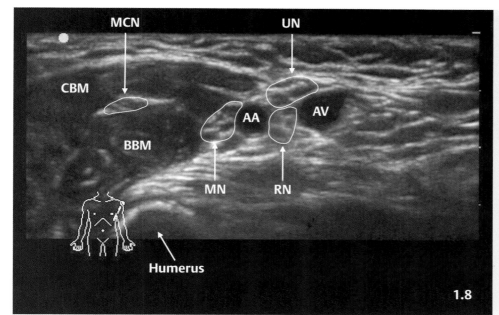

Fig. 16.5 Sonographic visualization of the left axillary brachial plexus in the short axis in a 3-year-old child. The nerves of the brachial plexus (white borders, MN: median nerve, UN: ulnar nerve, RN: radial nerve) are distributed around the axillary artery (AA). The musculo-cutaneous nerve (MCN) is located within a double fascia between the biceps brachii muscle (BBM) and the coracobrachialis muscle (CBM). AV, axillary vein.

## 16.2.2 Technique of Axillary Brachial Plexus Block

### Landmarks

Intersection of the pectoralis major muscle over the short head of the biceps brachii muscle and the coracobrachialis muscle, axillary artery in the ultrasound image.

### Position

The child is placed supine and the head is turned slightly to the contralateral side. The arm to be blocked is abducted to 90° and the elbow is flexed 90° and securely fixed on an arm support.

### Procedure

The transducer is placed at the intersection of the pectoralis major muscle over the short head of the biceps brachii muscle and the coracobrachialis muscle (▶ Fig. 16.4). After the axillary artery and axillary veins are identified by ultrasound, the nerves of the brachial plexus are visualized in the short axis (▶ Fig. 16.5). Then the region is disinfected, draped, and a sterile sleeve is placed on the transducer. The transducer is placed again at the previously determined position.

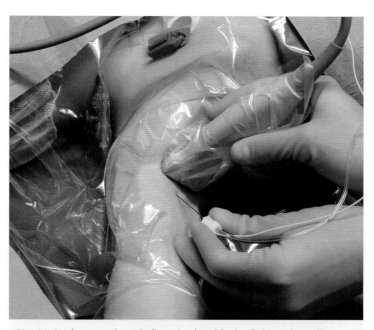

Fig. 16.6 Ultrasound-guided single-shot block of the right axillary brachial plexus in a 5-year-old child. The plexus is displayed in the short axis; the needle-transducer alignment is out of plane.

> **Practical Note**
>
> It is important to check the pressure of the transducer so that the axillary vein (several veins are sometimes present) is not completely compressed and remains detectable to avoid an accidental intravascular injection of the local anesthetic (see below).

After a stab incision with a lancet, the regional anesthesia needle is advanced toward the plexus under repeated aspiration in an out-of-plane technique (▶ Fig. 16.6). An in-plane technique is also possible. The local anesthetic is then applied either around the artery or the median, ulnar, and radial nerves are blocked separately. Then the transducer is slid slightly to the biceps brachii muscle and the musculocutaneous nerve is sought in the double fascia between the biceps brachii and coracobrachialis muscles. The needle is then advanced from the same puncture point toward the musculocutaneous nerve and, after negative aspiration, the block is performed.

If a continuous technique is planned, the catheter is then advanced about 2 to 3 cm beyond the end of the needle and is placed on the parts of the nerves of the brachial plexus that are most significant for the postoperative pain therapy, for example, near the radial nerve in a radius fracture.

### Local Anesthetic, Dosage

▶ **Single-shot block.** Administer a long-acting local anesthetic (e.g., ropivacaine 0.2–0.5% [2–5 mg/mL]), 0.4 to 1 mL/kg body weight, maximum 20 mL.

▶ **Continuous block.** Maximum dose for infants, toddlers, and children older than 6 months is 0.4 mg/kg body weight per hour of ropivacaine.

## 16.2.3 Indications and Contraindications

### Indications

The indications are described in Chapter 6.

### Contraindications

General contraindications (Chapter 20.2).

## 16.2.4 Complications, Side Effects, Method-Specific Problems

### Complications

Temporary vascular insufficiency with no pulse in the ipsilateral arm after conventional axillary plexus block (Bhat 2004).

The following complications have been reported only in adult patients:

• Accidental intravascular local anesthetic injection during ultrasound-guided block despite negative aspiration (Loubert et al 2008, Robards et al 2008).

• Accidental nerve puncture and local anesthetic application during ultrasound-guided block without subsequent neurological deficit (Russon and Blanco 2007).

### Method-Specific Problems

Due to strong pressure of the transducer, axillary veins can be compressed so that they can no longer be visualized by ultrasound. A local anesthetic injection after accidental puncture is still possible despite negative aspiration (Robards et al 2008).

## 16.2.5 Remarks on the Technique

Due to the very superficial location of the axillary brachial plexus, the lowest penetration depth of the ultrasound should be selected and the highest possible transducer frequency (≥ 10 MHz) should be set.

In principle, axillary catheter placement is also possible. However, the location is only conditionally suitable for hygiene reasons, especially in adolescents. Moreover, the risk of a catheter dislocation is relatively high, so that if there is an appropriate indication, a supraclavicular access for continuous techniques is preferable. The brachial plexus is also very superficial in the axillary region. It is therefore also useful here to tunnel the catheter subcutaneously (see above).

## References

Bhat R. Transient vascular insufficiency after axillary brachial plexus block in a child. Anesth Analg 2004; 98: 1284–1285

Bhatia A, Lai J, Chan VW, Brull R. Case report: pneumothorax as a complication of the ultrasound-guided supraclavicular approach for brachial plexus block. Anesth Analg 2010; 111: 817–819

Hillmann R, Döffert J. Praxis der anästhesiologischen Sonografie. Interventionelle Verfahren bei Erwachsenen und Kindern. 1st ed. Munich: Elsevier; Urban: 2009

Lichtenstein DA. Ultrasound examination of the lungs in the intensive care unit. Pediatr Crit Care Med 2009; 10: 693–698

Loubert C, Williams SR, Hélie F, Arcand G. Complication during ultrasound-guided regional block: accidental intravascular injection of local anesthetic. Anesthesiology 2008; 108: 759–760

Pande R, Pande M, Bhadani U, Pandey CK, Bhattacharya A. Supraclavicular brachial plexus block as a sole anaesthetic technique in children: an analysis of 200 cases. Anaesthesia 2000; 55: 798–802

Perlas A, Lobo G, Lo N, Brull R, Chan VW, Karkhanis R. Ultrasound-guided supraclavicular block: outcome of 510 consecutive cases. Reg Anesth Pain Med 2009; 34: 171–176

Reiss W, Kurapati S, Shariat A, Hadzic A. Nerve injury complicating ultrasound/electrostimulation-guided supraclavicular brachial plexus block. Reg Anesth Pain Med 2010; 35: 400–401

Renes SH, Spoormans HH, Gielen MJ, Rettig HC, van Geffen GJ. Hemidiaphragmatic paresis can be avoided in ultrasound-guided supraclavicular brachial plexus block. Reg Anesth Pain Med 2009; 34: 595–599

Robards C, Clendenen S, Greengrass R. Intravascular injection during ultrasound-guided axillary block: negative aspiration can be misleading. Anesth Analg 2008; 107: 1754–1755

Russon K, Blanco R. Accidental intraneural injection into the musculocutaneous nerve visualized with ultrasound. Anesth Analg 2007; 105: 1504–1505

Solanki SL, Jain A, Makkar JK, Nikhar SA. Severe stridor and marked respiratory difficulty after right-sided supraclavicular brachial plexus block. J Anesth 2011; 25: 305–307

Tsui B, Suresh S. Ultrasound imaging for regional anesthesia in infants, children, and adolescents: a review of current literature and its application in the practice of extremity and trunk blocks. Anesthesiology 2010; 112: 473–492

# 17 Lower Limb

Analgesia of the entire leg can be achieved through a combined block of the femoral nerve and the sciatic nerve. An advantage of this combined block is the significantly longer effect compared to caudal anesthesia.

## 17.1 Femoral Nerve Block

### 17.1.1 Anatomy

The anatomy is described in Chapter 10.

### 17.1.2 Sonoanatomy

A linear transducer is placed directly caudal and parallel to the inguinal ligament (▶ Fig. 17.1). The femoral neurovascular bundle is visualized in the short axis.

In the short axis, the femoral nerve has an oval shape and appears hyperechoic with hypoechoic fascicular ("honeycomb-like") internal structure (▶ Fig. 17.2). The femoral nerve is usually directly lateral to the femoral artery. The fascia lata is very echogenic and runs at the top of the ultrasound image, closer to the transducer than the nerve and vessels. The iliac fascia can be seen as a delicate hyperechoic band immediately above the femoral nerve (▶ Fig. 17.2) surrounding the iliopsoas muscle and the nerve. The femoral nerve is usually located in the angle between the artery and the iliac fascia, from which it can be well defined by controlled transducer pressure.

Below the nerve, more distant to the probe, runs the iliopsoas muscle. It can be identified by its typical hypoechoic structure.

### 17.1.3 Technique of Femoral Nerve Block

#### Landmarks

Inguinal ligament, femoral artery, and iliac fascia in the ultrasound image.

## Position

The child is positioned supine; the affected leg is externally rotated and slightly abducted.

## Procedure

The inguinal ligament is palpated and the transducer is placed parallel and just distal to the inguinal ligament (▶ Fig. 17.1). After sonographic identification of the femoral nerve located lateral to the artery in the short axis (▶ Fig. 17.2) the region is disinfected, draped, and a sterile sleeve is placed in the transducer. The transducer is placed again at the previously determined position.

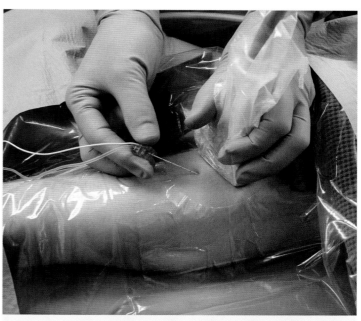

**Fig. 17.1** Transducer position and out-of-plane needle alignment for an ultrasound-guided single-shot block of the femoral nerve in a 2-year-old child. The linear probe is placed just distal and parallel to the inguinal ligament. The nerve is displayed in the short axis.

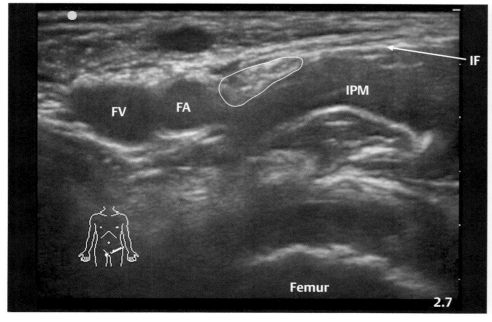

**Fig. 17.2** Ultrasound image of the left inguinal region in the short axis in a 5-year-old child. The femoral nerve (white outline) is located lateral to the femoral artery (FA). The iliac fascia (IF) is above the nerve and can be seen as a hyperechoic band and below it is the iliopsoas muscle (IPM). FV, femoral vein.

After a stab incision with a lancet, the regional anesthesia needle is advanced toward the nerve under repeated aspiration. After negative aspiration, the local anesthetic is spread around the nerve so that the nerve is surrounded as completely as possible.

If a continuous technique is planned, the catheter is then advanced 2 to 3 cm beyond the tip of the needle.

### Local Anesthetic, Dosage

▶ **Single-shot block.** Administration of 0.5 to 1 mL/kg body weight of a long-acting local anesthetic (e.g., ropivacaine 0.2–0.5% [2–5 mg/mL]), maximum 20 mL.

▶ **Continuous block.** Give infants, toddlers, and children older than 6 months a maximum 0.4 mg/kg per hour of ropivacaine.

## 17.1.4 Indications and Contraindications

### Indications

Indications are described in Chapter 10.

### Contraindications

General contraindications (Chapter 20.2).

## 17.1.5 Complications, Side Effects, Method-Specific Problems

### Complications

In the literature up to now, complications have been described only after conventional, landmark-based block techniques:
• Vascular punctures, as the femoral artery is located just medial to the nerve (Dalens et al 1989). There is a risk of intravascular local anesthetic application.
• Nerve damage.

## 17.1.6 Remarks on the Technique

It is usually easier to identify the nerve when it is visualized before the femoral artery divides into the femoral artery and the deep femoral artery. If it is visualized too far distally, the femoral nerve has already divided and is therefore often difficult to identify.

In children, the femoral nerve is often very superficial, so a catheter should be tunneled subcutaneously. Otherwise there is a risk of retrograde flow of the local anesthetic into the penetration

canal of the catheter and it will not adequately reach the nerve (Hillmann and Döffert 2009).

## 17.2 Distal Sciatic Nerve Block

### 17.2.1 Anatomy

The anatomy is described in Chapter 12.

### Sonoanatomy

A linear transducer is placed approximately the width of the patient's hand cranial to the popliteal crease in the region of the back of the lateral distal thigh and the sciatic nerve is visualized in the short axis (▶ Fig. 17.3).

The sciatic nerve is visualized in the short axis as a hyperechoic oval structure with a hypoechoic fascicular ("honeycomb-like") internal structure (▶ Fig. 17.4). The popliteal artery is located in the ultrasound image at the bottom, or away from the transducer and medial to the nerve and serves as a landmark. The biceps femoris muscle is at the top in the ultrasound image, or close to the transducer, and covers the sciatic nerve laterally.

## 17.2.2 Technique of Distal Sciatic Nerve Block

### Landmarks

Popliteal crease, in the ultrasound image: the popliteal artery is located medial to the nerve and farther from the transducer.

### Position

The patient is positioned on the side so that the leg to be blocked is on top. For a bilateral block, prone positioning is also possible,

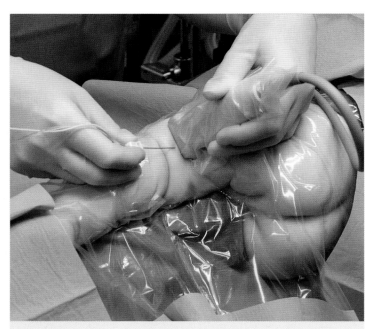

**Fig. 17.3** Transducer position and out-of-plane needle alignment in an ultrasound-guided single-shot block of the distal sciatic nerve in a 13-month-old child. The child is placed on the side and the linear transducer is placed above the popliteal crease in the region of the back of the lateral thigh. The nerve is displayed in the short axis.

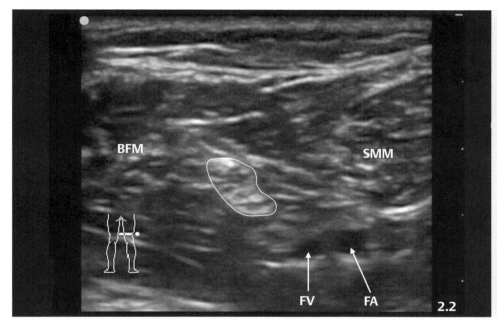

**Fig. 17.4** Ultrasound image of the back of the right distal thigh in the short axis in a 14-month-old child. The sciatic nerve (white outline) is identified lateral to and above the popliteal vessels (FA, femoral artery; FV, femoral vein). Medial to the nerve is the semimembranosus muscle (SMM) and lateral to it is the biceps femoris muscle (BFM).

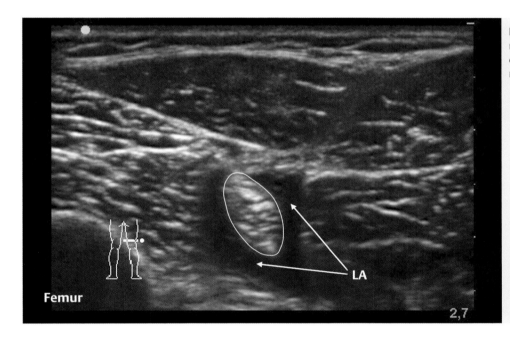

**Fig. 17.5** Ultrasound image of the distal sciatic nerve after ultrasound-guided block in a 6-year-old child. The nerve (white outline) is surrounded by the local anesthetic (LA).

but especially in an anesthetized child it is associated with a significantly greater effort.

## Procedure

The transducer is positioned slightly lateral in the region of the back of the distal thigh, a patient's handbreadth above the popliteal crease (▶ Fig. 17.3). In the ultrasound image, the sciatic nerve is located laterally and above the popliteal vessels, close to the transducer head. After sonographic identification of the nerve in the short axis (▶ Fig. 17.4), the bifurcation into the common fibular nerve and the tibial nerve should be visualized (see below). Then the region is disinfected, draped, and a sterile sleeve is placed on the transducer. The transducer is placed again at the previously determined position.

**Practical Note**

For a catheter technique, an out-of-plane needle direction is particularly suitable (▶ Fig. 17.3); for a single-shot method either an out-of-plane or an in-plane technique may be used.

After a stab incision with a lancet, the regional anesthesia needle is advanced toward the nerve under repeated aspiration. After negative aspiration, the local anesthetic is spread around the nerve so that it is surrounded as completely as possible (▶ Fig. 17.5)

If a continuous technique is planned, the catheter is advanced 2 to 3 cm beyond the tip of the needle.

## Local Anesthetic, Dosage

▶ **Single-shot block.** Administer a long-acting local anesthetic (e.g., ropivacaine 0.2–0.5% [2–5 mg/mL]), 0.5–1 mL/kg body weight, maximum 20 mL.

> **Caution**
>
> The maximum permissible local anesthetic dose per kilogram body weight must not be exceeded!

▶ **Continuous block.** Give infants, toddlers, and children older than 6 months a maximum of 0.4 mg/kg per hour of ropivacaine.

## 17.2.3 Indications and Contraindications

### Indications

The indications are described in Chapter 12.

### Contraindications

General contraindications (Chapter 20.2).

## 17.2.4 Complications, Side Effects, Method-Specific Problems

### Complications

In contrast to the subgluteal approach, the sciatic nerve is not fixated by bony structures in the region of the distal thigh, so that the risk of nerve damage and intraneural local anesthetic application is reduced (Ross 2006).

### Method-Specific Problems

A particular difficulty in scanning the sciatic nerve is anisotropy; this describes the directional dependence of the sound waves in the sonographic visualization of the nerve (Grechenig et al 2000). The nerve can be clearly visualized only when insonation is vertical. Just a few degrees deviation from the vertical angle of insonation can make the nerve invisible. Therefore, it is advisable to tilt the transducer during the examination slightly (about 10–15°) proximally so that the scanning plane is directed distally. This usually allows good visualization of the sciatic nerve (Hillmann and Döffert 2009).

## 17.2.5 Remarks on the Technique

The bifurcation of the sciatic nerve into the common fibular nerve and the tibial nerve should be visualized prior to performing the procedure to avoid an incomplete block due to the highly variable course of the sciatic bifurcation in the thigh (Schwemmer et al 2004).

> **Practical Note**
>
> If the sciatic nerve is not identified with certainty in a child using the above method, the transducer should be placed directly on the popliteal crease. In this location the tibial nerve is very superficial (close to the transducer), and "rides" on the vascular bundle and can easily be found. After identification, the nerve is then followed proximally until the sciatic bifurcation is visualized.

The so-called "seesaw" sign may be a further aid in identifying the nerve (Schafhalter-Zoppoth et al 2004). In the sonographic visualization of the sciatic nerve in the short axis at the level of the popliteal fossa, alternating active or passive dorsiflexion and plantar flexion of the foot at the upper ankle joint causes a seesaw motion of the tibial nerve and fibular nerve against each other. On dorsiflexion of the foot, the tibial nerve moves toward the skin of the popliteal fossa, while the common fibular nerve makes this movement on plantar flexion of the foot.

## References

Dalens B, Vanneuville G, Tanguy A. Comparison of the fascia iliaca compartment block with the 3-in-1 block in children. Anesth Analg 1989; 69: 705–713

Grechenig W, Clement HG, Peicha G, Klein A, Weiglein A. Ultrasound anatomy of the sciatic nerve of the thigh. [Article in German] Biomed Tech (Berl) 2000; 45: 298–303

Hillmann R, Döffert J. Praxis der anästhesiologischen Sonografie. Interventionelle Verfahren bei Erwachsenen und Kindern. 1st ed. Munich: Elsevier, Urban; 2009

Ross AK. Pediatric regional anesthesia. In: Motoyama EK, Davis PJ, eds. Smith's Anesthesia for Infants and Children. Philadelphia: Mosby/Elsevier; 2006

Schafhalter-Zoppoth I, Younger SJ, Collins AB, Gray AT. The "seesaw" sign: improved sonographic identification of the sciatic nerve. Anesthesiology 2004; 101: 808–809

Schwemmer U, Markus CK, Greim CA, Brederlau J, Trautner H, Roewer N. Sonographic imaging of the sciatic nerve and its division in the popliteal fossa in children. Paediatr Anaesth 2004; 14: 1005–1008

# 18 Abdominal Wall

## 18.1 Penile Root Block

### 18.1.1 Anatomy

In a penile root block, the two dorsal nerves of penis are blocked. The dorsal nerves of the penis are terminal branches of the pudendal nerve (S2–S4), which run through the subpubic space caudal to the symphysis slightly paramedian up to the dorsal side of the penis. This subpubic space is bordered cranially by the symphysis, caudally by the corpora cavernosa penis, and anteriorly by the fascia of Scarpa (inner membranous layer of the superficial abdominal fascia; ▶ Fig. 18.1). The nerves are located lateral to the dorsal arteries of penis and the unpaired deep dorsal vein of penis. This neurovascular bundle runs between the fascia of Buck (deep fascia of penis) and the tunica albuginea (▶ Fig. 18.2). Cranially, there is a connection between the fascia of Buck and the fascia of Scarpa.

The dorsal penile nerves supply sensory innervation to the glans penis and the distal two thirds of the penile skin. The proximal third of the penile skin receives its sensory supply from the genitofemoral nerves and iliohypogastric nerves.

### 18.1.2 Technique of Penile Root Block

#### Landmarks

Symphysis, penile root.

#### Position

The child is in the supine position.

### Procedure

The skin caudal to the symphysis is disinfected, then the symphysis is palpated and the penis is pulled slightly caudally or alternatively fixed caudally with an adhesive bandage across the thigh. An incision is made with a short-bevel needle (25 or 27 G) paramedian (0.5–1 cm lateral to the midline) just caudal to the symphysis (Dalens et al 1989). The needle is advanced in a slight mediocaudal direction (▶ Fig. 18.3) into the subpubic space until the fascia of Scarpa is perforated (clear "fascia click"). After negative aspiration, the local anesthetic is injected. Then a further injection is made on the opposite side using the same technique.

### Local Anesthetic, Dosage

Bupivacaine 0.5% (5 mg/mL), 1 mL/kg body weight per side (total volume 0.2 mL/kg body weight).

> **Caution**
>
> No epinephrine is added to the local anesthetic since the arterial blood supply of the penis is an end-arterial blood supply.

### 18.1.3 Indications and Contraindications

#### Indications

Pain after circumcision and interventions in the area of the front half of the penis (e.g., uncomplicated hypospadias repair).

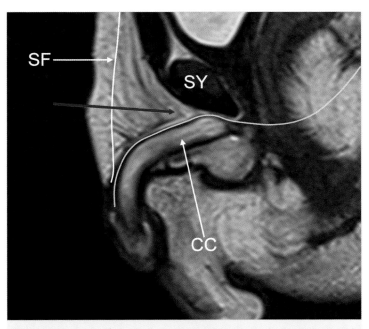

Fig. 18.1 MRI image of the anatomy of the genital area in the medial sagittal plane in a 7-month-old infant. The dorsal penile nerves (yellow) run caudally to the symphysis through the subpubic space (blue arrow). This space is bordered cranially by the symphysis (SY), caudally by the corpora cavernosa (CC), and ventrally by the fascia of Scarpa (SF). (Source: courtesy of Radiological Institute of Olga Hospital, Klinikum Stuttgart, Medical Director: Prof. Dr. P. Winkler.)

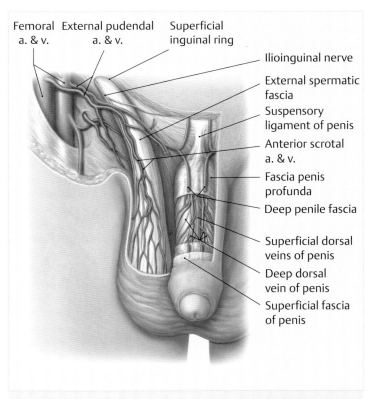

Fig. 18.2 Anatomical image of the male external genitalia. (Source: Schünke et al 2011.)

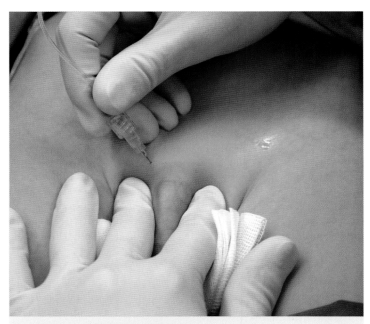

**Fig. 18.3** Paramedian penile block, Dalens technique, in a 5-year-old child. The regional anesthesia needle is inserted on both sides paramedian, just caudal to the symphysis and is advanced in a slightly mediocaudal direction in the subpubic space until the fascia of Scarpa is perforated.

## Contraindications

General contraindications (Chapter 20.2).

## 18.1.4 Complications, Side Effects, Method-Specific Problems

### Complications

- If the injection direction is too medial and too caudal, a hematoma may form due to perforating the fascia of Buck and injuring the dorsal vessel. Necrosis of the glans penis may develop from compression of the hematoma on the vessels (Sara and Lowry 1985). The risk of a hematoma is increased in a median puncture (Dalens et al 1989).
- If the injection direction is too caudal, accidental perforation of the tunica albuginea may occur with puncture of the corpora cavernosa und injection of the local anesthetic into the corpora cavernosa. The result is similar to an intravascular local anesthetic injection.
- Puncture of the urethra if the injection direction is too median and too caudal (Soh et al 2003).
- Osteomyelitis of the ischium (Abaci et al 2006).

### Method-Specific Problems

Analgesia gaps may occur in the area of the frenulum. The meatus is not anesthetized in the penile root block.

## 18.1.5 Remarks on the Technique

Burke et al (2000) report on temporary ischemia of the glans penis after using ropivacaine 0.75% (7.5 mg/mL). Due to the vasoconstrictive properties of ropivacaine, the scientific working group for pediatric anesthesia of the German Society of Anesthesia and Intensive Medicine (DGAI) has currently reached no

conclusive assessment of the use of ropivacaine in end-arterial areas (Mader et al 2007).

As an alternative to the technique described above, the block can also be made by a single median puncture (Bacon 1977). After bone contact with the symphysis, the needle is withdrawn slightly and advanced directly caudal to the symphysis. After aspiration, the local anesthetic is applied. This technique increases the risk of a hematoma (see above).

## 18.2 Ilioinguinal Nerve Block

### 18.2.1 Anatomy

The iliohypogastric nerve (T12, L1) and ilioinguinal nerve (L1) descend from the lateral border of the psoas major muscle between the renal capsule and the quadratus lumborum muscle. Both nerves run parallel and cranial to the iliac crest between the internal oblique muscle and the transversus abdominis muscle (► Fig. 18.4) and supply sensory innervation to the skin of the lateral hip region, the mons pubis, and the anterior upper part of the scrotum or the labia majora.

### 18.2.2 Sonoanatomy

A linear transducer is placed on the lateral abdominal wall medial or slightly craniomedial to the anterior superior iliac spine and the iliohypogastric and the ilioinguinal nerves are visualized in the short axis (► Fig. 18.5). The nerves can be visualized within a "lenticular" double fascia between the internal oblique muscle and the transversus abdominis muscle as hypoechoic structures surrounded by the hyperechoic fascia (► Fig. 18.6).

### 18.2.3 Technique of Ilioinguinal Nerve Block

#### Landmarks

Anterior superior iliac spine, muscles of the abdominal wall in the ultrasound image (see TAP block; Chapter 13.3), double fascia between the transversus abdominis muscle and the internal oblique muscle.

#### Position

The child is in the supine position.

#### Procedure

The anterior superior iliac spine is palpated and the transducer is placed medially or craniomedially to it (► Fig. 18.5). After ultrasound identification of the nerve within the double fascia between the internal oblique muscle and the transversus abdominis muscle (► Fig. 18.6), the region is disinfected, draped, and a sterile sleeve is put on the transducer. The transducer is placed again at the previously determined position.

After a stab incision of the skin with a lancet, a short-bevel regional anesthesia needle is inserted in an in-plane technique on the medial side of the transducer. The needle is advanced laterally in the direction of the iliac wing toward the nerve (► Fig. 18.7). After negative aspiration, the local anesthetic is injected around the nerves between the internal oblique and the transversus abdominis muscles.

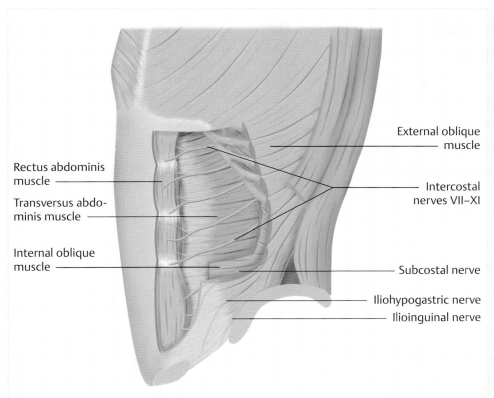

Fig. 18.4 Anatomical image of the lateral and anterior abdominal wall. The lateral and anterior cutaneous branches of the anterior rami of the caudal six intercostal nerves and the iliohypogastric and the ilioinguinal nerves run on the muscle fascia between the internal oblique muscle and the transversus abdominis muscle.

Rectus abdominis muscle

Transversus abdominis muscle

Internal oblique muscle

External oblique muscle

Intercostal nerves VII–XI

Subcostal nerve

Iliohypogastric nerve

Ilioinguinal nerve

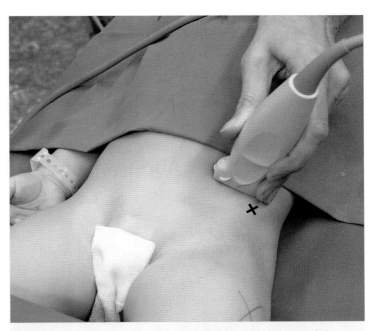

Fig. 18.5 Transducer position for sonographic visualization of the iliohypogastric nerve and the ilioinguinal nerve on the left side in a 20-month-old child. The linear probe is placed craniomedial to the anterior superior iliac spine (X) and the nerves are visualized in the short axis.

**Note**

Due to the very small distance of the nerves to the peritoneum, there is a risk of peritoneal penetration and injury to intra-abdominal organs. This risk is minimized with the in-plane puncture technique from medial direction because the entire regional anesthesia needle is visualized and the needle approaches the peritoneum tangentially.

## Local Anesthetic, Dosage

Ropivacaine 0.2% (2 mg/mL), 0.2 (–0.5) mL/kg body weight for each side.

## 18.2.4 Indications and Contraindications

### Indications

Adjuvant to general anesthesia and for postoperative analgesia after inguinal procedures (e.g., herniotomy, testicular displacement).

### Contraindications

General contraindications (Chapter 20.2).

## 18.2.5 Complications, Side Effects, Method-Specific Problems

### Complications

Until now, complications have been described in the literature only after a conventional, landmark-based block technique:

- The distance between the nerves and the peritoneum in children is sometimes only 1 mm (Willschke et al 2005, Hong et al 2010). Perforations of the abdominal wall with puncture of the intestine have been described (Jöhr and Sossai 1999, Frigon et al 2006).
- Small retroperitoneal hematoma in an adult patient (Vaisman 2001).
- Accidental simultaneous block of the ipsilateral femoral nerve (Lipp et al 2004). If the injection of the local anesthetic between the transversus abdominis muscle and the transverse fascia is too deep, the local anesthetic reaches the femoral nerve directly (Rosario et al 1997).

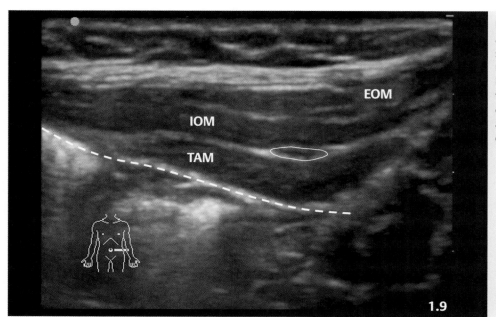

**Fig. 18.6** Ultrasound image of the left lateral abdominal wall craniomedial to the anterior superior iliac spine in a 20-month-old child. The nerves (white outline) are in a double fascia between the internal oblique muscle (IOM) and the transversus abdominis muscle (TAM). The distance between the peritoneum (dashed line) and the nerves is approximately 3 mm. EOM, external oblique muscle.

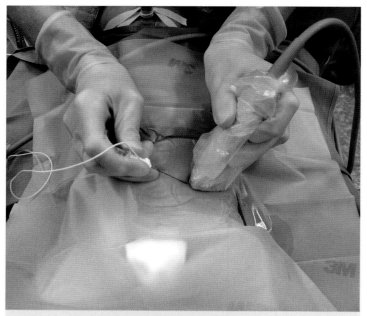

**Fig. 18.7** Ultrasound-guided single-shot block of the iliohypogastric and ilioinguinal nerves on the left side in a 20-month-old child. The nerves are visualized in the short axis; the needle-transducer alignment is in plane.

## Method-Specific Problems

Failure rates of up to 45% have been described using the landmark-based technique. Correct injection of the local anesthetic is required for the success of the block. Injections not around the nerves or directly into the adjacent muscles (internal oblique muscle, transversus abdominis muscle) usually lead to failure (Weintraud et al 2008).

The injected local anesthetic is rapidly absorbed from the abdominal wall and high plasma levels may occur, particularly in smaller children (< 15 kg), but without signs of intoxication (Smith et al 1996). Interestingly, Weintraud et al (2009) found a significantly more rapid absorption and higher maximum ropivacaine plasma levels after ultrasound-guided block in comparison with the conventional technique, but none of the children developed clinical signs of local anesthetic intoxication.

## 18.2.6 Remarks on the Technique

In an ultrasound-guided block, the amount of local anesthetic necessary for a successful block can be reduced, so that local anesthetic doses of 0.075 mL/kg body weight have been described in the literature (Willschke et al 2006). The author considers a minimum local anesthetic dose of 0.2 mL/kg body weight to be useful, because the success of the block is most important.

In approximately 50% of children, only two layers of muscle—the internal oblique muscle and the transversus abdominis muscle—can be visualized by ultrasound at the block site. In these cases only the aponeurosis of the external oblique muscle is present at the puncture site (Willschke et al 2005).

## 18.3 Transversus Abdominis Plane Block

### 18.3.1 Anatomy

The sensory innervation of the lateral and anterior abdominal wall is supplied by the lateral and anterior cutaneous branches of the anterior rami of the caudal six intercostal nerves (T7–T12). The sensory innervation of the inguinal area is supplied by the iliohypogastric nerve (T12 and L1) and ilioinguinal nerve (L1; see ► Fig. 18.4).

The anterior rami of the intercostal nerves and the iliohypogastric and ilioinguinal nerves run anteriorly on the muscle fascia between the internal oblique muscle and the transversus abdominis muscle (► Fig. 18.4). At the level of the mid-axillary line, the lateral cutaneous branches leave the anterior rami and move toward the skin. The anterior cutaneous branches finally pass through the lamina posterior into the rectus sheath and further to the skin.

### 18.3.2 Sonoanatomy

A linear transducer is placed on the lateral abdominal wall in the region of the mid-axillary line directly cranial and parallel to the iliac crest, and the three layers of the lateral abdominal wall

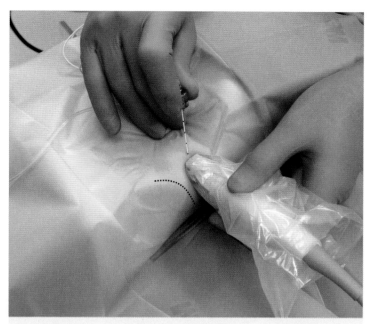

**Fig. 18.8** Transducer position and in-plane needle alignment for an ultrasound-guided TAP block in a 22-month-old child. The linear transducer is placed cranial to the iliac crest (dashed line) and the three layers of lateral abdominal wall muscles are visualized by ultrasound.

muscles are visualized by ultrasound (▶ Fig. 18.8). Close to the transducer is first the external oblique muscle, then the internal oblique muscle, and further away from the transducer is the transversus abdominis muscle (▶ Fig. 18.9). The transversus abdominis plane / fascia layer, where the anterior rami of the intercostal nerves and the iliohypogastric and ilioinguinal nerves run, is located between the internal oblique and the transversus abdominis muscles. In contrast to the iliohypogastric and ilioinguinal nerves (see above), the anterior rami are not visualized by ultrasound.

### 18.3.3 Technique of Transversus Abdominis Plane Block

#### Landmarks

Iliac crest, three layers of lateral abdominal wall muscles in the ultrasound image (from outside to inside): external oblique muscle, internal oblique muscle, transversus abdominis muscle.

#### Position

The child is in supine position and the ipsilateral arm is abducted, so that the region cranial to the iliac crest is easily accessible and the transducer can be placed accurately.

#### Procedure

The iliac crest is palpated. The transducer is placed in the mid-axillary line directly cranial and parallel to the iliac crest (▶ Fig. 18.8). After the three layers of the lateral abdominal wall muscles have been identified in the ultrasound scan (▶ Fig. 18.9), the region is disinfected, draped, and a sterile sleeve is placed on the transducer. The transducer is placed again at the previously determined position. After a stab incision in the skin with a lancet, a short-bevel regional anesthesia needle is inserted using an in-plane technique on the medial side of the transducer and is advanced slowly in posterolateral direction toward the fascia between internal oblique muscle and transversus abdominis muscle (▶ Fig. 18.8). After negative aspiration, the local anesthetic is injected so that the depot is formed above the muscle fascia (▶ Fig. 18.10). Since the lateral cutaneous branches of the anterior rami exit in the region of the mid-axillary line, the local anesthetic should be injected behind the mid-axillary line.

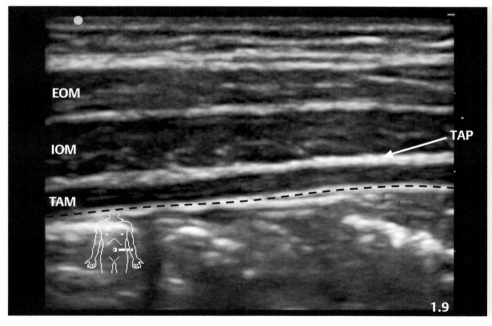

**Fig. 18.9** Ultrasound image of the left lateral abdominal wall cranial to the iliac crest in a 22-month-old child. The transversus abdominis plane (TAP) is located between the internal oblique muscle (IOM) and the transversus abdominis muscle (TAM). The distance between the peritoneum (dashed line) and the nerve is 2 to 3 mm. EOM, external oblique muscle.

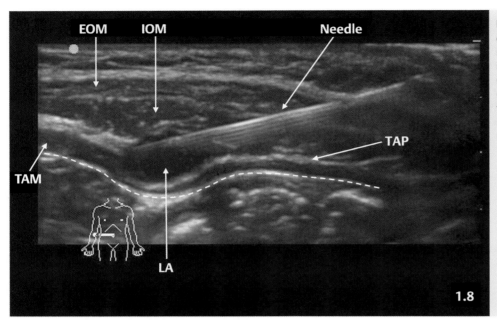

**Fig. 18.10** Sonographic image of ultrasound-guided TAP block on the right side in an 18-month-old child. The local anesthetic (LA) is injected between the internal oblique muscle (IOM) and the transversus abdominis muscle (TAM), so the depot is formed above the muscle fascia of the transversus abdominis muscle. Dotted line: peritoneum; EOM, external oblique muscle; TAP, transversus abdominis plane.

**Practical Note**

Due to the very small distance between the fascial layers and the peritoneum, which can be only about 2 mm, depending on the age of the child, an in-plane technique should be used to visualize the entire length of the needle and accurately locate and monitor the needle tip (▶ Fig. 18.10).

A continuous technique is possible, but should be used only in rare exceptions. The catheter is then advanced 1 to 2 cm beyond the tip of the needle.

## Local Anesthetic, Dosage

▶ **Single-shot block.** Long-acting local anesthetic (e.g., ropivacaine 0.1–0.2% [1–2 mg/mL]), 0.2 to 0.4 mL/kg body weight (Fredrickson and Seal 2009, Suresh and Chan 2009).

▶ **Continuous block.** Infants younger than 6 months, 0.2 mg/kg per hour of ropivacaine; infants, toddlers, and children older than 6 months, 0.4 mg/kg per hour of ropivacaine.

## 18.3.4 Indications and Contraindications

### Indications

Pain therapy after surgery in the abdominal wall caudal to the navel (e.g., open appendectomy, creation and relocation of an enterostomy).

**Caution**

A bilateral block is necessary for incisions that go beyond the midline.

### Contraindications

General contraindications (Chapter 20.2).

## 18.3.5 Complications, Side Effects, Method-Specific Problems

### Complications

The distance between the muscle fascia and the peritoneum is sometimes only a few millimeters in children, so that an accidental puncture of the abdominal cavity and injury of intra-abdominal organs is conceivable and possible.

Until now, complications have been reported in the literature only in adult patients:
- Accidental liver puncture (Farooq and Carey 2008, Lancaster and Chadwick 2010).
- Puncture of the abdominal cavity and intra-abdominal catheter placement without organ injury (Jankovic et al 2008).
- Simultaneous block of the ipsilateral femoral nerve (Walker 2010).
- Risk of high local anesthetic levels due to rapid absorption (see ilioinguinal block).
- The upper incidence of overall complications associated with the TAP (transversus abdominis plane) block in children is very low (0.3%), considering that all complications have been very minor and did not require any additional interventions (Long et al 2014).

### Method-Specific Problems

The accurate sonographic identification of the fascial layer between the internal oblique muscle and the transversus abdominis muscle is a precondition for proper injection of the local anesthetic to achieve sufficient block effect.

## 18.3.6 Remarks on the Technique

The technique of TAP block described here is more suitable for abdominal interventions caudal to the navel. Some studies reported no analgesia at all or sufficient analgesia and spread of local anesthetic cranial to T10 (Tran et al 2009, Lee et al 2010). If an analgesia level is sought above T10, a subcostal injection ("*subcostal TAP*") should be performed (Hebbard et al 2010, Lee et al 2010).

# References

Abaci A, Makay B, Unsal E, Mustafa O, Aktug T. An unusual complication of dorsal penile nerve block for circumcision. Paediatr Anaesth 2006; 16: 1094–1095

Bacon AK. An alternative block for post circumcision analgesia. Anaesth Intensive Care 1977; 5: 63–64

Burke D, Joypaul V, Thomson MF. Circumcision supplemented by dorsal penile nerve block with 0.75% ropivacaine: a complication. Reg Anesth Pain Med 2000; 25: 424–427

Dalens B, Vanneuville G, Dechelotte P. Penile block via the subpubic space in 100 children. Anesth Analg 1989; 69: 41–45

Farooq M, Carey M. A case of liver trauma with a blunt regional anesthesia needle while performing transversus abdominis plane block. Reg Anesth Pain Med 2008; 33: 274–275

Fredrickson MJ, Seal P. Ultrasound-guided transversus abdominis plane block for neonatal abdominal surgery. Anaesth Intensive Care 2009; 37: 469–472

Frigon C, Mai R, Valois-Gomez T, Desparmet J. Bowel hematoma following an iliohypogastric-ilioinguinal nerve block. Paediatr Anaesth 2006; 16: 993–996

Hebbard PD, Barrington MJ, Vasey C. Ultrasound-guided continuous oblique subcostal transversus abdominis plane blockade: description of anatomy and clinical technique. Reg Anesth Pain Med 2010; 35: 436–441

Hong JY, Kim WO, Koo BN, Kim YA, Jo YY, Kil HK. The relative position of ilioinguinal and iliohypogastric nerves in different age groups of pediatric patients. Acta Anaesthesiol Scand 2010; 54: 566–570

Jankovic Z, Ahmad N, Ravishankar N, Archer F. Transversus abdominis plane block: how safe is it? Anesth Analg 2008; 107: 1758–1759

Jöhr M, Sossai R. Colonic puncture during ilioinguinal nerve block in a child. Anesth Analg 1999; 88: 1051–1052

Lancaster P, Chadwick M. Liver trauma secondary to ultrasound-guided transversus abdominis plane block. Br J Anaesth 2010; 104: 509–510

Lee TH, Barrington MJ, Tran TM, Wong D, Hebbard PD. Comparison of extent of sensory block following posterior and subcostal approaches to ultrasound-guided transversus abdominis plane block. Anaesth Intensive Care 2010; 38: 452–460

Lipp AK, Woodcock J, Hensman B, Wilkinson K. Leg weakness is a complication of ilio-inguinal nerve block in children. Br J Anaesth 2004; 92: 273–274

Long JB, Birmingham PK, De Oliveira GS Jr, Schaldenbrand KM, Suresh S. Transversus abdominis plane block in children: a multicenter safety analysis of 1994 cases from the PRAN (Pediatric Regional Anesthesia Network) database. Anesth Analg 2014; 119: 395–399

Mader T, Hornung M, Boos K et al. Handlungsempfehlungen zur Regionalanästhesie bei Kindern. Anästh Intensivmed 2007; 48: 79–85

Rosario DJ, Jacob S, Luntley J, Skinner PP, Raftery AT. Mechanism of femoral nerve palsy complicating percutaneous ilioinguinal field block. Br J Anaesth 1997; 78: 314–316

Sara CA, Lowry CJ. A complication of circumcision and dorsal nerve block of the penis. Anaesth Intensive Care 1985; 13: 79–82

Schünke M, Schulte E, Schumacher U. Prometheus. LernAtlas der Anatomie. Allgemeine Anatomie und Bewegungssystem. Illustrations by M. Voll and K. Wesker. 3rd ed. Stuttgart: Thieme; 2011: 228

Smith T, Moratin P, Wulf H. Smaller children have greater bupivacaine plasma concentrations after ilioinguinal block. Br J Anaesth 1996; 76: 452–455

Soh CR, Ng SB, Lim SL. Dorsal penile nerve block. Paediatr Anaesth 2003; 13: 329–333

Suresh S, Chan VW. Ultrasound guided transversus abdominis plane block in infants, children and adolescents: a simple procedural guidance for their performance. Paediatr Anaesth 2009; 19: 296–299

Tran TM, Ivanusic JJ, Hebbard P, Barrington MJ. Determination of spread of injectate after ultrasound-guided transversus abdominis plane block: a cadaveric study. Br J Anaesth 2009; 102: 123–127

Vaisman J. Pelvic hematoma after an ilioinguinal nerve block for orchialgia. Anesth Analg 2001; 92: 1048–1049

Walker G. Transversus abdominis plane block: a note of caution! Br J Anaesth 2010; 104: 265

Weintraud M, Marhofer P, Bösenberg A et al. Ilioinguinal/iliohypogastric blocks in children: where do we administer the local anesthetic without direct visualization? Anesth Analg 2008; 106: 89–93

Weintraud M, Lundblad M, Kettner SC et al. Ultrasound versus landmark-based technique for ilioinguinal-iliohypogastric nerve blockade in children: the implications on plasma levels of ropivacaine. Anesth Analg 2009; 108: 1488–1492

Willschke H, Marhofer P, Bösenberg A et al. Ultrasonography for ilioinguinal/iliohypogastric nerve blocks in children. Br J Anaesth 2005; 95: 226–230

Willschke H, Bösenberg A, Marhofer P et al. Ultrasonographic-guided ilioinguinal/iliohypogastric nerve block in pediatric anesthesia: what is the optimal volume? Anesth Analg 2006; 102: 1680–1684

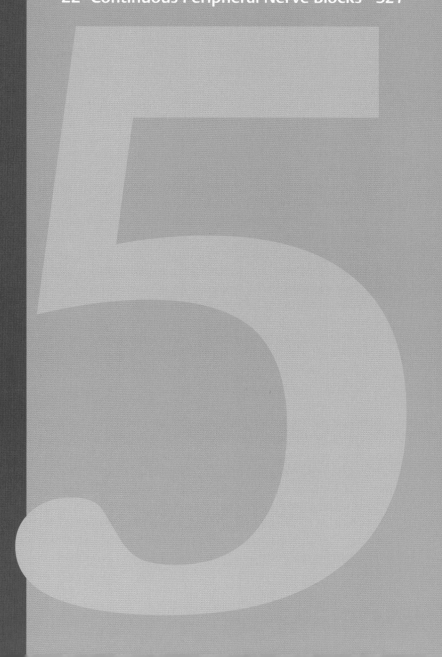

# Part 5

## General Aspects of Peripheral Nerve Blocks of the Extremities

# 19 Special Features of Peripheral Nerve Blocks

## 19.1 Advantages of Peripheral Nerve Blocks

According to a meta analysis of Rodgers et al (2000) central neuraxial blocks (CNB) are associated with a reduction in postoperative mortality and morbidity. There are no comparable studies regarding peripheral nerve blocks. However, it can be inferred that peripheral nerve blocks offer advantages in at-risk patients compared with general anesthesia and also compared with neuraxial blocks.

While peripheral blocks are performed quite frequently on the upper limb, they are still not used as frequently for operations on the lower limb. One reason for this may be that parts of both the lumbar and sacral plexuses always have to be anesthetized for a complete block of the lower limb (two injections).

Considerable drops in blood pressure can occur with central neuraxial blocks. The major advantage of peripheral nerve blocks is therefore the lower interference with the circulation. Thus, cardiac arrest was seen significantly less often after peripheral blocks than after spinal anesthesia (Auroy et al 1997). Furthermore, possible complications (infections, hemorrhage, nerve injury) are less serious than the complications of CNB blocks.

While intact coagulation is an absolute requirement for neuraxial blocks, the criteria for peripheral nerve blocks are less strict. Normal coagulation clinically and in the patient's medical records is usually sufficient for performing a peripheral nerve block (see below).

Under certain circumstances, peripheral blocks are the procedure of choice for surgical anesthesia. In the nonfasting patient, regional anesthesia procedures should be preferred; for the upper limb, only peripheral nerve blocks should be considered.

Many patients with rheumatic diseases have severely limited mouth opening, often combined with extreme deformity of the entire spine. Both general anesthesia and neuraxial blocks are associated with considerable technical difficulties and risks in these patients.

Postoperative nausea and vomiting (PONV) often poses unbearable problems for patients in the perioperative phase, caused for the most part by intra- and postoperative application of opioids, but also by cardiovascular instability resulting from regional blocks in the locality of the spinal cord. Small amounts of remifentanil (e.g., 0.05 µg/kg/min) in addition to peripheral regional anesthesia evidently do not increase a patient's risk of nausea and vomiting. Peripheral blocks have been shown to significantly reduce the rate of PONV, especially when applied in postoperative pain management (Borgeat et al 2003).

In the outpatient sector, peripheral blocks offer numerous benefits compared to other anesthesia procedures, for example, a patient recovers from surgery more quickly (Hadzic et al 2005).

Thanks to the development of the (single-use) elastomer pump, continuous blocks can now also be performed in an outpatient setting. This means that procedures that could formerly be performed in an outpatient setting to a limited extent only because of expected postoperative pain can now be performed on outpatients due to adequate pain therapy (Ilfeld and Enneking 2005).

> **Note**
>
> In general, continuous regional anesthesia should always be part of a multimodal concept for postoperative pain control (Meier 2005).

Numerous other examples could be cited where peripheral nerve blocks represent the procedure of choice.

> **Note**
>
> Every anesthetist should master the standard techniques of peripheral block of the upper and lower limbs in order to be able to make an individual decision on the best anesthetic procedure in the individual case.

## 19.2 Problems of Peripheral Nerve Blocks

### 19.2.1 Incomplete Block

Although small, the possible risk of an incomplete block should be anticipated and prepared for.

The reported incidence of incomplete block varies greatly. Failure rates of up to 30% are reported for axillary plexus anesthesia. Such problems should be explained to the patient and strategies for further procedure must be discussed. The time needed for a complete block to develop may vary with the technique and the local anesthetic employed; some blocks may require up to 40 minutes (or more) to achieve full effect. The logistics of peripheral nerve blocks should therefore be well planned.

However, with some experience an early prognosis can be made as to whether a completely successful block can be expected. The first evidence of onset of the block is a rise in skin temperature caused by sympathetic block, followed by hypoesthesia and motor weakness. These signs of incipient success of the block should appear within 10 to 15 minutes; if this is not the case, there is no point in waiting any longer.

### Procedure in Case of Incomplete Block

The following aspects should be considered in case of an incomplete regional block for intraoperative anesthesia:

- Patients are often irritated by the fact that they still "feel" something but do not actually complain of pain. In this case, mild analgosedation is adequate to solve the problem. The patient should be given an oxygen mask; monitoring of oxygenation (pulse oximetry) is mandatory, and monitoring of the patient's ventilation by capnometry or EEG monitoring of sedation may be indicated (Chapter 21.2).
- If the block is absolutely inadequate for surgical purposes, no attempt should be made to increase a patient's pain tolerance by giving higher doses of analgesics and sedatives, unless the airway is appropriately secured. If there are no contraindications, general anesthesia (e.g., propofol and a laryngeal mask) is

indicated in these cases. In most cases, a partial block exists and only a small supplementary amount of an opiate may be sufficient to achieve surgical tolerance (e.g., 10 µg sufentanil).

- If there are contraindications to general anesthesia or reservations on the part of the patient, most peripheral nerve blocks offer the option of selective nerve block supplementation distal to the already-performed block. The following are examples:
  - Incomplete interscalene plexus anesthesia for shoulder operation: supplementation by block of the suprascapular nerve and the supraclavicular nerves
  - Incomplete supraclavicular, infraclavicular, or axillary plexus anesthesia: supplementation by selective nerve blocks in the upper arm, elbow, or wrist region
  - Incomplete femoral and sciatic nerve block for operations on the ankle or foot: supplementation by distal sciatic nerve block, saphenous nerve block, or foot block

> **Caution**
>
> After a peripheral nerve block has been performed resulting in a partial effect, supplementary blocks should be performed only distal to the previous block and only with an "atraumatic" needle (Chapter 21.3) and using a nerve stimulator and/or ultrasound guidance. Blocks should not be repeated in the area already infiltrated with local anesthetic.

## 19.2.2 Dosages of Local Anesthetic

A greater volume of local anesthetic is required for peripheral blocks.

Peripheral nerve blocks are associated with seizures significantly more often than are neuraxial blocks (Auroy et al 1997). In peripheral nerve blocks where larger volumes of local anesthetic are used or when there is a risk of injection into an artery leading to the brain, all safety precautions required for dealing with such an incident must be taken (peripheral venous access, possibility of intubation and ventilation with 100% oxygen, emergency medications). Moreover, it is necessary to ensure patient safety by selecting the least toxic local anesthetic and not exceeding the recommended maximum doses. The injection must always be given slowly while observing the patient.

# References

Auroy Y, Narchi P, Messiah A, Litt L, Rouvier B, Samii K. Serious complications related to regional anesthesia: results of a prospective survey in France. Anesthesiology 1997; 87: 479–486

Borgeat A, Ekatodramis G, Schenker CA. Postoperative nausea and vomiting in regional anesthesia: a review. Anesthesiology 2003; 98: 530–547

Hadzic A, Karaca PE, Hobeika P et al. Peripheral nerve blocks result in superior recovery profile compared with general anesthesia in outpatient knee arthroscopy. Anesth Analg 2005; 100: 976–981

Ilfeld BM, Enneking FK. Continuous peripheral nerve blocks at home: a review. Anesth Analg 2005; 100: 1822–1833

Meier G. Medikamentöse Schmerztherapie. In: Stein V, Greitemann B, eds. Rehabilitation in Orthopädie und Unfallchirurgie. Heidelberg: Springer; 2005

Rodgers A, Walker N, Schug S et al. Reduction of postoperative mortality and morbidity with epidural or spinal anaesthesia: results from overview of randomized trials. BMJ 2000; 321: 1493

# 20 Complications and General Contraindications of Peripheral Blocks

## 20.1 Complications of Peripheral Nerve Blocks

Besides the specific complications described for the individual techniques, the following complications of peripheral nerve blocks are possible:

- Toxic reactions caused by the local anesthetic (LAST: Local Anesthetic Systemic Toxicity)
- Neurological injuries (neuropathy)

### 20.1.1 Toxic Reactions Caused by the Local Anesthetic

▶ **Overdose.** Toxic reactions can be due to overdose at a correct initial injection site. The symptoms do not occur immediately at the time the injection is made, but can be expected to develop later, at the time of maximum blood levels depending on the rate of absorption.

▶ **Accidental intravascular injection.** In the event of accidental intravascular injection of the local anesthetic, small amounts may be enough to cause a toxic reaction (see above). For this reason, the maximum doses for many local anesthetics recommended by the manufacturer should be regarded with a degree of skepticism, since much smaller doses can lead to major incidents in the event of accidental intravascular injection, while much higher doses may be tolerated with correct injection.

▶ **Systemic intoxication.** Systemic intoxication by local anesthetics is expressed in cerebral and cardiac effects; the cerebral effects usually precede the cardiac effects (▶ Fig. 20.1). Early symptoms are a metallic taste on the tongue, tinnitus, dizziness,

and acoustic phenomena, followed by muscle twitching, confusion, unconsciousness, seizure, and coma. The cardiac changes occur in parallel with correspondingly higher blood levels. First there is tachycardia and hypertension, followed by bradycardia and hypotension possibly progressing to asystole.

---

**Practical Note**

When injecting the local anesthetic it is important to watch for early symptoms of intoxication in order to stop administration immediately in case of accidental intravascular injection. For this reason, in addition to repeated aspiration to rule out intravascular injection, the local anesthetic must be given slowly with constant verbal communication with the patient ("verbal monitoring") to ensure that the patient still responds lucidly and has no symptoms (Mulroy and Hejtmanek 2010).

Intoxication symptoms are enhanced by hypoxia and acidosis, so prophylactic oxygen administration is recommended.

---

▶ **Cerebral intoxication.** In case of cerebral intoxication, oxygen must be given immediately and if there is a seizure, the patient must also be ventilated adequately (if necessary with intubation and mechanical ventilation) and benzodiazepines (midazolam, diazepam) or barbiturates should be administered.

▶ **Cardiotoxic effect.** The cardiac effects are differentiated between indirect effects (tachycardia, hypertension) that can be explained by the central inhibition of the "inhibitory effects" and the direct cardiotoxic effect, which occurs in the form of bradycardia up to complete cardiopulmonary arrest associated with impairment of contractility.

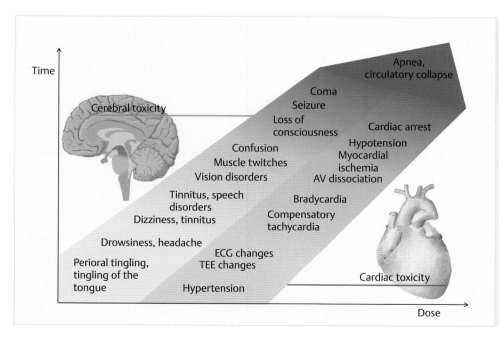

**Fig. 20.1** Cerebral and cardiac symptoms of systemic intoxication by local anesthetics. (Source: Graf and Niesel 2010.)

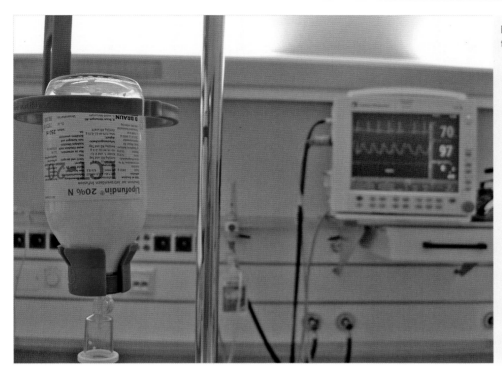

Fig. 20.2 Administration of a 20% lipid emulsion to treat severe local anesthetic intoxication.

After successful ventilation and oxygenation, a lipid infusion should be considered at the first sign of intoxication (▶ Fig. 20.2; Weinberg 2010). Propofol is not a substitute for administering a 20% lipid solution.

## Treatment of Systemic Intoxication with Local Anesthetics (LAST)

**Recommendation for the treatment** of systemic intoxication with local anesthetics (dosages for adults; Weinberg 2010):

- *Secure airways:* Avoid hypoxia and acidosis (sufficient ventilation, administration of 100% $O_2$).
- *Treatment of a seizure:* Benzodiazepines, if necessary propofol or thiopental (fractionated), lipid infusion (see below).
- *Treatment of circulatory arrest:* Resuscitation according to standard protocol: epinephrine fractionated (10–100 µg). *Avoid:* calcium channel blockers, beta receptor blockers. If the patient has ventricular arrhythmia: amiodarone.
- *Treatment with a 20% lipid emulsion:*
  - Initial bolus: 1.5 mL/kg body weight within 1 minute (equivalent to about 100 mL); continuous: 0.25 mL/kg body weight per minute (equivalent to 400 mL in 20 min).
  - If adequate circulation cannot be restored:
    - 2 repetitions of the bolus at 5-minute intervals (equivalent to 2 further boli of 100 mL)

- If necessary, double the infusion rate (0.5 mL/kg/min, 400 mL within 10 min)
- Continue infusion until stable circulation is restored.

The American Society of Regional Anesthesia and Pain Therapy (ASRA) published a checklist for the treatment of systemic intoxication with local anesthetics (Neal et al 2012).

## Selecting the Local Anesthetic

When selecting the local anesthetic, consideration must be given to its potential toxicity, especially in the event of accidental intravascular injection.

Medium-acting local anesthetics are less toxic than the long-acting drugs; prilocaine compares positively to the other medium-acting local anesthetics mainly due to its high spread volume. The formation of methemoglobin by prilocaine is a disadvantage. For this reason, doses higher than 600 mg should be avoided. Repeated doses of prilocaine should not be given.

Of the currently employed long-acting local anesthetics—namely, racemic bupivacaine, levobupivacaine, S(–) isomer of bupivacaine, and the S(–) isomer ropivacaine—the least cardiotoxic is ropivacaine. With regard to intracellular energy metabolism also, it has clear advantages compared to levobupivacaine.

In contrast to ropivacaine and the medium-acting local anesthetics, levobupivacaine and bupivacaine may lead to a complete block of ATP synthesis in the myocardium at toxic concentrations (Sztark et al 1998, 2000).

Allergic reactions are extremely rare with the amide local anesthetics that are used almost exclusively today.

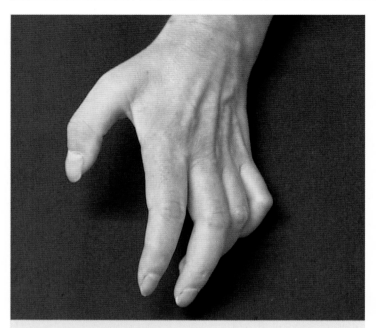

**Fig. 20.3** Permanent nerve damage after peripheral regional anesthesia (ulnar nerve damage with typical claw hand).

## 20.1.2 Neurological Injuries (Neuropathy)

Neurological injuries (▶ Fig. 20.3) after peripheral nerve blocks are reported with an incidence between 0.019% (Auroy et al 1997), 0.04% (Barrington et al 2009), 1.7% (Fanelli et al 1999), and 3% (Brull et al 2007).

Not all postoperative nerve lesions are due to a nerve block; other causes such as position-induced injury or injury caused by the operation must be considered (Cheney et al 1999, Fanelli et al 1999, Barrington et al 2009).

> **Note**
>
> Permanent or severe nerve damage in connection with peripheral blocks is considered to be extremely rare (Brull et al 2007, Neal 2008).
> The incidence is reported to be 0.019% (Auroy et al 1997) and 0.04% (Barrington et al 2009).

A subfascial hematoma can lead to mechanical nerve compression (Jöhr 1987). Occasionally brachial plexus neuropathy or "idiopathic neuritis" or "idiopathic plexitis" occurs in association with an interscalene brachial plexus block (Tetzlaff et al 1997, Horlocker et al 2000, Hebl et al 2001). This is associated with severe nerve pain, numbness, and motor weakness. Characteristically, this complication will become manifest only after complete disappearance of the block in the meantime. An immediate injury due to the injection has not taken place here; accordingly, the neurological picture cannot be attributed to injury of individual cords or nerves. The syndrome is due to an inflammatory immunological process. Postoperative plexus neuropathy can also occur spontaneously independently of the anesthesia procedure performed. This makes it difficult to make a causal distinction from regional anesthesia (Malamut et al 1994).

▶ **Classification of Nerve Injuries.** Nerve injuries are classified into one of three groups: neurapraxia, axonotmesis, and neurotmesis (Sawyer et al 2000):
- *Neurapraxia* is a functional paralysis without any evident anatomical lesion.
- In *axonotmesis* the axons are disrupted while the myelin sheath is still intact.
- In *neurotmesis* there is complete (mechanical) disruption of both axon and myelin sheath.

Usually, neurapraxia and axonotmesis have a good prognosis (Stan et al 1995, Fanelli et al 1999). After weeks to months, complete or extensive resolution of the paresis and pain can be expected (Stöhr 1996). However, in individual cases (neurotmesis), residual paresis interfering with function—sometimes associated with causalgiform pain syndromes—can persist.

> **Note**
>
> Very little data is available on which measures are best for avoiding nerve damage (Neal 2008).

▶ **Avoiding nerve damage.** Recommendations to use atraumatic needles and avoid deliberately triggering paresthesia and giving injections with unexpectedly high injection pressure are based mainly on the opinions of experts and animal experiments (Shah et al 2005, Neal 2001). The superiority of nerve stimulation or ultrasound guidance for finding peripheral nerves compared with inducing paresthesia to avoid nerve damage has not been proven in human studies (Neal 2008).

There are no evidence-based recommendations even for the question of whether the patient must be awake, mildly sedated, strongly sedated, or anesthetized in order to avoid nerve damage when a peripheral nerve block is performed (Neal 2008). Also unanswered is the question of whether and to what extent pre-existing nerve damage increases the risk of traumatic nerve damage due to peripheral nerve blocks (Sinner and Graf 2010). There is insufficient information to answer this.

The risks must be weighed against the benefits compared with other available anesthesia and analgesia techniques (Neal 2008). In general, the authors of this book do not consider pre-existing nerve damage to be a limitation for conducting a peripheral nerve block (Büttner 2010).

Animal experiments have confirmed the theory that the nerve must be approached with caution (Steinfeldt et al 2011). Even without penetrating the nerve, strong mechanical stress can lead to a morphological change in the form of temporary nerve damage.

> **Practical Note**
>
> The direction of the needle is also considered to be a factor in nerve injuries. The needle direction should be at a shallow angle and parallel to the course of the nerve if anatomically possible (Hempel and Baur 1982). For needles with a 15° bevel, the combination with a nerve stimulator (Hirasawa et al 1990) and/or ultrasound is recommended in any case.

▶ **Recommendations.** Based on current information, the authors of this book make the following recommendations to avoid nerve damage that could arise as a result of conducting peripheral nerve blocks:

- Peripheral blocks should be performed with the aid of the nerve stimulator and/or under ultrasound guidance.
- If the patient reports paresthesia during the injection, the needle position must be changed.
- If strong resistance is encountered unexpectedly the injection should not be forced. Therefore, the first few milliliters must be administered with a light touch ("test dose").
- Whenever possible, the block should be performed on a lightly sedated, cooperative patient.
- In children and uncooperative patients, the block can be performed under heavy sedation or general anesthesia, weighing the risks and benefits (Neal 2008, Taenzer et al 2014).
- The patient under general anesthesia may not be relaxed if a nerve stimulator is used, as in this case no response can be expected from nerve stimulation.

The nerve must always be approached cautiously (Steinfeldt et al 2011).

# 20.2 General Contraindications to Peripheral Nerve Blocks

(▶ Table 20.1)

## 20.2.1 Infections

Infections in the region of the puncture site constitute an absolute contraindication to every kind of regional anesthesia. Infections in the area of innervation of the limb to be blocked are not an absolute contraindication as long as the insertion site itself is not affected. Bacteremia is not a contraindication for "single-shot" blocks.

However, an indwelling catheter should be avoided, as any foreign body may promote septic colonization (Hempel 1998, Reisig et al 2009). For medicolegal reasons, the patient must be informed about the potentially greater infection risk when an indwelling catheter is placed.

## 20.2.2 Coagulation Disorders

The patient history and medical examination are the most important measures for clarifying coagulation disorders before performing a regional block. Blocks in the neck, head, and trunk regions should not be performed if there is a history and/or clinical confirmation of a coagulation disorder.

**Table 20.1** General contraindications to peripheral nerve blocks

| Absolute | Relative |
|---|---|
| Infections in the region of the puncture site | Neurological deficits (prior documentation required) |
| Manifest coagulation disorders with blocks in the head, neck, and trunk regions | |
| Refusal by the patient | |

> **Note**
>
> Techniques in which vascular puncture is knowingly accepted (e.g., transarterial technique) should be avoided.

Taking acetylsalicylic acid (ASS) and low-dose heparinization with unfractionated or low-molecular-weight heparin do not contraindicate use of peripheral nerve blocks as long as there is no evidence of an obvious coagulation disorder. There are no reports of serious complications with respect to the antithrombotic agents (fondaparinux, rivaroxaban, dabigatran) and platelet aggregation inhibitors (ticlopidine, clopidogrel, prasugrel, tigrelor, cilostazol), particularly in association with peripheral blocks.

> **Note**
>
> With the exception of the psoas block, few major complications of peripheral nerve blocks have been described in association with medications affecting coagulation.

Bickler et al (2006) report three cases of hematoma after combined femoral nerve / sciatic nerve block with no further serious consequences. In particular, there have been no reports of persistent nerve injury in this connection. Performing peripheral nerve blocks during medication with antithrombotic medication and/or platelet aggregation inhibitors can therefore be justified after careful analysis of the risks and benefits (German Society of Anesthesia and Intensive Care Medicine [DGAI] recommendation 2005).

Monitoring should be ensured following the block for prompt identification of a nerve compression syndrome as a result of a developing hematoma. In this case, the catheter should be removed according to the procedure for neuraxial blocks (Gogarten et al 2007, 2010).

The interscalene block using the Meier approach, the axillary block, and the "midhumeral approach" in the upper limb, and femoral nerve block and distal sciatic nerve block in the lower limb, are considered to be *safer techniques*. Under the conditions listed above and after careful consideration, plexus blocks in the proximity of the clavicle (upper limb) and proximal sciatic nerve blocks (lower limb) can be performed.

> **Note**
>
> Because of several serious case reports in association with medications affecting coagulation (Klein et al 1997, Weller et al 2003) and the close proximity to the spine, the psoas block and paravertebral blocks should be performed under the same strict conditions as neuraxial blocks (Gogarten et al 2007, 2010;
> ▶ Table 20.2 and ▶ Table 20.3, ▶ Fig. 20.4). This also applies to removal of those catheters.

Preoperative coagulation diagnostics should be made only in case of doubt.

▶ **Cockgraft formula.** Many of the drugs listed above accumulate if kidney function is impaired. Impaired kidney function, which often remains undetected in daily routine, is considered to be a

**Table 20.2** Recommended time intervals before and after neuraxial puncture or catheter removal when taking coagulation inhibitory substances (Waurick et al 2014)

|  | Before puncture/ catheter removal* | After puncture/ catheter removal* | Laboratory control |
|---|---|---|---|
| Unfractionated heparins (prophylaxis, <15,000 IU/d) | 4 h | 1 h | Platelets under treatment>5 d |
| Unfractionated heparins (treatment) | 4–6 h (IV) | 1 h (no i. bolus) | aPTT, (ACT), platelets |
| Low-molecular-weight heparins (prophylaxis) | 12 h | 4 h | Platelets under treatment>5 d |
| Low-molecular-weight heparins (treatment) | 24 h | 4 h | Platelets, (anti-Xa) |
| Fondaparinux (prophylaxis, 1 × 2.5 mg/dL) | 36–42 h | 6–12 h | (anti-Xa) |
| Vitamin-K antagonists | INR<1.4 | After catheter removal | INR |
| Hirudins (lepirudin, desirudin) | 8–10 h | 2–4 h | aPTT, ECT |
| Argatroban** (prophylaxis) | 4 h | 5–7 h | aPTT, ECT, ACT |
| Acetylsalicylic acid (100 mg)*** | None | None |  |
| Clopidogrel | 7–10 d | After catheter removal |  |
| Ticlopidine | 7–10 d | After catheter removal |  |
| Prasugrel | 7–10 d | 6 h after removal |  |
| Ticagrelor | 5 d | 6 h after removal |  |
| NSAR | None | None |  |

Abbreviations: aPTT, activated partial thromboplastin time; ECT, ecarin clotting time; ACT, activated clotting time; INR, international normalized ratio; IV, intravenous.

\* All data refer to patients with normal renal function

\*\* Prolonged time interval in hepatic failure

\*\*\* No additional anticoagulants 4–5 half-life periods before puncture/catheter removal (e.g., no LMH 36–42 h before puncture or catheter removal). ASS can be continued.

**Table 20.3** Recommended time intervals before and after neuraxial puncture or catheter removal when taking coagulation inhibiting substances. Supplement for the newer oral antithrombotic agents (information only for prophylactic dosage regimen)

|  | Last administration before puncture/ catheter removal | First administration after puncture/ catheter removal |
|---|---|---|
| Rivaroxaban (1 × 10 mg/d) | 22–26 h | 6 h |
| Dabigatran (1 × 150–220 mg/d) | 28–34 h | 6 h |
| Apixaban (2 × 2.5 mg/d) | 26–30 h | 5–7 h |

Applies only to patients with normal renal function (extended time interval in renal impairment)

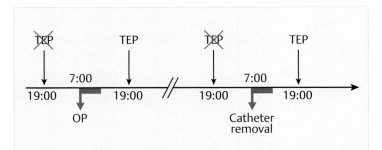

**Fig. 20.4** Procedure in patients under prophylaxis with fondaparinux or simultaneous administration of acetylsalicylic acid and low-molecular-weight heparins: the last thromboembolism prophylaxis (TEP) should be administered 36–42 h before neuraxial puncture / catheter removal, the next administration no sooner than 6 h after puncture / catheter removal. (Source: courtesy of Gogarten W et al 2007.)
TEP: Time interval for placement and/or removal of the catheter

major factor for epidural hematomas in older patients. The Cockgraft formula makes it possible to estimate creatinine clearance (mL/min) based on body weight, serum creatinine, and gender.

The Cockgraft formula:

$$\frac{(140 - \text{age}) \times \text{body weight (kg)}}{72 \times \text{serum creatinine (mg/dL)}}$$

The factor 0.85 is applied to women (men 1.0).

## 20.2.3 Pre-existing Neurological Deficits

Previous neurological disease or peripheral nerve lesions of acute or chronic origin do not represent per se a contraindication to a peripheral regional procedure, but should be well documented before the block is performed.

# References

Auroy Y, Narchi P, Messiah A, Litt L, Rouvier B, Samii K. Serious complications related to regional anesthesia: results of a prospective survey in France. Anesthesiology 1997; 87: 479–486

Barrington MJ, Watts SA, Gledhill SR et al. Preliminary results of the Australasian Regional Anaesthesia Collaboration: a prospective audit of more than 7000 peripheral nerve and plexus blocks for neurologic and other complications. Reg Anesth Pain Med 2009; 34: 534–541

Bickler P, Brandes J, Lee M, Bozic K, Chesbro B, Claassen J. Bleeding complications from femoral and sciatic nerve catheters in patients receiving low molecular weight heparin. Anesth Analg 2006; 103: 1036–1037

Brull R, McCartney CJL, Chan VWS, El-Beheiry H. Neurological complications after regional anesthesia: contemporary estimates of risk. Anesth Analg 2007; 104: 965–974

Büttner J. Primum nil nocere. Regional anesthesia in neurologic diseases. [Article in German] Anaesthesist 2010; 59: 777–778

Cheney FW, Domino KB, Caplan RA, Posner KL. Nerve injury associated with anesthesia: a closed claims analysis. Anesthesiology 1999; 90: 1062–1069

Fanelli G, Casati A, Garancini P, Torri G Study Group on Regional Anesthesia. Nerve stimulator and multiple injection technique for upper and lower limb blockade: failure rate, patient acceptance, and neurologic complications. Anesth Analg 1999; 88: 847–852

Gogarten W, Van Aken H, Büttner J et al. Rückenmarknahe Regionalanästhesie und Thromboembolieprophylaxe/antithrombotische Medikation. Anästh Intensivmed 2007; 48: S109–S124

Gogarten W, Vandermeulen E, Van Aken H, Kozek S, Llau JV, Samama CM European Scoeity of Anaesthesiology. Regional anaesthesia and antithrombotic agents: recommendations of the European Society of Anaesthesiology. Eur J Anaesthesiol 2010; 27: 999–1015

Graf BM, Niesel HC. Pharmakologie der Lokalanästhetika. In: Van Aken H, Wulf H, eds. Lokalanästhesie, Regionalanästhesie, Regionale Schmerztherapie. 3rd ed. Stuttgart: Thieme; 2010: 56–105

Hebl JR, Horlocker TT, Pritchard DJ. Diffuse brachial plexopathy after interscalene blockade in a patient receiving cisplatin chemotherapy: the pharmacologic double crush syndrome. Anesth Analg 2001; 92: 249–251

Hempel V, Baur KF. Regionalanästhesie für Schulter, Arm und Hand. Munich: Urban & Schwarzenberg; 1982

Hempel V. Interscalene block and infections of the shoulder. [Article in German] Anaesthesist 1998; 47: 940

Hirasawa Y, Katsuni Y, Küsswetter W, Sprotte G. Experimentelle Untersuchungen zu peripheren Nervenverletzungen durch Injektionsnadeln. Reg Anästhesie 1990; 13: 11–15

Horlocker TT, O'Driscoll SW, Dinapoli RP. Recurring brachial plexus neuropathy in a diabetic patient after shoulder surgery and continuous interscalene block. Anesth Analg 2000; 91: 688–690

Jöhr M. A complication of continuous blockade of the femoral nerve. [Article in German] Reg Anaesth 1987; 10: 37–38

Klein SM, D'Ercole F, Greengrass RA, Warner DS. Enoxaparin associated with psoas hematoma and lumbar plexopathy after lumbar plexus block. Anesthesiology 1997; 87: 1576–1579

Malamut RI, Marques W, England JD, Sumner AJ. Postsurgical idiopathic brachial neuritis. Muscle Nerve 1994; 17: 320–324

Mulroy MF, Hejtmanek MR. Prevention of local anesthetic systemic toxicity. Reg Anesth Pain Med 2010; 35: 177–180

Neal JM. How close is close enough? Defining the "paresthesia chad". Reg Anesth Pain Med 2001; 26: 97–99

Neal JM, Mulroy MF, Weinberg GL American Society of Regional Anesthesia and Pain Medicine. American Society of Regional Anesthesia and Pain Medicine checklist for managing local anesthetic systemic toxicity: 2012 version. Reg Anesth Pain Med 2012; 37: 16–18

Reisig F, Neuburger M, Breitbarth J, Buettner J. Identification of six predictive factors for infectious complications in peripheral regional anaesthesia. Reg Anesth Pain Med 2009; 34: 61

Sawyer RJ, Richmond MN, Hickey JD, Jarrratt JA. Peripheral nerve injuries associated with anaesthesia. Anaesthesia 2000; 55: 980–991

Shah S, Hadzic A, Vloka JD, Cafferty MS, Moucha CS, Santos AC. Neurologic complication after anterior sciatic nerve block. Anesth Analg 2005; 100: 1515–1517

Sinner B, Graf BM. Regional anesthesia and neurological diseases. [Article in German] Anaesthesist 2010; 59: 781–805

Stan TC, Krantz MA, Solomon DL, Poulos JG, Chaouki K. The incidence of neurovascular complications following axillary brachial plexus block using a transarterial approach. A prospective study of 1,000 consecutive patients. Reg Anesth 1995; 20: 486–492

Steinfeldt T, Poeschl S, Nimphius W et al. Forced needle advancement during needle-nerve contact in a porcine model: histological outcome. Anesth Analg 2011; 113: 417–420

Stöhr M. Iatrogene Nervenläsionen. 2nd ed. Stuttgart: Thieme; 1996

Sztark F, Malgat M, Dabadie P, Mazat JP. Comparison of the effects of bupivacaine and ropivacaine on heart cell mitochondrial bioenergetics. Anesthesiology 1998; 88: 1340–1349

Sztark F, Nouette-Gaulain K, Malgat M, Dabadie P, Mazat JP. Absence of stereospecific effects of bupivacaine isomers on heart mitochondrial bioenergetics. Anesthesiology 2000; 93: 456–462

Tetzlaff JE, Dilger J, Yap E, Brems J. Idiopathic brachial plexitis after total shoulder replacement with interscalene brachial plexus block. Anesth Analg 1997; 85: 644–646

Weinberg GL. Treatment of local anesthetic systemic toxicity (LAST). Reg Anesth Pain Med 2010; 35: 188–193

Weller RS, Gerancher JC, Crews JC, Wade KL. Extensive retroperitoneal hematoma without neurologic deficit in two patients who underwent lumbar plexus block and were later anticoagulated. Anesthesiology 2003; 98: 581–585

Waurick K, Riess H, Van Aken H, Kessler P, Gogarten W, Volk T. S1-Leitlinie: Rückenmarknahe Regionalanästhesie und Thromboseprophylaxe/antithrombotische Medikation. Anästhesiologie Intensivmed 2014; 9: 464–492

# 21 General Principles for Performing Peripheral Blocks

## 21.1 Essential Components Necessary for Proper Aseptic Technique

Although the risk of infection with "single-shot" nerve blocks is relatively small, a strictly sterile technique must nevertheless be observed. There has been one documented case of a fatal necrotizing fasciitis due to single-shot axillary block (Nseir et al 2004). Mandatory preparation for the therapist includes as a minimum hand scrub, mask, cap, and sterile surgical gloves and carefully spraying and wiping the skin with alcoholic disinfectants, paying meticulous attention to the prescribed contact time.

Much higher demands must be made when placing peripheral nerve catheters for continuous administration of local anesthetic. Peripheral regional pain catheters carry a substantial risk of infection (see Chapter 22).

> **Note**
>
> The strictest hygienic standards are required for dealing with continuous regional pain catheters.

▶ **Hygiene recommendations.** The guidelines on hygiene in the administration and subsequent care of regional block techniques are clearly defined (Morin et al 2006). Essential aspects are:
- Hand-washing is mandatory for all personnel involved before starting the procedure.
- Wearing a mask and cap is mandatory for all personnel involved in the procedure wearing a sterile gown is recommended.
- For skin areas rich in sebaceous glands (neck, axilla, groin), the alcoholic disinfectant must have a contact time of 10 minutes; alcohol solutions with a higher percentage of ethanol achieve the required reduction of bacteria on the skin in areas rich in sebaceous glands after 2.5 minutes (Cutasept med F, see manufacturer's information)
  - After patient positioning, it is recommended to use generous spray disinfection of the puncture site before starting the other preparations for placing a continuous block.
  - The site chosen must be kept wet with the disinfectant for the entire contact time.
  - After another hand-washing, sterile gowning and gloving, and preparation of the sterile field, the initial spray disinfection must be repeated as a wipe disinfection several times.
- Sterile draping of the planned insertion site should include a widespread area and should not obscure anatomical landmarks and a clear view of the expected response (▶ Fig. 21.1).
- After fixation of the catheter, the insertion site must be covered with a sterile dressing. The date and time of catheter placement must be noted (see "Complications of Peripheral Nerve Catheters for Pain Management" in Chapter 22).

Strict adherence to these guidelines on hygiene has resulted in a significantly lower infection rate in continuous peripheral regional anesthesia procedures (Reisig et al 2005, 2013).

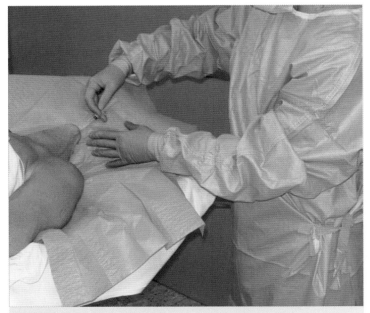

**Fig. 21.1** Particularly when placing continuous peripheral nerve blocks, the strictest hygiene requirements should be followed: cap, sterile gown, facemask, extensive skin disinfection, and sterile draping. The draping must ensure that a view of the anatomical landmarks and the expected muscle responses is not obscured.

## 21.2 General Principles of Informed Consent, Positioning and Monitoring

Anesthesia-related mortality has fallen markedly in recent decades and is today estimated at 1 death per 10,000 anesthesia procedures. Many incidents of complications during both general and regional anesthesia can be avoided. An important requirement is judicious preparation and monitoring and early identification of a problematic situation.

A requirement for every regional anesthesia is the patient's legally effective informed consent. In day surgery or in the outpatient pain clinic, continuous peripheral block techniques can be performed and continued successfully on an outpatient basis (Rawal et al 1997, Rawal 2000). However, the basic conditions (getting home, side effects, etc.) must be carefully discussed and evaluated with the patient and if necessary the relatives or family doctor should also be involved. Besides the anesthetist's competence, the facilities and equipment are of fundamental importance in regional anesthesia. The treatment room should have a calm atmosphere, be of adequate size, and allow the patient to be placed in suitable positions.

Emergency medications, the possibility of ventilation and intubation, and also a defibrillator must be available. Every patient should have an IV line and basic monitoring (ECG, blood pressure monitoring).

In addition to monitoring of the vital parameters, assessment and monitoring of the onset, distribution, and quality of the nerve block is required. The procedure and sequence should be documented.

## 21.2.1 Patient Informed Consent before Peripheral Nerve Blocks

The procedure of a peripheral nerve block must be explained to the patient. It is important also to mention the possibility of an incomplete block and discuss further procedures in this case. General anesthesia should always be considered, so information must also be provided about this.

A regional block can be planned as a supplement to general anesthesia in major surgery, particularly when continuous peripheral nerve analgesia is planned or for postoperative pain management. Whether sedation is desired for performance of the block must be discussed.

As well as specific complications of the technique (e.g., Horner syndrome, pneumothorax), the patient must be generally informed about toxic reactions caused by the local anesthetic and about possible nerve injuries. Hematomas and false aneurysms can also occur after vascular puncture. If continuous peripheral techniques are planned, the risk of infection must be described. It must be pointed out to the patient that some problems can become apparent only after the end of the block (e.g., infection, pneumothorax). The patient should be instructed to report problems of any kind.

For continuous procedures of the lower limb, the patient must be informed of the possible *risk of falling* on getting up as a result of the impaired motor and sensory function and depth perception (Muraskin et al 2007, Ilfeld et al 2010). There is a risk of injury (see also Chapter 22). The patient should get up only with assistance at the start!

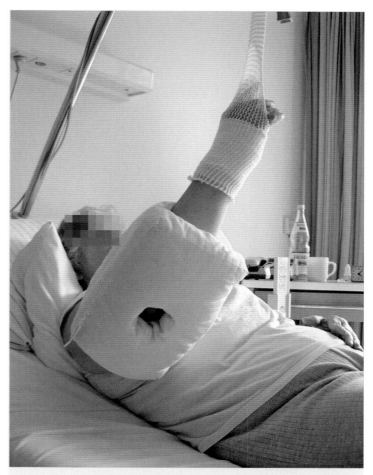

**Fig. 21.2** Special pads help to prevent nerve injury in the (partially) anesthetized arm.

## 21.2.2 Position

The most comfortable position possible should be ensured for the patient. Positioning aids (cushions, pads, etc.) can facilitate the procedure. Position-related injuries in particular must be avoided. Attention must be paid to regions particularly at risk (e.g., ulnar nerve in the ulnar sulcus; common fibular nerve distal to the head of the fibula). Pressure-free positioning of the limb must also be ensured in the postoperative period. This applies especially to continuous techniques. Special pads and splints are available (▶ Fig. 21.2).

In premedicated or sedated patients, an additional (abdominal) positioning strap may be useful in the operative area to secure the patient in order to avoid unintended falls.

## 21.2.3 Monitoring

▶ **Consciousness.** Many patients want sedation and this requires special attention and monitoring by the anesthetist. Pulse oximetry should be ensured in sedated patients in addition to ECG and blood pressure monitoring; ECG monitoring of the depth of sedation may be useful (▶ Fig. 21.3).

▶ **Circulation.** Oscillometric automatic blood pressure measurement has become well established in clinical practice. Monitoring of circulation during regional anesthesia can be expanded, depending on the risk classification of the patient and the type of operation.

▶ **Electrocardiography.** There should be continuous ECG monitoring during the performance of a regional anesthesia block and

perioperatively. Together with blood pressure monitoring and pulse oximetry, the ECG is the basis of monitoring patients under regional anesthesia.

▶ **Ventilation.** Perioperative monitoring of ventilation during regional anesthesia is usually just clinical (visual and acoustic). With indirect measurement of ventilation by means of pulse oximetry, the consequences of reduced alveolar ventilation are identified with a marked delay, particularly when oxygen is being given (hypercapnic normoxia). Additional monitoring of spontaneous respiration (at least as a trend) can be performed by measuring end-expiratory $CO_2$. To do this, a $CO_2$ line is placed close to the patient's nose under the oxygen mask. Transcutaneous monitoring and $CO_2$ measurement is now possible (TOSCA) (▶ Fig. 21.4).

▶ **Oxygenation.** The importance of pulse oximetry during regional anesthesia is uncontroversial. It has a key position in the monitoring of vital functions through the indirect monitoring of circulation and ventilation. Low oxygen levels that are not consistent with the clinical impression may indicate methemoglobinemia if prilocaine was used as local anesthetic. Vasoconstriction is a limiting factor of pulse oximetry.

▶ **Temperature.** Monitoring of body temperature is indicated particularly in elderly patients, in prolonged operations, and when there is increased blood loss. In regional anesthesia with a marked sympathetic block, heat redistribution occurs and the

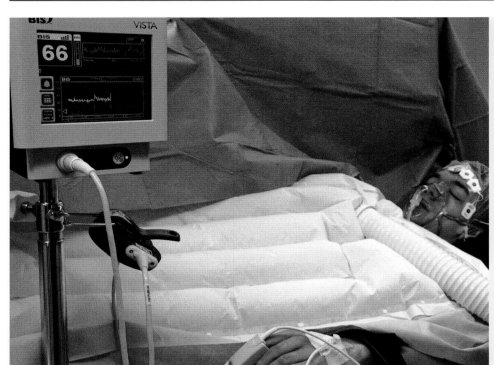

**Fig. 21.3** Measuring depth of sedation by ECG monitoring.

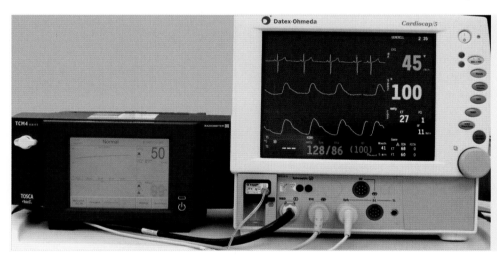

**Fig. 21.4** Monitoring the depth of sedation using transcutaneous $CO_2$ measurement (TOSCA).

insulating function of the periphery (vasoconstriction) is eliminated. In addition, the patient finds the cool room temperature (air conditioning) unpleasant. Adequate warming is therefore recommended during prolonged operations. Convection warming systems are regarded as particularly suitable (e.g., Warm Touch from Covidien GmbH; Bair Hugger from Arizant).

# 21.3 Technical Aids for Performing Peripheral Nerve Blocks ▶

## 21.3.1 Vascular Doppler Sonography

Doppler ultrasound is used in regional anesthesia for orientation of the course of blood vessels and to avoid vascular puncture. It can be extremely helpful especially in difficult anatomical situations. With different acoustic transducers, the small and very handy devices that are now available can show both superficial (8 MHz) and very deep (4 MHz) veins and arteries (▶ Fig. 21.5).

Example of suitable Doppler devices: handydop by Kranzbühler, Huntleigh, Elcat.

## 21.3.2 Ultrasonography

Ultrasound scanning is described in detail in Chapter 1.

## 21.3.3 Surface Thermometer

Depending on the proportion of sympathetic fibers, blockade of peripheral nerves leads to regional sympathetic block. The proportion of sympathetic fibers is very high in the brachial plexus and the sciatic nerve, for instance. The effects of the block can be checked very well by monitoring the skin temperature. As the C-fibers (postganglionic sympathetic fibers) are blocked first, a rise in skin temperature distal to the site of the block is an early indication of the onset of the block. The rise in skin temperature is 2 to 8° Celsius depending on the baseline and can be measured quickly and easily with a surface thermometer.

A suitable thermometer (adjustable to surface temperature) is, for example, First Temp Genius, Sherwood Medical (▶ Fig. 21.6).

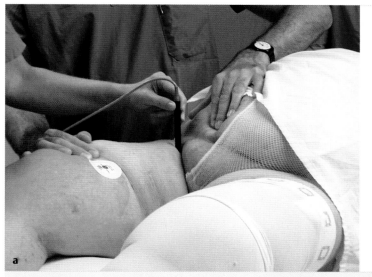
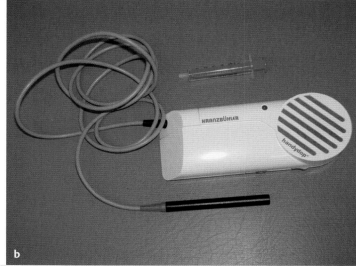

**Fig. 21.5** Vascular Doppler ultrasound to visualize the course of vessels in difficult anatomical situations.

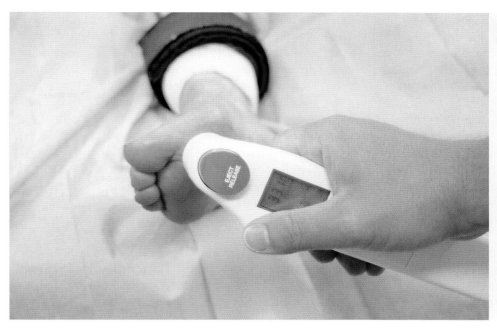

**Fig. 21.6** Suitable surface thermometer to objectify the success of the block.

## 21.3.4 Peripheral Nerve Stimulation

The need for peripheral nerve stimulation (PNS) in performing conduction anesthesia continues to be controversial (Schwarz et al 1998). Regional anesthesia can also be performed successfully without nerve stimulation. This applies particularly for techniques that for anatomical reasons (common fascial sheath around the nerves) allow a loss-of-resistance technique (e.g., axillary plexus anesthesia). PNS can then be used for additional orientation.

However, use of a nerve stimulator should be mandatory in difficult anatomical situations and in nerve blocks involving a large skin–nerve distance (e.g., sciatic nerve). PNS is particularly indicated for nerves with predominantly motor fibers (e.g., femoral nerve), as paresthesia cannot always be produced because of lack of sensory fibers, which means an increased risk of injuries to the nerve. In purely motor neurons, an overproportionate incidence of intraneural injection can be expected (Urmey 1997, Graf and Martin 2001). In these structures, the block can be performed in combination with ultrasound guidance.

PNS cannot be regarded as a substitute for anatomical knowledge, but it is a valuable aid for precise localization of the nerve.

The following are the minimum requirements for a nerve stimulator (Kaiser and Neuburger 2010; ▶ Fig. 21.7).

Electrical design:
- Adjustable constant current
- Monophasic rectangular output pulse
- Adjustable pulse duration (0.1–1.0 ms)
- Adjustable current intensity (0–5.0 mA)
- Precisely adjustable
- Digital display of actual current value
- Stimulating frequency 1–2 Hz

Device safety:
- Alarm when circuit is interrupted
- Alarm when impedance is too high
- Alarm on internal device error
- Outputs clearly assigned
- Reliable instructions for use, stating tolerated deviations

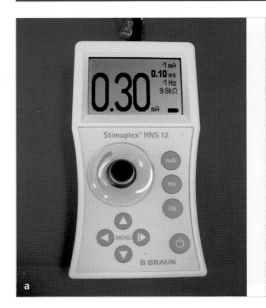
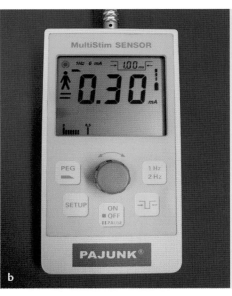

**Fig. 21.7** Nerve stimulators for performing peripheral nerve blocks.
**a** (B. Braun Melsungen AG.)
**b** (Source: courtesy of Pajunk GmbH, Geisingen, Germany.)

Numerous animal experiments and clinical trials using ultrasound have shown that the concept of a clear relationship between the level of stimulus current and the pulse width, on the one hand, and the distance of the needle to the nerve on the other hand, must be reconsidered (Gurnaney et al 2007, Rigaud et al 2008, Tsai et al 2008, Tsui et al 2008, Robards et al 2009, Li et al 2011).

It has been shown that a response at less than 0.2 mA/0.1 ms was always associated with an intraneural needle position, but on the other hand no response was produced despite intraneural needle position up to a stimulation current of 1.7 mA/0.1 ms in some cases (Tsai et al 2008). Several studies show that stimulation at lower levels (<0.5 mA/0.1 ms) offers no advantage with respect to the position of the needle in comparison with higher stimulation currents. An intraneural injection cannot be definitely ruled out even at stimulation currents greater than 0.5 mA/0.1 ms, but is less likely than at lower stimulation currents less than 0.5 mA/0.1 ms (Gurnaney et al 2007, Rigaud et al 2008, Robards et al 2009).

A dramatic increase in electrical resistance can be an indication of an intraneural needle position (Tsui et al 2008). Experimental reversal of the current flow (the cathode is conventionally used for stimulation) leads to a valid correlation between stimulation current and needle–nerve distance (Li et al 2011).

## Practical Notes on the Use of the Nerve Stimulator

- The pulse duration is given as "ms" for millisecond. Note: In Anglo-American usage, the pulse duration is sometimes given as μsec (0.1 ms = 100 μsec).
- When the nerve stimulator is operated after perforation of the skin, it should first be ensured, using a low amplitude, that the needle tip is not already in the vicinity of the nerve, as uncontrolled muscle contractions might occur otherwise. The subsequent search for the nerve begins at a current amplitude of 1.0 mA and a pulse width of 1.0 ms or 0.1 ms with decreasing current.
- As soon as contractions in the key muscle are produced, the nerve stimulator is switched to the shorter pulse (0.1 ms). The

current concept that the pulse width of 1 ms inherently would be substantially more uncomfortable has not been confirmed. Rather, it is the total energy applied (i.e., the product of current times pulse width: $E\,[nC] = I\,[mA] \times t\,[\mu s]$) which is responsible for the discomfort felt by the patient (Hadzic et al 2004). Nevertheless, if at all possible the pulse width should be kept at 0.1 ms since only this level permits fine-tuning of the distance between needle tip and nerve (Neuburger et al 2001).

- Injection at a response below 0.5 mA and a pulse width of 0.1 ms should be avoided.
- Practical clinical experience has shown that a response at 0.2 to 0.3 mA/1.0 ms often corresponds to a response of 1 mA/0.1 ms (Neuburger et al 2001).
- In patients with polyneuropathy (e.g., diabetes mellitus), it is useful to select a longer pulse (1.0 ms).
- A minimum distance between the electrode and stimulation needle has not been established. When nerve stimulators with adjustable stabilized current output are used, the site of placement of the cutaneous electrode appears to be unimportant for the function of the nerve stimulator (Hadzic 2004).
- For the stimulation level desired (≤0.5–0.7 mA, 0.1 ms), the administration of saline or local anesthetics will change the electric field and, compared with the administration of glucose 5%, will therefore result in immediate adverse effects on, or even loss of, the response (Tsui et al 2004, Neuburger et al 2005, Tsui and Kropelin 2005). Knowing this, so-called "multiple injection" techniques have to be regarded critically, since the response of the nerve stimulator may be significantly impaired after an initial injection of saline or local anesthetic at the puncture site (Neuburger et al 2005).
- Contrary to the statements of the manufacturers, PNS can also be used in patients with implanted cardiac pacemakers/defibrillators (Kaiser and Neuburger 2010). However, it should be ensured that the pacemaker aggregate, the cardiac electrodes, and the heart are not on the line connecting the skin electrode to the stimulation needle. The indication should be made strictly and the options of nerve stimulation / ultrasound should be weighed. Cardiac arrest was reported in one case study (Engelhardt et al 2006).

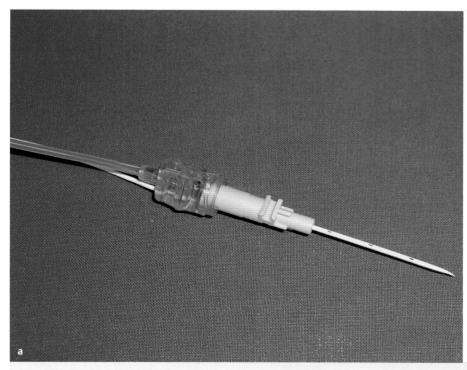
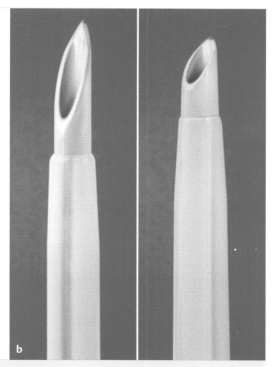

**Fig. 21.8** Contiplex-D needle, unipolar needle with a 15° or 30° bevel and indwelling needle (B. Braun Melsungen AG).

## 21.3.5 Needles and Catheters

Needles insulated on the shaft and conductive at the tip (monopolar or unipolar) are used as stimulation needles with the nerve stimulator. For ultrasound-guided blocks, specially processed surfaces allow better visualization with ultrasound even at steeper puncture angles (Chapter 1). There are needles for single-shot techniques and for continuous techniques.

► **Needle tips.** The major difference in the design of the tip of the needle is between needles with a bevel (15°, 30°; ► Fig. 21.8), Tuohy needles, and pencil-point needles. Pencil-point and Tuohy needles make it possible to advance the catheter in a certain direction in continuous techniques.

► **Potential trauma.** Statements on the advantages and disadvantages of different types of needles with respect to potential injuries are limited mainly to animal tests (Selander et al 1977, Hirasawa et al 1990, Selander 1993, Steinfeldt et al 2010a, 2010b, 2011).

---

**Note**

There are no clinical trials on advantages and disadvantages of different types of needles with respect to potential nerve damage. The decision as to which type of needle to use therefore remains at the discretion of the user.

Needles with a so-called sharp or long bevel (15°) slide best through the tissue, but the potential risk of injuring the nerve is greater (Selander et al 1977, Hirasawa et al 1990, Selander 1993).

---

► **Catheter techniques.** There are two techniques, which differ in both material and procedure, for catheter insertion:

• Needles with a surrounding plastic cannula (► Fig. 21.8): These are needles inside a plastic indwelling cannula that make it possible to guide the indwelling cannula to the nerve. After successful placement and removal of the needle, a catheter is advanced 3 to 5 cm beyond the tip of the indwelling cannula. The indwelling cannula is then removed.
• Needles for the "catheter-through-needle" technique (► Fig. 21.9): These are needles through which, after successful placement, a catheter can be advanced directly about 3 cm beyond the tip of the needle. The needle is then removed.

► **Needle with steel stylet.** A needle with a plastic indwelling part is a special type of needle with a not hollow bored, solid steel stylet and 45° bevel and rounded edges (18 G/20 G) (Kombi-Plex B, Pajunk; ► Fig. 21.10). This needle can be used for a single-shot perivascular plexus block or femoral nerve block as well as to place a catheter for a continuous procedure. For a single-shot block, the indwelling plastic part can be left until the end of the operation; for a continuous block, the indwelling plastic part must be removed after the catheter is advanced.

Due to the solid stylet with the 45° bevel, the loss of resistance when the connective tissue is penetrated is felt clearly (► Fig. 21.10).

## Examples of Needles for Single-Shot Blocks with Electrical Insulation (Noninsulated Needle Tips as "Contact Point")

Stimuplex D needles (B. Braun) with 15° bevel (20 G/22 G/23 G/25 G, 35/40/55/70/80/120/150 mm) and 30° bevel (22 G, 40/50/80 mm).

Stimuplex Ultra needles (B. Braun) with 30° bevel (20 G/22 G, 35/50/80/150 mm) with echogenic marking (suitable for ultrasound).

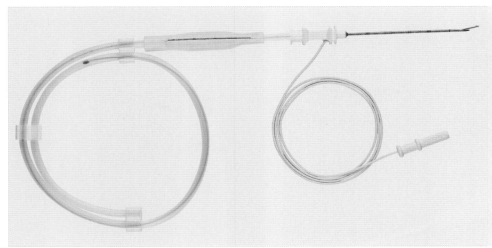

**Fig. 21.9** Insulated needles (with catheter-through-needle technique), PlexoLong catheter set. (Source: courtesy of Pajunk GmbH, Geisingen, Germany.) The needle comes in various lengths (5–15 cm) and with different tips (bevel, pencil-point with lateral opening, and Tuohy needle). For better visualization in ultrasound, it is also available with a specially processed surface ("cornerstone" needle).

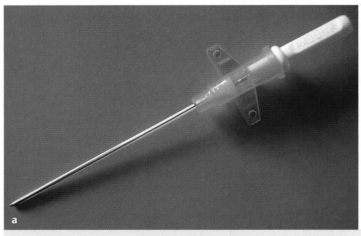
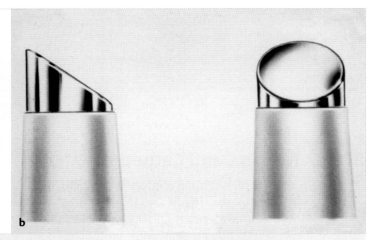

**Fig. 21.10** Needle with steel stylet (source: courtesy of Pajunk GmbH, Geisingen, Germany).
**a** Combination needle for axillary plexus anesthesia (18 G, 51 mm).
**b** Enlarged needle tip.

UniPlex needles (Pajunk, UPK) with Sprotte tip (22G/24G/25G, 40/50/70/90/150 mm) or bevel (20 G/21 G/24 G/25 G, 25/35/40/50/80/100/120/150 mm).

SonoPlex needles (Pajunk) with Sprotte tip (22 G/24 G, 40/50/70/90 mm) or bevel tip (20 G/21 G/22 G/24 G, 25/40/50/80/100/120/150 mm) with "cornerstone" reflectors and NanoLine coating (suitable for ultrasound).

## Examples of Needles for Continuous Blocks with Electrical Insulation Coating (Noninsulated Needle Tip as "Contact Point")

- Needles with plastic indwelling part (catheter through indwelling needle):
  - Contiplex D (B. Braun) with 15° bevel (18 G/20 G, 33/55/80/110 mm) and 30° bevel (18 G, 55 mm) ("Braunula system")
  - MultiSet NanoLine (UniPlex [UPK] or UniPlexSono [UPKS] needle in indwelling needle; Pajunk) with Sprotte or facet tip (UPK 21 G, indwelling needle 18 G, 51/75 mm)
- Needles for "catheter-through-needle" technique:
  - Contiplex Tuohy (B. Braun; 18 G, 40/50/100/150 mm)
  - Contiplex Tuohy Ultra set (B. Braun; 18 G, 40/50/100/150 mm; especially suited for ultrasound)
  - Contiplex S (B. Braun; with 20° bevel and rounded edges; 18 G, 50/100/150 mm)
  - Contiplex S Ultra set (B. Braun; with 20° bevel and rounded edges; 18 G, 50/100/150 mm; especially suited for ultrasound)
  - PlexoLong NanoLine with facet tip (19 G, 30/50/100/150 mm), Sprotte tip (19 G/21 G, 30/60/120/150 mm), Tuohy tip (18 G/21 G, 30/50/100/150 mm)
  - PlexoLong Sono NanoLine with facet tip (19 G, 50/100/150 mm), Sprotte tip (19 G, 60/120 mm), Tuohy tip (especially suited for ultrasound, 18 G, 50/100 mm)

## Stimulation Catheters

Special catheters are available that have a stimulation tip for checking their position.

Whether or not stimulation catheters result in better blocks when used in long-term administration of local anesthetics is still the subject of discussion. Casati et al (2005), Pham-Dang et al (2003), and Salinas et al (2004) reported some advantages of the stimulation catheters compared with conventional models (higher success rate, less need for analgesics). In contrast, the prospective blind study by Morin et al (2005) did not find any advantages of stimulation catheters when compared with femoral nerve block catheters in major knee surgery. Nevertheless, these catheters can be employed for precise placement of the catheter,

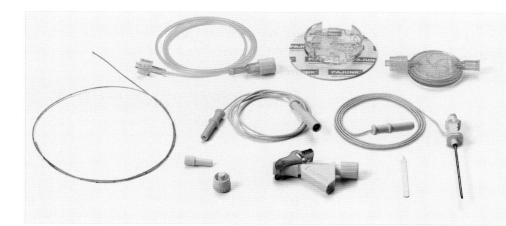

**Fig. 21.11** A stimulation catheter enables the position of the catheter tip to be checked by electrostimulation with a nerve stimulator. (Source: courtesy of Pajunk GmbH, Geisingen, Germany.)

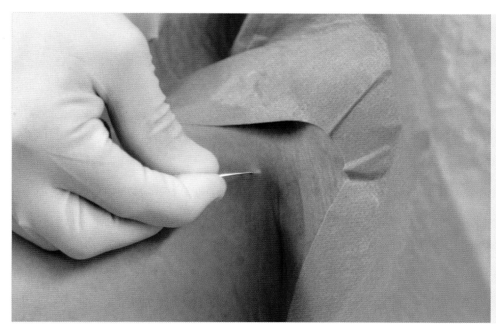

**Fig. 21.12** An incision with a lancet is necessary, especially with an "atraumatic" needle to allow it to penetrate the skin; at the same time it prevents skin particles from entering the tissue.

for instance, in difficult anatomical situations. A stimulation catheter is also suitable for the differential diagnosis of dislocation/tachyphylaxis (e.g., StimuLong Plus, Pajunk, Geisingen, Germany; ▶ Fig. 21.11).

**Practical Note**

Successful stimulation at a sufficient interval since the last administration of local anesthetic indicates that there is no catheter dislocation. In this case, a higher concentration or change of the local anesthetic can lead to an adequate effect. If it is inadequate, an attempt can be made to correct the catheter position by withdrawing it.

# 21.4 General Principles for Performing Regional Anesthesia

## 21.4.1 With Nerve Stimulator ▶

- The insertion site and its surrounding area are disinfected and (for continuous techniques) draped with sterile drapes.
- Infiltration anesthesia with a 26 G needle should not be too deep to avoid premature block of superficial parts of the plexus.

- A skin puncture is then made with a lancet or sharp needle. This is recommended especially when using a short-bevel needle in order to advance it through the tissue with minimal force. At the same time, this prevents punched-out material from being carried inward (▶ Fig. 21.12).
- The needle is advanced subcutaneously with slight rotation of the needle tip (if necessary slightly "shaking" the needle tip to loosen it from the surrounding tissue).
- In the loss-of-resistance technique: advance the needle until there is a "fascial click."
- The nerve stimulator is then attached.
- A longer pulse (1.0 ms) should be selected when stimulating sensory nerves.
- The distance of the skin electrode from the site of stimulation is not important, but the distance must be adequate to ensure sterility.
- Maximum muscle contractions should be avoided as the patient can find these unpleasant.
- The stimulation needle is advanced carefully. When using the "immobile needle" technique, perform intermittent aspirations to detect an intravascular position.
- Continuous aspiration should not be performed as the cannula lumen can become occluded by tissue.

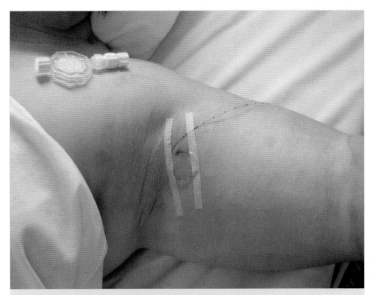

**Fig. 21.13** The catheter can be fixated with a sterile adhesive strip (Steristrip).

- When there is a motor response, the current is reduced gradually until muscle contractions in the region of the key muscles are still just visible at a pulse amplitude of 0.5 to 0.7 mA and 0.1 ms pulse width. The local anesthetic is then injected.
- The catheter should usually be placed after expanding the perineural space with a certain proportion of volume (e.g. local anesthetic or 5% glucose solution), as experience has shown that the catheter can then be advanced more easily (Pham-Dang et al 2006).
- The catheter is usually advanced approximately 3 cm beyond the distal end of the needle. If the catheter position is found to be incorrect, it should be withdrawn to the original stimulation position.
- Check of catheter position: The position of the tip of the catheter can be checked using a stimulation catheter (see above) and corrected if necessary.
- The catheter can be fixated by a sterile adhesive dressing (▶ Fig. 21.13).
- A sterile dressing should include an absorbent dressing for the first 24 hours. This can then be replaced by a transparent adhesive bandage.
- Document the depth of puncture and the skin level of the catheter.

## 21.4.2 With Ultrasound ▶

(See also Chapter 1):
- Orienting visualization of the puncture region
- Optimization of the ultrasound settings (penetration depth, focus, frequency, etc.)
- Disinfection and generous draping (for continuous blocks)
- Sterile sleeve on the transducer
- Local anesthesia (see above), skin incision
- Puncture in plane or out of plane under ultrasound guidance
- Good visualization of spread of local anesthetic in the target area
- Catheter advanced after injecting 10 to 20 mL of glucose 5% or local anesthetic
- Check spread of local anesthetic over the catheter tip, correction if needed

The position of the catheter can be checked using ultrasound. Visualize the position of the tip of the catheter in ultrasound and, if necessary, correct the injection of the local anesthetic with respect to the nerve.

> **Note**
>
> A combination of nerve stimulator with ultrasound is possible and sometimes useful.

With respect to avoiding complications, the use of the nerve stimulator for performing peripheral blocks is still considered to be an equally valuable procedure despite the increasingly widespread use of ultrasound.

# 21.5 Analgosedation
## 21.5.1 For Peripheral Nerve Blocks

Regional blocks for postoperative pain therapy can be performed in the anesthetized patient or under spinal anesthesia if they are placed with correct use of a nerve stimulator and employing atraumatic insulated needles.

> **Practical Note**
>
> However, the awake, cooperative patient may help to avoid nerve injury.

Under sedation with midazolam or propofol, patients are often restless and difficult to control (Morin et al 2004). Evidently, it is more the analgesic rather than the sedative component in analgosedation that improves patient comfort while keeping them cooperative (Morin et al 2004). For example, in regional blocks, 0.1 mg fentanyl resulted in better patient acceptance than midazolam (3 mg) or placebo (0.9% saline).

The following recommendations for analgosedation enable performance of a regional peripheral nerve block in a sedated but cooperative patient:
- Sufentanil 5 µg + midazolam 1 mg (Gentili et al 1999)
- Alternative: remifentanil 0.05 µg/kg body weight per minute, if necessary after a "loading dose" of 0.3 µg/kg.

> **Practical Note**
>
> This dose of remifentanil provides ideal conditions for placement of a nerve block but requires monitoring of ventilation. It is advisable to give oxygen through a mask during placement of the block. After a successful block, a patient on a remifentanil infusion must be adequately monitored!

## 21.5.2 Concomitant Medication during Surgery under Regional Anesthesia

Remifentanil has also proved effective at the above dosage for analgosedation during surgery (Lauwers et al 1999).

Intraoperative sedation with remifentanil under regional anesthesia:
- Remifentanil 0.05 µg/kg body weight per minute (Graf and Martin 2001).

**Table 21.1** Overview of commonly used local anesthetics

| Substance | Potency in vitro (procaine = 1) | Molecular weight | pK$_a$ (25°C) | Distribution coefficient | Protein binding | Duration of action |
|---|---|---|---|---|---|---|
| Mepivacaine | 3–4 | 246 | 7.6 | 0.8 | 77% | 1.5–3 h |
| Prilocaine | 3–4 | 220 | 7.9 | 0.9 | 56% | 1–3 h |
| Bupivacaine | 16 | 288 | 8.16 | 27.5 | 96% | 1.5–8 h |
| Ropivacaine | 14–16 | 276 | 8.05 | 6.7 | 95% | 3–6 h |

Weighing the desired effect and the side effects, Holas et al (1999) recommend the combination of propofol and remifentanil at the following dosage:

- Remifentanil 0.03 µg/kg body weight per minute + propofol 0.7 mg/kg body weight per hour (Ford et al 1984).

Target-controlled infusion with propofol is recommended for sedation during regional blocks (Janzen et al 2000, Sutcliffe 2000). This can also be patient-controlled (Irwin et al 1997).

# 21.6 General Principles for Administration of Local Anesthetics in Peripheral Nerve Block

## 21.6.1 Local Anesthetics

Medium-acting and long-acting amide local anesthetics are most frequently used in regional anesthesia today (▶ Table 21.1).

The choice of a local anesthetic for a peripheral block is influenced by the following considerations:

Peripheral blocks have a relatively long onset time, so a local anesthetic with a rapid onset is desirable. Because of their chemical structure, medium-acting local anesthetics have advantages in this respect. However, the latency time obtained in a combined femoral–sciatic nerve block with 0.75% (7.5 mg/mL) ropivacaine was found to be similar to 2% (20 mg/mL) mepivacaine (Casati et al 1999).

When the "single-shot" technique is used, a long-acting local anesthetic is often required depending on the anticipated duration of surgery; moreover, the long-acting local anesthetic may provide correspondingly long-lasting postoperative analgesia. With ropivacaine, an average duration of analgesia of 12 to 14 hours can be expected (Casati et al 1999, Wank et al 2002), and in individual cases the effect may last up to 20 hours. A partial motor block can be observed for almost the same period. Patients must be informed about the probable duration of the block, so that they do not worry unnecessarily.

Relatively high doses of local anesthetic are administered in peripheral blocks. Many peripheral techniques include the risk of accidental intravascular injection. For this reason, the local anesthetic with the lowest toxicity should be preferred. Medium-acting local anesthetics are less toxic than long-acting ones. Among the long-acting local anesthetics, ropivacaine is less toxic than bupivacaine. Currently, it is not known if local anesthetics are myotoxic at a clinically relevant level. However, ropivacaine exhibits considerably less myotoxicity than bupivacaine (Zink and Graf 2004). While it is argued that ropivacaine is of lower potency for central blocks compared with bupivacaine (D'Angelo

and James 1999), numerous studies confirm the equipotency of ropivacaine to bupivacaine in peripheral blocks (Hilgier 1985, Hickey et al 1992, Greengrass et al 1998, Klein et al 1998, Casati et al 2000a, 2001, Eroglu et al 2004). Being less lipophilic than bupivacaine, ropivacaine provides a better differential block at lower concentrations than bupivacaine (Borgeat et al 2001).

*Mixtures* of a long-acting local anesthetic with a medium-acting one are occasionally used. This combines the relatively short onset of the medium-acting local anesthetic with the long duration of the long-acting one.

> **Note**
>
> It must be remembered that the toxicity of mixtures of local anesthetics is additive.

## 21.6.2 Dosage

Depending on age and physical constitution, a volume of 20 to 50 mL of a 1% (10 mg/mL) solution of a medium-acting local anesthetic can be recommended for all peripheral nerve blocks close to the trunk (▶ Table 21.2). Blocks performed using ultrasound permit lower volumes to be used.

▶ **Prilocaine.** The recommended maximum dose of prilocaine is 600 mg.

> **Note**
>
> Due to methemoglobinemia caused by prilocaine, no repeat doses should be given after the maximum dose has been administered.

▶ **Mepivacaine.** The recommended maximum dose of mepivacaine is 500 mg.

Dosages of up to 750 mg in adults of normal weight are tolerated without problems (Cockings et al 1987, Simon et al 1990).

After an initial dose of 400 mg of mepivacaine, repeat doses of up to 400 mg can be given up to three times at two-hour intervals for axillary continuous plexus anesthesia without fear of toxic blood levels or clinical signs of overdose (Büttner et al 1989).

**Table 21.2** Dosage of local anesthetics in peripheral blocks close to the trunk (normal-weight adult)

| Duration of action | Volume (single shot): 30–50 mL |
|---|---|
| Medium-acting local anesthetic | Prilocaine 1%<br>Alternative: mepivacaine 1% |
| Long-acting local anesthetic (max. 40 mL) | Ropivacaine 0.75%<br>Alternative: bupivacaine 0.5% |

▶ **Ropivacaine.** As a long-acting local anesthetic, ropivacaine has proved to be less toxic than bupivacaine and to have similar potency in peripheral nerve blocks (see above). For axillary plexus block, a dose of up to 300 mg of ropivacaine 0.75% (7.5 mg/mL) has proved to be effective without side effects (Wank et al 2002).

▶ **Combined blocks (e.g., femoral–sciatic nerve block).** In combined femoral–sciatic nerve block, the established maximum doses will have to be exceeded to achieve an adequate effect for the two techniques. Normally, the toxicity of the local anesthetic presents no clinically relevant problem in such cases because of the delayed absorption of local anesthetic in lower-limb nerve blocks (Magistris et al 2000), provided accidental intravascular injection does not occur. When continuous techniques are performed, the two blocks can be initiated with a medium-acting local anesthetic. If a continuous technique is not used and longer-lasting analgesia is desired, a combination of a medium-acting local anesthetic (prilocaine or mepivacaine) with ropivacaine can be given. The total dose in this case should not be more than 150 mg of ropivacaine and 300 to 400 mg of mepivacaine.

Addition of epinephrine can generally be omitted in peripheral blocks.

## 21.6.3 Measures to Shorten the Latency Time

A problem of peripheral nerve blocks is their relatively long onset time. Numerous attempts have been made to shorten it. There are essentially three approaches:
- Carbonization of the local anesthetic
- Alkalinization of the local anesthetic
- Warming of the local anesthetic

### Carbonization of the Local Anesthetic

The anticipated advantage of using a local anesthetic in the carbonic acid salt formulation instead of the HCl preparation (e.g., mepivacaine-$CO_2$ vs. mepivacaine-HCl) has not been confirmed (Krebs and Hempel 1985, Dreesen et al 1986). Shorter onset times were not found with peripheral blocks, although high blood levels did indicate a faster absorption of the $CO_2$-containing formulation.

### Alkalinization of the Local Anesthetic

Numerous randomized, mostly double-blind, studies were able to show a faster onset of peripheral nerve blocks as a result of alkalinization of the local anesthetic solution (Hilgier 1985, DiOrio and Ellis 1988, Coventry and Todd 1989, Tetzlaff et al 1990, 1995, Büttner and Klose 1991, Quinlan et al 1992, Capogna et al 1995, Gormley et al 1996). Moreover, better tolerance of the blood-free field tourniquet (Tetzlaff et al 1993), more profound motor block (Tetzlaff et al 1995), and a better overall block effect (Quinlan et al 1992) were observed. Only a few studies showed no beneficial effect of alkalinization on the onset time (Candido et al 1995, Auroy et al 1997, Chow et al 1998), probably as a result of too great an increase in the pH (Candido et al 1995, Auroy et al 1997), which may have resulted in precipitation of the local anesthetic.

The optimal proportions of local anesthetic and added sodium bicarbonate that are influenced by the local anesthetic used and its concentration must be maintained. The following proportions are well tested and recommended:
- Mepivacaine 1% (10 mg/mL) (or 1.5% [15 mg/ mL])
  10 mL + NaHCO₃ 8.4% 1 mL.

This proportion can also be applied to prilocaine. The alkalinization of ropivacaine is theoretically possible (e.g., 0.1 mL bicarbonate / 20 mL ropivacaine; Fulling and Peterfreund 2000) but is not recommended for routine clinical use because of the risk of precipitation (Milner et al 2000).

## Warming of the Local Anesthetic

Warming the local anesthetic to body temperature leads to a significantly faster onset (Heath et al 1990). The mechanism is unclear. Overheating must be ruled out.

## 21.6.4 Adjuvants

Attempts to improve the quality of the block and prolong the duration of action by adding various adjuvants have been reported.

### Clonidine, Dexmedetomidine

When added to different local anesthetics, clonidine leads to a significant prolongation of postoperative analgesia (Büttner et al 1992, Casati et al 2000b, El Saied et al 2000). For surgery in infected tissue (paronychia) the administration of 400 mg of mepivacaine combined with 100 μg of clonidine will result in a more profound axillary brachial plexus block than mepivacaine alone (Iohom et al 2005). However, no effect could be demonstrated in conjunction with 0.75% (7.5 mg/mL) ropivacaine for axillary plexus block (Erlacher et al 2000). The optimal dosage appears to be 0.5 to 1 μg clonidine/kg body weight added to the local anesthetic solution (Singelyn et al 1996, Bernard and Macaire 1997). Higher dosages are accompanied by systemic side effects such as sedation and hypotension (Büttner et al 1992). In intravenous regional anesthesia there was better toleration of a tourniquet with the addition of 150 μg of clonidine (Gentili et al 1999).

Addition of clonidine (2 μg/mL) to a continuous peripheral nerve block for postoperative pain control evidently does not offer any clinically relevant benefits (Ilfeld et al 2005).

> **Practical Note**
>
> Clonidine 0.5 to 1.0 μg/kg bodyweight added to the local anesthetic leads to prolongation of the block; an intensification of the block is sometimes also seen in patients with chronic pain.

Similar effects were found when using dexmedetomidine, another alpha-2 agonist, combined with local anesthetics (e.g., levobupivacaine) for peripheral regional blocks (Biswas et al 2014).

# Opioids

Any anticipated benefit of adding opioids to local anesthetics for peripheral nerve block has not been confirmed (Bouaziz et al 2000, Magistris et al 2000, Murphy et al 2000, Nishikawa et al 2000).

# Neostigmine

Neostigmine appears to have some beneficial effects on postoperative analgesia but does not lead to a faster block (Bone et al 1999).

# References

Auroy Y, Narchi P, Messiah A, Litt L, Rouvier B, Samii K. Serious complications related to regional anesthesia: results of a prospective survey in France. Anesthesiology 1997; 87: 479–486

Bernard JM, Macaire P. Dose-range effects of clonidine added to lidocaine for brachial plexus block. Anesthesiology 1997; 87: 277–284

Biswas S, Das RK, Mukherjee G, Ghose T. Dexmedetomidine an adjuvant to levobupivacaine in supraclavicular brachial plexus block: a randomized double blind prospective study. Ethiop J Health Sci 2014; 24: 203–208

Bone HG, Van Aken H, Booke M, Bürkle H. Enhancement of axillary brachial plexus block anesthesia by coadministration of neostigmine. Reg Anesth Pain Med 1999; 24: 405–410

Borgeat A, Kalberer F, Jacob H, Ruetsch YA, Gerber C. Patient-controlled interscalene analgesia with ropivacaine 0.2% versus bupivacaine 0.15% after major open shoulder surgery: the effects on hand motor function. Anesth Analg 2001; 92: 218–223

Bouaziz H, Kinirons BP, Macalou D et al. Sufentanil does not prolong the duration of analgesia in a mepivacaine brachial plexus block: a dose response study. Anesth Analg 2000; 90: 383–387

Büttner J, Klose R, Hammer H. Continuous axillary catheter plexus anesthesia—a method of postoperative analgesia and sympathetic nerve block following hand surgery. [Article in German] Handchir Mikrochir Plast Chir 1989; 21: 29–32

Büttner J, Klose R. Alkalinization of mepivacaine for axillary plexus anesthesia using a catheter. [Article in German] Reg Anaesth 1991; 14: 17–24

Büttner J, Ott B, Klose R. The effect of adding clonidine to mepivacaine. Axillary brachial plexus blockade. [Article in German] Anaesthesist 1992; 41: 548–554

Candido KD, Winnie AP, Covino BG, Raza SM, Vasireddy AR, Masters RW. Addition of bicarbonate to plain bupivacaine does not significantly alter the onset or duration of plexus anesthesia. Reg Anesth 1995; 20: 133–138

Capogna G, Celleno D, Laudano D, Giunta F. Alkalinization of local anesthetics. Which block, which local anesthetic? Reg Anesth 1995; 20: 369–377

Casati A, Fanelli G, Borghi B, Torri G. Ropivacaine or 2% mepivacaine for lower limb peripheral nerve blocks. Anesthesiology 1999; 90: 1047–1052

Casati A, Fanelli G, Albertin A et al. Interscalene brachial plexus anesthesia with either 0.5% ropivacaine or 0.5% bupivacaine. Minerva Anestesiol 2000a; 66: 39–44

Casati A, Magistris L, Fanelli G et al. Small-dose clonidine prolongs postoperative analgesia after sciatic-femoral nerve block with 0.75% ropivacaine for foot surgery. Anesth Analg 2000b; 91: 388–392

Casati A, Fanelli G, Magistris L, Beccaria P, Berti M, Torri G. Minimum local anesthetic volume blocking the femoral nerve in 50% of cases: a double-blinded comparison between 0.5% ropivacaine and 0.5% bupivacaine. Anesth Analg 2001; 92: 205–208

Casati A, Fanelli G, Koscielniak-Nielsen Z et al. Using stimulating catheters for continuous sciatic nerve block shortens onset time of surgical block and minimizes postoperative consumption of pain medication after halux valgus repair as compared with conventional nonstimulating catheters. Anesth Analg 2005; 101: 1192–1197

Chow MY, Sia ATH, Koay CK, Chan YW. Alkalinization of lidocaine does not hasten the onset of axillary brachial plexus block. Anesth Analg 1998; 86: 566–568

Cockings E, Moore PL, Lewis RC. Transarterial brachial plexus blockade using high doses of 1, 5% mepivacaine. Reg Anesth 1987; 12: 159–164

Coventry DM, Todd JG. Alkalinisation of bupivacaine for sciatic nerve blockade. Anaesthesia 1989; 44: 467–470

D'Angelo R, James RL. Is ropivacaine less potent than bupivacaine? Editorial Anesthesiology 1999; 90: 941–943

DiOrio S, Ellis R. Comparison of pH-adjusted and plain solutions of mepivacaine for brachial plexus anaesthesia. Reg Anesth 1988; 13: 1S–3(abstract)

Dreesen H, Büttner J, Klose R. Comparison of the effect and serum level of mepivacaine HCL and mepivacaine CO2 in axillary brachial plexus anesthesia. [Article in German] Reg Anaesth 1986; 9: 42–45

El Saied AH, Steyn MP, Ansermino JM. Clonidine prolongs the effect of ropivacaine for axillary brachial plexus blockade. Can J Anaesth 2000; 47: 962–967

Engelhardt L, Große J, Birnbaum J, Volk T. Inhibition of a pacemaker during nerve stimulation for peripheral regional anaesthesia. Anaesthesia 2007; 62: 1071–1074

Erlacher W, Schuschnig C, Orlicek F, Marhofer P, Koinig H, Kapral S. The effects of clonidine on ropivacaine 0.75% in axillary perivascular brachial plexus block. Acta Anaesthesiol Scand 2000; 44: 53–57

Eroglu A, Uzunlar H, Sener M, Akinturk Y, Erciyes N. A clinical comparison of equal concentration and volume of ropivacaine and bupivacaine for interscalene brachial plexus anesthesia and analgesia in shoulder surgery. Reg Anesth Pain Med 2004; 29: 539–543

Ford DJ, Pither CE, Raj P. Comparison of insulated and uninsulated needles for locating peripheral nerves with a peripheral nerve stimulator. Anesth Analg 1984; 63: 925–928

Fulling PD, Peterfreund RA. Alkalinization and precipitation characteristics of 0.2% ropivacaine. Reg Anesth Pain Med 2000; 25: 518–521

Gentili M, Bernard JM, Bonnet F. Adding clonidine to lidocaine for intravenous regional anesthesia prevents tourniquet pain. Anesth Analg 1999; 88: 1327–1330

Gormley WP, Hill DA, Murray JM, Fee JP. The effect of alkalinisation of lignocaine on axillary brachial plexus anaesthesia. Anaesthesia 1996; 51: 185–188

Graf BM, Martin E. Peripheral nerve block. An overview of new developments in an old technique. [Article in German] Anaesthesist 2001; 50: 312–322

Greengrass RA, Klein SM, D'Ercole FJ, Gleason DG, Shimer CL, Steele SM. Lumbar plexus and sciatic nerve block for knee arthroplasty: comparison of ropivacaine and bupivacaine. Can J Anaesth 1998; 45: 1094–1096

Gurnaney H, Ganesh A, Cucchiaro G. The relationship between current intensity for nerve stimulation and success of peripheral nerve blocks performed in pediatric patients under general anesthesia. Anesth Analg 2007; 105: 1605–1609

Hadzic A, Vloka JD, Claudio RE, Hadzic N, Thys DM, Santos AC. Electrical nerve localization: effects of cutaneous electrode placement and duration of the stimulus on motor response. Anesthesiology 2004; 100: 1526–1530

Heath PJ, Brownlie GS, Herrick MJ. Latency of brachial plexus block. The effect on onset time of warming local anaesthetic solutions. Anaesthesia 1990; 45: 297–301

Hickey R, Rowley CL, Candido KD, Hoffman J, Ramamurthy S, Winnie AP. A comparative study of 0.25% ropivacaine and 0.25% bupivacaine for brachial plexus block. Anesth Analg 1992; 75: 602–606

Hilgier M. Alkalinization of bupivacaine for brachial plexus block. Reg Anesth 1985; 8: 59–61

Hirasawa Y, Katsuni Y, Küsswetter W, Sprotte G. Experimentelle Untersuchungen zu peripheren Nervenverletzungen durch Injektionsnadeln. Reg Anästhesie 1990; 13: 11–15

Holas A, Krafft P, Marcovic M, Quehenberger F. Remifentanil, propofol or both for conscious sedation during eye surgery under regional anaesthesia. Eur J Anaesthesiol 1999; 16: 741–748

Ilfeld BM, Morey TE, Thannikary LJ, Wright TW, Enneking FK. Clonidine added to a continuous interscalene ropivacaine perineural infusion to improve postoperative analgesia: a randomized, double-blind, controlled study. Anesth Analg 2005; 100: 1172–1178

Ilfeld BM, Duke KB, Donohue MC. The association between lower extremity continuous peripheral nerve blocks and patient falls after knee and hip arthroplasty. Anesth Analg 2010; 111: 1552–1554

Iohom G, Machmachi A, Diarra DP et al. The effects of clonidine added to mepivacaine for paronychia surgery under axillary brachial plexus block. Anesth Analg 2005; 100: 1179–1183

Irwin MG, Thompson N, Kenny GNC. Patient-maintained propofol sedation. Assessment of a target-controlled infusion system. Anaesthesia 1997; 52: 525–530

Janzen PRM, Hall WJ, Hopkins PM. Setting targets for sedation with a target-controlled propofol infusion. Anaesthesia 2000; 55: 666–669

Kaiser H, Neuburger M. Periphere elektrische Nervenstimulation. In: Van Aken H, Wulf H, eds. Lokalanästhesie, Regionalanästhesie, Regionale Schmerztherapie. 3rd ed. Stuttgart: Thieme; 2010: 130–148

Klein SM, Greengrass RA, Steele SM et al. A comparison of 0.5% bupivacaine, 0.5% ropivacaine, and 0.75% ropivacaine for interscalene brachial plexus block. Anesth Analg 1998; 87: 1316–1319

Krebs P, Hempel V. Mepivacaine for axillary plexus anesthesia. Comparison of mepivacaine-CO2 and mepivacaine-HCl. [Article in German] Reg Anaesth 1985; 8: 33–35

Lauwers M, Camu F, Breivik H et al. The safety and effectiveness of remifentanil as an adjunct sedative for regional anesthesia. Anesth Analg 1999; 88: 134–140

Li J, Kong X, Gozani SN, Shi R, Borgens RB. Current-distance relationships for peripheral nerve stimulation localization. Anesth Analg 2011; 112: 236–241

Magistris L, Casati A, Albertin A et al. Combined sciatic-femoral nerve block with 0.75% ropivacaine: effects of adding a systemically inactive dose of fentanyl. Eur J Anaesthiol 2000; 17: 348–353

Milner QJ, Guard BC, Allen JG. Alkalinization of amide local anaesthetics by addition of 1% sodium bicarbonate solution. Eur J Anaesthiol 2000; 17: 38–42

Morin AM, Vasters FG, Wulf H et al. Does fentanyl or midazolam improve patient's comfort and cooperation when given for regional catheter placement? A randomized, controlled and double-blind trial. [Article in German] Anaesthesist 2004; 53: 944–949

Morin AM, Eberhart LHJ, Behnke HKE et al. Does femoral nerve catheter placement with stimulating catheters improve effective placement? A randomized, controlled, and observer-blinded trial. Anesth Analg 2005; 100: 1503–1510

Morin AM, Kerwat KM, Buettner J et al. Hygieneempfehlungen für die Anlage und weiterführende Versorgung von Regionalanästhesie-Verfahren. Anaesth Intensivmed 2006; 47: 372–379

Muraskin SI, Conrad B, Zheng N, Morey TE, Enneking FK. Falls associated with lower-extremity-nerve blocks: a pilot investigation of mechanisms. Reg Anesth Pain Med 2007; 32: 67–72

Murphy DB, McCartney CJ, Chan VW. Novel analgesic adjuncts for brachial plexus block: a systematic review. Anesth Analg 2000; 90: 1122–1128

Neuburger M, Rotzinger M, Kaiser H. Electric nerve stimulation in relation to impulse strength. A quantitative study of the distance of the electrode point to the nerve. [Article in German] Anaesthesist 2001; 50: 181–186

Neuburger M, Gültlinger O, Ass B, Büttner J, Kaiser H. Influence of blockades with local anesthetics on the stimulation ability of a nerve by peripheral nerve stimulation. Results of a randomized study. [Article in German] Anaesthesist 2005; 54: 575–577

Nishikawa K, Kanaya N, Nakayama M, Igarashi M, Tsunoda K, Namiki A. Fentanyl improves analgesia but prolongs the onset of axillary brachial plexus block by peripheral mechanism. Anesth Analg 2000; 91: 384–387

Nseir S, Pronnier P, Soubrier S et al. Fatal streptococcal necrotizing fasciitis as a complication of axillary brachial plexus block. Br J Anaesth 2004; 92: 427–429

Pham-Dang C, Kick O, Collet T, Gouin F, Pinaud M. Continuous peripheral nerve blocks with stimulating catheters. Reg Anesth Pain Med 2003; 28: 83–88

Pham-Dang C, Guilley J, Dernis L et al. Is there any need for expanding the perineural space before catheter placement in continuous femoral nerve blocks? Reg Anesth Pain Med 2006; 31: 393–400

Quinlan JJ, Oleksey K, Murphy FL. Alkalinization of mepivacaine for axillary block. Anesth Analg 1992; 74: 371–374

Rawal N, Hylander J, Nydahl PA, Olofsson I, Gupta A. Survey of postoperative analgesia following ambulatory surgery. Acta Anaesthesiol Scand 1997; 41: 1017–1022

Rawal N. Patient-controlled regional analgesia at home. Tech Reg Anesth Pain Manage 2000; 4: 62–66

Reisig F, Neuburger M, Breitbarth J, et al. Erfolgreiche Etablierung der neuen DGAI-Leitlinien für die Anlage kontinuierlicher peripherer Regionalanästhesien. Vorläufige Ergebnisse einer prospektiven Untersuchung aus dem Jahr 2005. Garmisch-Partenkirchen: Poster BAT; 2005

Reisig F, Neuburger M, Zausig YA, Graf BM, Büttner J; Deutsche Gesellschaft für Anästhesiologie und Intensivmedizin. Successful infection control in regional anesthesia procedures: observational survey after introduction of the DGAI hygiene recommendations. [Article in German] Anaesthesist 2013; 62: 105–112

Rigaud M, Filip P, Lirk P, Fuchs A, Gemes G, Hogan Q. Guidance of block needle insertion by electrical nerve stimulation: a pilot study of the resulting distribution of injected solution in dogs. Anesthesiology 2008; 109: 473–478

Robards C, Hadzic A, Somasundaram L et al. Intraneural injection with low-current stimulation during popliteal sciatic nerve block. Anesth Analg 2009; 109: 673–677

Salinas FV, Neal JM, Sueda LA, Kopacz DJ, Liu SS. Prospective comparison of continuous femoral nerve block with nonstimulating catheter placement versus stimulating catheter-guided perineural placement in volunteers. Reg Anesth Pain Med 2004; 29: 212–220

Schwarz U, Zenz M, Strumpf M. Junger P. Braucht man wirklich einen Nervenstimulator für regionale Blockaden? Anästhesiol Intensivmed 1998; 12: 609–615

Selander D, Dhuner KG, Lundborg G. Peripheral nerve injury due to injection needles used for regional anaesthesia. An experimental study of the acute effects of needle point trauma. Acta Anaesthesiol Scand 1977; 21: 182–188

Selander D. Peripheral nerve injury caused by injection needles. Br J Anaesth 1993; 71: 323–325

Simon MA, Gielen MJ, Lagerwerf AJ, Vree TB. Plasma concentrations after high doses of mepivacaine with epinephrine in the combined psoas compartment/sciatic nerve block. Reg Anesth 1990; 15: 256–260

Singelyn FJ, Gouverneur JM, Robert A. A minimum dose of clonidine added to mepivacaine prolongs the duration of anesthesia and analgesia after axillary brachial plexus block. Anesth Analg 1996; 83: 1046–1050

Steinfeldt T, Nimphius W, Werner T et al. Nerve injury by needle nerve perforation in regional anaesthesia: does size matter? Br J Anaesth 2010a; 104: 245–253

Steinfeldt T, Nimphius W, Wurps M et al. Nerve perforation with pencil point or short bevelled needles: histological outcome. Acta Anaesthesiol Scand 2010b; 54: 993–999

Steinfeldt T, Werner T, Nimphius W et al. Histological analysis after peripheral nerve puncture with pencil-point or Tuohy needletip. Anesth Analg 2011; 112: 465–470

Sutcliffe N. Sedation during loco-regional anaesthesia. Acta Anaesth Belg 2000; 51:153–156

Taenzer A, Walker BJ, Bosenberg AT et al. Interscalene brachial plexus blocks under general anesthesia in children: Is this safe practice?: A report from the Pediatric Regional Anesthesia Network (PRAN). Reg Anesth Pain Med 2014; 39: 502–505

Tetzlaff JE, Yoon HJ, O'Hara J, Reaney J, Stein D, Grimes-Rice M. Alkalinization of mepivacaine accelerates onset of interscalene block for shoulder surgery. Reg Anesth 1990; 15: 242–244

Tetzlaff JE, Yoon HJ, Brems J et al. Alkalinization of mepivacaine improves the quality of interscalene brachial plexus block for shoulder surgery. Anesth Analg 1993; 76: S432(abstract)

Tetzlaff JE, Yoon HJ, Brems J, Javorsky T. Alkalinization of mepivacaine improves the quality of motor block associated with interscalene brachial plexus anesthesia for shoulder surgery. Reg Anesth 1995; 20: 128–132

Tsai TP, Vuckovic I, Dilberovic F et al. Intensity of the stimulating current may not be a reliable indicator of intraneural needle placement. Reg Anesth Pain Med 2008; 33: 207–210

Tsui BC, Wagner A, Finucane B. Electrophysiologic effect of injectates on peripheral nerve stimulation. Reg Anesth Pain Med 2004; 29: 189–193

Tsui BC, Kropelin B. The electrophysiological effect of dextrose 5% in water on single-shot peripheral nerve stimulation. Anesth Analg 2005; 100: 1837–1839

Tsui BCH, Pillay JJ, Chu KT, Dillane D. Electrical impedance to distinguish intraneural from extraneural needle placement in porcine nerves during direct exposure and ultrasound guidance. Anesthesiology 2008; 109: 479–483

Urmey FW. Femoral nerve block for the management of postoperative pain. In: Urmey FW, ed. Techniques in Regional Anesthesia and Pain Management. Philadelphia: Saunders; 1997: 2: 88–92

Wank W, Büttner J, Maier KR, Emanuelson BM, Selander D. Pharmacokinetics and efficacy of 40 ml ropivacaine 7.5 mg/ml (300 mg), for axillary brachial plexus block—an open pilot study. Eur J Drug Metab Pharmacokinet 2002; 27: 53–59

Zink W, Graf BM. Local anesthetic myotoxicity. Reg Anesth Pain Med 2004; 29: 333–340

# 22 Continuous Peripheral Nerve Blocks

## 22.1 Advantages

The superiority of peripheral nerve blocks for postoperative analgesia after major shoulder and knee surgery compared to systemic intravenous patient-controlled analgesia (PCA) with opioids has been demonstrated clearly (Borgeat et al 1997, Singelyn et al 1998, Capdevila et al 1999). Continuous epidural analgesia and a continuous femoral nerve block via catheter are considered to be equally effective for postoperative analgesia after extensive knee surgery; because of the lower risk, the peripheral block should be preferred (see below). However, apart from the superiority with regard to the analgesic effect, a significant benefit on the duration of rehabilitation and on the quality of the rehabilitation is also achieved (Capdevila et al 1999).

With the aid of a continuous peripheral nerve block, possible major complications in association with neuraxial blocks can be avoided.

Selective nerve block of the affected lower limb can be reliably achieved with a continuous peripheral block, enabling early mobilization as only one limb is affected. However, it must be borne in mind that motor weakness is present in the affected limb.

In contrast to epidural block, prolonged urinary diversion is not required.

The contraindications with regard to neuraxial techniques are much wider than for peripheral blocks, so that a peripheral nerve catheter for continuous pain management can be placed in cases where a neuraxial procedure is contraindicated or not technically feasible.

## 22.2 Indications

Indications are:
- Severe postoperative pain
- Posttraumatic pain states
- Physiotherapy treatment
- Sympathetic block
- Prevention and treatment of amputation stump and phantom pain

### 22.2.1 Differential Indications

The following are examples of indications for continuous peripheral nerve blocks and suitable catheters for regional pain management.

### Shoulder

In arthroscopy of the shoulder, postoperative analgesia by continuous interscalene brachial plexus block is clearly superior to the intra-articular administration of local anesthetics plus suprascapular nerve block. There is no difference between the intra-articular administration of local anesthetics and placebo (Singelyn et al 2004).

Continuous subacromial infusion of local anesthetics for postoperative pain control after reconstructive surgery of the rotator cuff is also clearly less effective than interscalene brachial plexus block (Delaunay et al 2005).

Continuous suprascapular nerve block is well suited for physiotherapy in frozen shoulder syndrome, as long as there has not been any previous surgery. It carries less risk than interscalene brachial plexus block and results in significantly less impairment of the sensory and motor functions in the affected arm.

▶ **Conclusion.** Interscalene brachial plexus block is the treatment of choice for postoperative pain control after painful shoulder surgery. Continuous subacromial infusion of local anesthetics can be recommended only if there are contraindications to interscalene brachial plexus block. Suprascapular nerve block is the procedure of choice in nonsurgical indications (frozen shoulder syndrome).

### Elbow, Forearm, and Hand

Continuous axillary block is well suited for postoperative pain control after elbow surgery, one alternative being infraclavicular brachial plexus block.

### Hip
### Hip Replacement

Postoperative pain after total hip replacement can usually be controlled quite well by intravenous PCA with opioids (Biboulet et al 2004). In high-risk patients, continuous regional analgesia may be indicated, but peripheral regional nerve blocks should be preferred over neuraxial techniques due to the lower risk. Another option would be continuous femoral nerve block via catheter or psoas block (Capdevila et al 2005a). Due to the proximity of the catheter for continuous femoral nerve block to the surgical field and the greater effect of the psoas block, the latter has some advantages over the femoral nerve block. However, any decision for psoas block must be made considering the contraindications to this procedure.

### Proximal Femoral Fracture

A femoral nerve block will provide adequate pain control after proximal femoral fracture. If surgery must be delayed, a continuous block technique may be useful until the time of surgery. Because of the close proximity of the catheter to the surgical field, the surgeon should be consulted.

### Knee
### Total Knee Replacement

Apart from major shoulder surgery, total knee replacement is one of the most painful operations. The superiority of regional nerve blocks (continuous epidural analgesia; continuous femoral nerve block via catheter) over PCA with opioids has been demonstrated (Capdevila et al 1999, Singelyn et al 1998). Femoral nerve block without (Barrington et al 2005) as well as in combination with a continuous sciatic nerve block (Al-Zahrani et al 2014) has proven to be as effective as continuous epidural analgesia.

► **Spinal hematoma.** In female patients undergoing knee replacement surgery under epidural analgesia, the risk of spinal hematoma has been shown to be as great as 1:3,600 (Moen et al 2004). On the other hand, the risk of spinal hematoma under epidural analgesia in obstetrics has been found to be 1:200,000 (Moen et al 2004).

Although this retrospective Scandinavian study for the period 1990 to 1999 did not apply the strict guidelines for epidural block under concomitant anticoagulation, one third of the women still fulfilled these criteria. The publication points out that osteoporosis is one etiological factor of epidural hematoma in epidural analgesia which has not been focused on in the past. Particularly older patients undergoing knee replacement surgery fall into this high-risk group. Therefore, a peripheral regional nerve block should be selected for postoperative pain control.

► **Quality of anesthesia.** No difference for postoperative analgesia was found between continuous femoral nerve block and continuous psoas block (Capdevila et al 2005a), despite the fact that femoral nerve block does not affect the obturator nerve. In a few patients who underwent femoral nerve block for postoperative pain control after total knee replacement, single-shot obturator nerve block (Chapter 13.4) had to be added in the recovery room.

► **Risk.** From a risk point of view, continuous femoral nerve block via catheter should be preferred. However, this decision will also be influenced by the type of intraoperative anesthesia.

Note

If the operation is performed under a combined psoas/posterior sciatic nerve block, one option might be to continue the psoas block.

► **Weakness of the quadriceps femoris.** After lumbar plexus block after total knee replacement has worn off, a certain weakness of the quadriceps femoris muscles with impaired function is often observed. Sometimes this leads to the discussion that regional anesthesia might prolong the postoperative recovery. However, studies have demonstrated that the weakness of the quadriceps femoris muscles can usually be explained by the procedure itself, and not the block.

Even 4 weeks after total knee replacement, patients still display a 62% loss of maximum strength of the quadriceps femoris muscles, with a 17% drop in activation under maximum voluntary innervation. In addition, a 10% rate of muscle atrophy (measured at the maximum cross-sectional area of the quadriceps femoris muscles) was seen compared with the preoperative baseline. The impaired voluntary innervation is regarded as being far more responsible for the loss in muscle power than the atrophy itself. Evidently, pain does not play a central role. No patients in this study received perioperative regional nerve blocks (Mizner et al 2005).

► **Additional continuous sciatic nerve block.** There is increasing controversy over whether additional continuous sciatic nerve block might offer further postoperative benefits to patients with total knee replacement (Ben-David et al 2004, Geiger et al 2005, Morin et al 2005, Pham Dang et al 2005, Abdallah and Brull 2011, Cappelleri et al 2011, Wegener et al 2011).

About 70 to 85% of the patients will profit from sciatic nerve block in terms of a significant reduction in postoperative pain, this being particularly true for patients with preoperative flexion contracture (Ben-David et al 2004, Geiger et al 2005).

Single-shot administration of a long-acting local anesthetic is not sufficient, as the pain in the area innervated by the sciatic nerve persists for about 36 hours (Pham Dang et al 2005, Wegener et al 2011), and this period cannot be covered by one single-shot block. The combination of a femoral nerve block or a psoas block with a continuous sciatic nerve block offers superior analgesia compared with a continuous femoral nerve block or psoas block alone, but there is disagreement about the effect of an additional sciatic nerve block on the functional result (Ben-David et al 2004, Morin et al 2005, Wegener et al 2011).

It should be noted that intermittent monitoring of the motor function of the dorsal and plantar flexors of the foot is mandatory in order to detect any operative injury to the sciatic nerve at an early stage. This monitoring may be realized by intermittent bolus administration with appropriate neurologic windows or by a low concentration of the local anesthetic (e.g., 0.2% ropivacaine), which makes a differential block with analgesia possible while leaving motor function unaffected.

Note

An increase in nerve damage after total knee replacement due to the introduction of peripheral block techniques for postoperative analgesia has not been found (Jacob et al 2011).

► **Multimodal concept.** Hebl et al (2005) employed a multimodal concept for postoperative pain control after total hip/knee replacement, with continuous psoas block or femoral nerve block combined with sciatic nerve block being the central element. They were able to demonstrate that the 50% reduction in opioid use in the postoperative period resulted in earlier ambulation, shorter length of stay, significant reduction in PONV, less dysfunctional cognition, and less urinary retention compared with historical controls (Hebl et al 2005).

## Tibial Plateau Fracture, Tibial Plateau Osteotomy, Intramedullary Nail

Contrary to the assumption that it is primarily the sciatic nerve that innervates the bone of the tibial plateau, femoral nerve block is a highly efficient procedure for pain control in injuries and surgery at this level. The greatly feared compartment syndrome in connection with a tibial plateau fracture can be detected early, as the function of the sciatic nerve is not impaired. It is important that the surgeon is well aware of this fact. After intramedullary nailing of the lower leg, the substantial pain at the subpatellar point where the nail is inserted into the tibia can be well managed by femoral nerve block.

## Combined Continuous Peripheral Nerve Blocks

Combined continuous block of several peripheral nerves in one limb (e.g., femoral and sciatic nerve) is possible, as well as parallel blocks in two limbs (e.g., bilateral continuous axillary block, bilateral distal sciatic nerve block). Bilateral interscalene brachial plexus block is contraindicated! See below for dosages of the local anesthetic.

## 22.3 Local Anesthetics: Administration, Dosage

Different types of administration can be distinguished:
- Intermittent administration of a bolus
- Continuous administration
- Patient-controlled bolus delivery with or without basic continuous infusion

Which of the listed methods will be used depends, among other things, on the local conditions. Numerous variants of local anesthetic administration for postoperative pain therapy through continuous peripheral nerve catheters have been studied (Meyer and Hermann 1998, Singelyn et al 1999, Singelyn and Gouverneur 2000).

▶ **Dosage recommendations.** The following dosage recommendations can be given for the long-term use of local anesthetics:
- Ropivacaine 0.2 to 0.375% (2–3.75 mg/mL), 6 to 12 mL/h
- Alternative: bupivacaine 0.125 to 0.375% (1.25–3.75 mg/mL), 5 to 10 mL/h, max. 30 mg/h

When two blocks are to be performed in parallel, 0.33% (3.3 mg/mL) ropivacaine may be delivered continuously for each block at a dose of 6 mL/h, as long as there are no limiting factors on the patient's side (e.g., decompensated cardiac failure, severely impaired renal clearance). The authors of this atlas look back on substantial experience with this dosing regimen, without having seen any incidents that may be traced back to this dose of the local anesthetic. Under this regimen, intermittent additional bolus administration of 10 mL ropivacaine 0.33% (3.3 mg/mL) up to four times a day is tolerated without any problems.

Ropivacaine should be preferred because of the lower toxicity and reduced motor impairment in the low concentration ranges (Borgeat et al 2001). In the first 24 hours postoperatively, 0.2% (2 mg/mL) ropivacaine at a dosage of 0.25 mg/kg body weight per hour proved ineffective (Salonen et al 2000). Therefore, 0.33 to 0.375% (3.3–3.75 mg/mL) ropivacaine is often used in this situation.

▶ **Infusion or syringe pumps.** The use of infusion or syringe pumps has proved useful for techniques of continuous regional anesthesia. Continuous delivery can be provided through perfusor syringes. A disadvantage is that the syringes must be changed frequently at relatively high infusion rates (6–10 mL/h). However, syringe pumps with a freely selectable volume per bolus have been available for some years, and are suitable for greater volumes (60–100 mL).

Devices that enable both continuous and patient-controlled intermittent delivery (PCA) are well tried and tested. A commercially available plastic bag (Polybag) containing 200 mL of ropivacaine can be attached to these pumps. If a higher concentration of ropivacaine is desired, 240 mL of a 0.33% (3.3 mg/mL) solution can be made by adding 40 mL of 1% (10 mg/mL) ropivacaine (▶ Table 22.1). As well as the advantage of less frequent bag changes, which is important for hygiene reasons, these devices provide the patient with greater mobility. The use of large-volume infusion units leads to considerably improved organizational options.

The devices are subject to the medical devices act (MPG). The provisions of this law require among other things, that the user (physician, nurse, etc.) be instructed in its use. The legal requirements have contributed to optimal device safety and faulty operation or programming can be almost completely ruled out.

▶ **Elastomer pumps.** Elastomer pumps (▶ Fig. 22.1) are also gaining increasing interest; these are filled with a certain volume of local anesthetic (usually 250 mL) and infuse the local anesthetic solution at a fixed delivery rate (e.g., 5 or 10 mL/h). These systems work very reliably with few disruptions and a bolus delivery by the patient is now possible with some of the currently available systems.

## 22.3.1 Care of Peripheral Pain Catheters in a General Ward

The requirements for care of catheters for peripheral continuous nerve blocks are fundamentally the same as for neuraxial catheters. However, special features differing from neuraxial blockades must be taken into account.

> **Note**
>
> According to the local requirements of current rules, changing the syringes or local anesthetic bags and tubing or filters can theoretically be delegated to nursing personnel, provided they have sufficient knowledge and experience with regard to possible complications, side effects of drugs, and first aid in case of incidents (Van Aken et al 2001).

In Germany this is specified in the "Agreement on the Organization of Postoperative Pain Therapy" by the Professional Associa-

**Table 22.1** Suggestions for increasing the concentration of Naropin 2 mg/mL in the "Polybag"

| Ropivacaine (Naropin Polybag 200 mL / actual volume 210 mL) | Standard Milliliters additional volume | 420 mg Ropivacaine Total milligrams | 210 mL Volume Total volume (mL) | 2 mg/mL Ropivacaine Concentration (mg/mL) |
|---|---|---|---|---|
| Increase in concentration by addition of Naropin 10 mg/mL | 10 | 520 | 220 | 2.4 |
| | 20 | 620 | 230 | 2.7 |
| | 40 | 820 | 250 | 3.3 |
| | 60 | 1020 | 270 | 3.8 |

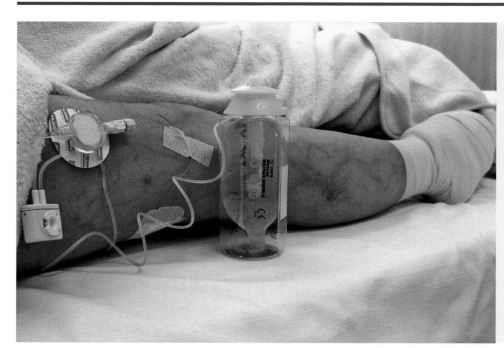

**Fig. 22.1** Mechanical elastomer pump (here, distal sciatic nerve catheter).

tion of German Anesthesiologists and the Professional Association of German Surgeons (Anästh Intensivmed 1993; 34: 28–32). Accordingly, approved training as a specialist nurse in anesthesia/intensive care is not required, but it is necessary to check qualifications before delegating tasks and to ensure the availability of a physician at short notice during all procedures. Which physician is responsible for instruction and checking qualifications depends on the organization of pain therapy in the individual hospital. A clear agreement between the specialist departments and nursing services management on competence and areas of responsibility is strongly recommended.

If analgesia is inadequate, the following is recommended:
• Possibility of a surgical complication should be considered.
• Possible catheter dislocation should be checked.
• If the catheter position is correct, after administration of a local anesthetic bolus, an increased dose can be given.

▶ **Surgical complications.** Experience has shown that complications such as compartment syndrome or infection at the site of surgery can be detected by an above-average requirement for local anesthetic or additional analgesics (Cometa et al 2011). Uncritical augmentation of analgesics and local anesthetic could be dangerous. The surgeon should be informed in order to assess the situation.

▶ **Catheter dislocation.** The original stimulation depth of the needle and the length of catheter inserted should be noted to facilitate detection of dislocation. Advancement of the catheter too far can also be the cause of inadequate analgesia.

For example, an interscalene plexus catheter that has been advanced too far can cause a complete motor and sensory block in the hand, but with persistent pain in the region of the operated shoulder.

Occasionally, a catheter that has been advanced too far beyond the tip of the needle may move away from the target nerves. In this case, too, withdrawal to about the depth at which the nerve was originally stimulated with the needle can lead to successful analgesia. If there are doubts about the correct position of a regional pain catheter, a single effective dose of local anesthetic

can be given to check whether a successful block occurs. If this is not the case, the catheter should be removed.

## 22.3.2 Peripheral Nerve Catheters for Outpatient Regional Pain Management

Operations associated with considerable postoperative pain are increasingly performed on an outpatient basis (Ilfeld and Enneking 2005). A precondition for this is, of course, adequate postoperative pain therapy. According to a survey, one of the main reasons for dissatisfaction with outpatient surgery is inadequate pain therapy after discharge (Ghosh and Sallam 1994, Wedderburn et al 1996). In addition to their high degree of effectiveness, the advantages of peripheral nerve catheters, particularly for outpatient postoperative pain therapy, include:
• the absence of respiratory depression (versus opioids), and
• significantly less nausea and vomiting.

If regional pain therapy is not available, these two factors often make early discharge impossible in an outpatient setting (Candido et al 2001, Grant et al 2001, Klein et al 2001, 2002, Krone et al 2001, Mulroy et al 2001, Rawal 2001, Ilfeld and Enneking 2002, Ilfeld et al 2002a, Rawal et al 2002, White et al 2003). Significant superiority compared with conventional pain therapy was shown in the outpatient setting for continuous brachial plexus block (Ilfeld et al 2002a, Rawal et al 2002) as well as for continuous distal sciatic nerve block (Ilfeld et al 2002b). These advantages were:
• Less pain
• Less sleep disturbance
• Less need for analgesics
• Fewer side effects (nausea, gastrointestinal symptoms, etc.)
• Greater general satisfaction.

In all these studies, no complications related to local anesthetic or catheters were observed.

▶ **Preconditions.** A precondition for continuous peripheral regional analgesia in an outpatient setting is a properly informed and cooperative patient. A competent contact person must be available around the clock and the distance to the responsible clinic should be reasonably short, so that the patient can easily go there in the event of problems that cannot be resolved by telephone.

▶ **Disposables.** For the outpatient setting, disposable elastomer pumps are available that allow continuous administration with a fixed basic rate (Infuser LV5/10, capacity 250 mL, Baxter). The advantage of these disposable infusion pumps is their low malfunction rate (Capdevila et al 2003). More and more (disposable) elastomer pumps are becoming commercially available, which not only offer a base rate, but also the option of intermittent patient-controlled bolus delivery (Ilfeld et al 2004a). The limiting factor seems to be their price. On the other hand, it is just this pain management that has made it possible to offer certain operations as outpatient surgery (White et al 2003).

▶ **Informed consent.** The patient must be given adequate detailed information, both oral and written, about risks and problems that can arise in connection with the continuous peripheral regional anesthesia.

▶ **Residual sensation.** It is important always to select a concentration of local anesthetic that enables the patient to preserve some residual sensation and ensure that motor function is preserved. The limb must be well padded to prevent any position-related nerve damage (ulnar nerve injury, fibular nerve injury). In blocks of the lower limb, patients must be capable of completely relieving the affected limb using crutches since there is a risk of falling when sensation and/or motor function is impaired.

▶ **Dosage.** The best results were obtained with a 2 mg/mL ropivacaine base rate of 8 mL/h and the option of a PCA-bolus of 2 mL once per hour for interscalene brachial plexus catheter block in shoulder surgery of moderate pain severity, and 4 mL once per hour for distal sciatic nerve catheter block in outpatient foot surgery of moderate pain severity (Ilfeld et al 2004b,c). In general, pain control should be multimodal here as well; that is, the patients should also have the option of taking additional NSAIDs and oxycodone, for example.

▶ **Aftercare.** Telephone contact should be made with the patient at least once a day. The patient must be informed about possible changes at the injection site that might indicate developing infection. In this case patients must be informed that they should contact their physician promptly. The catheter should be removed by a competent person who can make a correct assessment.

## 22.3.3 Complications of Peripheral Nerve Catheters for Pain Management

### Infection

The most feared and most significant complication of peripheral nerve catheters is infection. Superficial erythema of the injection site is observed with an incidence of 5 to 10% (Meier et al 1997).

The reported rate of clinically relevant moderate and severe infections (▶ Fig. 22.2) is 0.05 to 3% (Capdevila et al 2005b, Neuburger et al 2006). Since the rate clearly depends on the duration of indwelling, it should be kept as short as possible (but as long as needed)! Catheters placed in areas rich in sebaceous glands (neck, axilla, and groin) are subject to a higher rate of infection (Morin et al 2005, Neuburger et al 2006). Interscalene brachial plexus catheter is associated with the highest risk of infection (Neuburger et al 2006). A strict hygiene protocol allowed the rate of infection to be reduced from 3% to 1% (Reisig et al 2005; Chapter 21).

The following preventive measures should be observed:
• Absolute asepsis when placing the catheter
• Daily inspection of the injection site

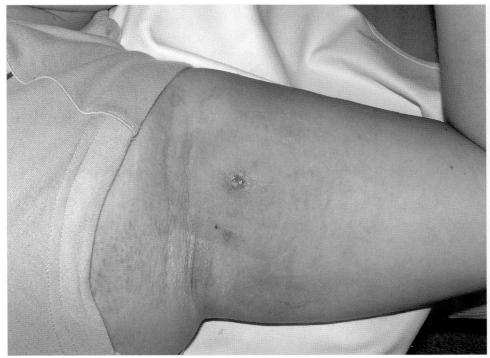

Fig. 22.2 Abscess after continuous peripheral nerve block; pain is often the first early sign of local inflammation and must be carefully investigated!

Crucial evidence is not so much redness but rather secretion that occasionally oozes from the injection site (not to be confused with local anesthetic that occasionally leaks from the injection site) and pain in the area.

> **Note**
>
> Pain in the area of the injection site is the most sensitive indicator of early infection. In case of doubt, the catheter should be removed immediately.

The patient should be continuously monitored in the following days as an abscess can develop even after removal of the catheter. If there are already signs of an infection (fever, elevated inflammation markers, local redness, hardness, tenderness), a culture should be taken if possible and calculated therapy with *3 × 1.5 g cefuroxime IV introduced*, as the pathogens are usually gram-positive cocci. If necessary, treatment must be switched, depending on the results of the culture. If an abscess is present, surgical intervention may be required.

## Nerve Injury Due to Peripheral Catheters

There is no information reported on the incidence of nerve injury due to peripheral nerve catheters for continuous pain treatment. Occasionally, the surgeon wants to perform an immediate postoperative neurological assessment. In this case it is advisable to perform the block with a medium-acting local anesthetic, and then, after postoperative neurological examination, start continuous infusion of the local anesthetic (after giving an adequate bolus).

## Catheter Tear, Looping

Rupture or accidental shearing of peripheral nerve catheters has been described (Lee and Goucke 2002). These complications can occur during catheter placement, particularly when the catheter with guide wire is withdrawn before removal of the needle through which the catheter was introduced. Accordingly, the needle must always be withdrawn before the guide wire is removed.

> **Note**
>
> Any catheter withdrawal through a needle, particularly one with a sharp-edged bevel, should be done with caution (light traction), if at all; if any resistance is encountered the catheter should be removed together with the needle, as otherwise there is a risk of the catheter being sheared off (Coventry and Timperley 2004).

When catheters have been secured with a skin suture, it is essential to ensure that the catheter is not severed when it is removed. If the catheter is tunneled with an indwelling venous cannula, the catheter may be sheared off by this procedure (Reisig et al 2011).

If the catheter has been sheared off or severed, surgical removal must be given careful consideration, because except for those cases where the catheter may be palpated immediately below the skin, this usually will involve an extensive surgical procedure requiring the operating room and appropriate anesthesia. A preoperative CT scan, MRI or ultrasound scan can be very helpful in locating the catheter.

In most cases in which removal of the catheter would involve a major surgical procedure (deep position), the catheter should be left in place after informed (written) consent of the patient and surgery should be considered only if the patient complains about problems.

When it is advanced too far, *knots and looping of the catheter* are possible (Krebs and Hempel 1984). If persistent resistance occurs during removal of the catheter, the procedure should be stopped and a radiograph with contrast performed. In this case the catheter may have to be removed surgically.

## Duration In Situ of Peripheral Nerve Catheters for Pain Management

The time that peripheral pain catheters are left in situ should be kept as short as possible because of the risk of infection. The average duration is generally reported as 4 to 6 days (Büttner et al 1989, Meier et al 1997). The necessity of the pain catheter must be re-evaluated daily. If in doubt, a "cessation trial" can clarify the question of further need for the catheter. For chronic pain therapy, average maintenance of 37.4 days with a maximum of 240 days has been reported (Schreiber et al 1997). In these cases, subcutaneous tunneling of the catheter is recommended. Subcutaneous implantation of a port system for axillary block for long-term analgesia in patients with CRPS 1 and 2 has also been described (Aguilar et al 1995, 1998). The longest duration was 16 months.

## Risk of Falling

Especially with femoral nerve catheters and proximal sciatic nerve catheters, there is an increased risk of falling that the patient should be informed of—with corresponding rules for the patient and ward personnel ("stand up only with assistance").

## Documentation

Full recording and documentation of all regional pain catheters is essential. A central record of all catheters currently in situ is required (e.g., recovery room, computer-assisted record). This enables daily monitoring of all patients and thus documentation of all problems and complications. To prevent any gaps arising in the information, each patient should receive a special form for documentation of dosages and special features.

# References

Abdallah FW, Brull R. Is sciatic nerve block advantageous when combined with femoral nerve block for postoperative analgesia following total knee arthroplasty? A systematic review. Reg Anesth Pain Med 2011; 36: 493–498

Aguilar JL, Domingo V, Samper D, Roca G, Vidal F. Long-term brachial plexus anesthesia using a subcutaneous implantable injection system. Case report. Reg Anesth 1995; 20: 242–245

Aguilar JL, Mendiola MA, Valdivia J. Long-term continuous axillary brachial plexus blockade using an implanted port. In: Urmey WF, ed. Techniques in Regional Anesthesia and Pain Management. Philadelphia: Saunders; 1998: 74–78

Barrington MJ, Olive D, Low K, Scott DA, Brittain J, Choong P. Continuous femoral nerve blockade or epidural analgesia after total knee replacement: a prospective randomized controlled trial. Anesth Analg 2005; 101: 1824–1829

Ben-David B, Schmalenberger K, Chelly JE. Analgesia after total knee arthroplasty: is continuous sciatic blockade needed in addition to continuous femoral blockade? Anesth Analg 2004; 98: 747–749

Biboulet P, Morau D, Aubas P, Bringuier-Branchereau S, Capdevila X. Postoperative analgesia after total-hip arthroplasty: Comparison of intravenous patient-controlled analgesia with morphine and single injection of femoral nerve or psoas compartment block. A prospective, randomized, double-blind study. Reg Anesth Pain Med 2004; 29: 102–109

Borgeat A, Schäppi B, Biasca N, Gerber C. Patient-controlled analgesia after major shoulder surgery: patient-controlled interscalene analgesia versus patient-controlled analgesia. Anesthesiology 1997; 87: 1343–1347

Borgeat A, Kalberer F, Jacob H, Ruetsch YA, Gerber C. Patient-controlled interscalene analgesia with ropivacaine 0.2% versus bupivacaine 0.15% after major open shoulder surgery: the effects on hand motor function. Anesth Analg 2001; 92: 218–223

Büttner J, Klose R, Hammer H. Continuous axillary catheter plexus anesthesia—a method of postoperative analgesia and sympathetic nerve block following hand surgery. [Article in German] Handchir Mikrochir Plast Chir 1989; 21: 29–32

Candido KD, Franco CD, Khan MA, Winnie AP, Raja DS. Buprenorphine added to the local anesthetic for brachial plexus block to provide postoperative analgesia in outpatients. Reg Anesth Pain Med 2001; 26: 352–356

Capdevila X, Barthelet Y, Biboulet P, Ryckwaert Y, Rubenovitch J, d'Athis F. Effects of perioperative analgesic technique on the surgical outcome and duration of rehabilitation after major knee surgery. Anesthesiology 1999; 91: 8–15

Capdevila X, Macaire P, Aknin P, Dadure C, Bernard N, Lopez S. Patient-controlled perineural analgesia after ambulatory orthopedic surgery: a comparison of electronic versus elastomeric pumps. Anesth Analg 2003; 96: 414–417

Capdevila X, Coimbra C, Choquet O. Approaches to the lumbar plexus: success, risks, and outcome. Reg Anesth Pain Med 2005a; 30: 150–162

Capdevila X, Pirat P, Bringuier S et al. French Study Group on Continuous Peripheral Nerve Blocks. Continuous peripheral nerve blocks in hospital wards after orthopedic surgery: a multicenter prospective analysis of the quality of postoperative analgesia and complications in 1,416 patients. Anesthesiology 2005b; 103: 1035–1045

Cappelleri G, Ghisi D, Fanelli A, Albertin A, Somalvico F, Aldegheri G. Does continuous sciatic nerve block improve postoperative analgesia and early rehabilitation after total knee arthroplasty? A prospective, randomized, double-blinded study. Reg Anesth Pain Med 2011; 36: 489–492

Cometa MA, Esch AT, Boezaart AP. Did continuous femoral and sciatic nerve block obscure the diagnosis or delay the treatment of acute lower leg compartment syndrome? A case report. Pain Med 2011; 12: 823–828

Coventry DM, Timperley J. Perineural catheter placement: another potential complication. Reg Anesth Pain Med 2004; 29: 174–175

Delaunay L, Souron V, Lafosse L, Marret E, Toussaint B. Analgesia after arthroscopic rotator cuff repair: subacromial versus interscalene continuous infusion of ropivacaine. Reg Anesth Pain Med 2005; 30: 117–122

Geiger P, Tisch-Rottensteiner K, Winckelmann J et al. Continuous sciatic nerve block for postoperative pain therapy after total knee arthroplasty—is it really necessary? Reg Anesth Pain Med 2005; 29 Suppl. 2: 34

Ghosh S, Sallam S. Patient satisfaction and postoperative demands on hospital and community services after day surgery. Br J Surg 1994; 81: 1635–1638

Grant SA, Nielsen KC, Greengrass RA, Steele SM, Klein SM. Continuous peripheral nerve block for ambulatory surgery. Reg Anesth Pain Med 2001; 26: 209–214

Hebl JR, Kopp SL, Ali MH et al. A comprehensive anesthesia protocol that emphasizes peripheral nerve blockade for total knee and total hip arthroplasty. J Bone Joint Surg Am 2005; 87 Suppl 2: 63–70

Ilfeld BM, Enneking FK. A portable mechanical pump providing over four days of patient-controlled analgesia by perineural infusion at home. Reg Anesth Pain Med 2002; 27: 100–104

Ilfeld BM, Morey TE, Enneking FK. Continuous infraclavicular brachial plexus block for postoperative pain control at home: a randomized, double-blinded, placebo-controlled study. Anesthesiology 2002a; 96: 1297–1304

Ilfeld BM, Morey TE, Wang RD, Enneking FK. Continuous popliteal sciatic nerve block for postoperative pain control at home: a randomized, double-blinded, placebo-controlled study. Anesthesiology 2002b; 97: 959–965

Ilfeld BM, Morey TE, Enneking FK. New portable infusion pumps: real advantages or just more of the same in a different package? Reg Anesth Pain Med 2004a; 29: 371–376

Ilfeld BM, Morey TE, Wright TW, Chidgey LK, Enneking FK. Interscalene perineural ropivacaine infusion: a comparison of two dosing regimens for postoperative analgesia. Reg Anesth Pain Med 2004b; 29: 9–16

Ilfeld BM, Thannikary LJ, Morey TE, Vander Griend RA, Enneking FK. Popliteal sciatic perineural local anesthetic infusion: a comparison of three dosing regimens for postoperative analgesia. Anesthesiology 2004c; 101: 970–977

Ilfeld BM, Enneking FK. Continuous peripheral nerve blocks at home: a review. Anesth Analg 2005; 100: 1822–1833

Jacob AK, Mantilla CB, Sviggum HP, Schroeder DR, Pagnano MW, Hebl JR. Perioperative nerve injury after total knee arthroplasty: regional anesthesia risk during a 20-year cohort study. Anesthesiology 2011; 114: 311–317

Klein SM, Nielsen KC, Martin A et al. Interscalene brachial plexus block with continuous intraarticular infusion of ropivacaine. Anesth Analg 2001; 93: 601–605

Klein SM. Beyond the hospital: continuous peripheral nerve blocks at home. [editorial] Anesthesiology 2002; 96: 1283–1285

Krebs P, Hempel V. Eine neue Kombinationsnadel für die hohe axilläre Plexusbrachialis-Anästhesie. Anästh Intensivmed 1984; 25: 219

Krone SC, Chan VW, Regan J et al. Analgesic effects of low-dose ropivacaine for interscalene brachial plexus block for outpatient shoulder surgery-a dose-finding study. Reg Anesth Pain Med 2001; 26: 439–443

Lee BH, Goucke CR. Shearing of a peripheral nerve catheter. Anesth Analg 2002; 95: 760–761

Meier G, Bauereis C, Heinrich C. Interscalene brachial plexus catheter for anesthesia and postoperative pain therapy. Experience with a modified technique. [Article in German] Anaesthesist 1997; 46: 715–719

Meyer J, Herrmann M. Interscalene brachial plexus catheter for anesthesia and postoperative pain therapy. Experience with a modified technique. [Article in German] Anaesthesist 1998; 47: 136–142

Mizner RL, Petterson SC, Stevens JE, Vandenborne K, Snyder-Mackler L. Early quadriceps strength loss after total knee arthroplasty. The contributions of muscle atrophy and failure of voluntary muscle activation. J Bone Joint Surg Am 2005; 87: 1047–1053

Moen V, Dahlgren N, Irestedt L. Severe neurological complications after central neuraxial blockades in Sweden 1990–1999. Anesthesiology 2004; 101: 950–959

Morin AM, Kratz CD, Eberhart LHJ et al. Postoperative analgesia and functional recovery after total-knee replacement: comparison of a continuous posterior lumbar plexus (psoas compartment) block, a continuous femoral nerve block, and the combination of a continuous femoral and sciatic nerve block. Reg Anesth Pain Med 2005; 30: 434–445

Mulroy MF, Larkin KL, Batra MS, Hodgson PS, Owens BD. Femoral nerve block with 0.25% or 0.5% bupivacaine improves postoperative analgesia following outpatient arthroscopic anterior cruciate ligament repair. Reg Anesth Pain Med 2001; 26: 24–29

Neuburger M, Breitbarth J, Reisig F, Lang D, Büttner J. Complications and adverse events in continuous peripheral regional anesthesia Results of investigations on 3,491 catheters. [Article in German] Anaesthesist 2006; 55: 33–40

Pham Dang C, Gautheron E, Guilley J et al. The value of adding sciatic block to continuous femoral block for analgesia after total knee replacement. Reg Anesth Pain Med 2005; 30: 128–133

Rawal N. Analgesia for day-case surgery. Br J Anaesth 2001; 87: 73–87

Rawal N, Allvin R, Axelsson K et al. Patient-controlled regional analgesia (PCRA) at home: controlled comparison between bupivacaine and ropivacaine brachial plexus analgesia. Anesthesiology 2002; 96: 1290–1296

Reisig F, Neuburger M, Breitbarth J, et al. Erfolgreiche Etablierung der neuen DGAI-Leitlinien für die Anlage kontinuierlicher peripherer Regionalanästhesien. Vorläufige Ergebnisse einer prospektiven Untersuchung aus dem Jahr 2005. Garmisch-Partenkirchen: Poster BAT; 2005

Reisig F, Breitbarth J, Ott B, Büttner J. Sheared catheter in regional anaesthesia: causes and follow-up of an axallary plexus catheter. [Article in German] Anaesthesist 2011; 60: 942–945

Salonen MH, Haasio J, Bachmann M, Xu M, Rosenberg PH. Evaluation of efficacy and plasma concentrations of ropivacaine in continuous axillary brachial plexus block: high dose for surgical anesthesia and low dose for postoperative analgesia. Reg Anesth Pain Med 2000; 25: 47–51

Schreiber T, Meissner W, Ullrich K. Continuous vertical infraclavicular brachial plexus block: an alternative to the axillary plexus catheter? Intern Monitor Reg Anaesth 1997; 9: 3, 49 (abstract)

Singelyn FJ, Deyaert M, Joris D, Pendeville E, Gouverneur JM. Effects of intravenous patient-controlled analgesia with morphine, continuous epidural analgesia, and continuous three-in-one block on postoperative pain and knee rehabilitation after unilateral total knee arthroplasty. Anesth Analg 1998; 87: 88–92

Singelyn FJ, Seguy S, Gouverneur JM. Interscalene brachial plexus analgesia after open shoulder surgery: continuous versus patient-controlled infusion. Anesth Analg 1999; 89: 1216–1220

Singelyn FJ, Gouverneur JM. Extended "three-in-one" block after total knee arthroplasty: continuous versus patient-controlled techniques. Anesth Analg 2000; 91: 176–180

Singelyn FJ, Lhotel L, Fabre B. Pain relief after arthroscopic shoulder surgery: a comparison of intraarticular analgesia, suprascapular nerve block, and interscalene brachial plexus block. Anesth Analg 2004; 99: 589–592

Van Aken H, Klose R, Wulf H. Zum täglichen Wechsel von Spritzenpumpe, Leitung und Filtern bei liegendem Periduralkatheter, Stellungnahme des wissenschaftlichen Arbeitskreises Regionalanästhesie der DGAI. Anästh Intesivmed 2001; 42: 973–974

Wedderburn AW, Dodds SR, Morris GE. A survey of post-operative care after day case surgery. Ann R Coll Surg Engl 1996; 78 Suppl: 70–71

Wegener JT, van Ooij B, van Dijk CN, Hollmann MW, Preckel B, Stevens MF. Value of single-injection or continuous sciatic nerve block in addition to a continuous femoral nerve block in patients undergoing total knee arthroplasty: a prospective, randomized, controlled trial. Reg Anesth Pain Med 2011; 36: 481–488

White PF, Issioui T, Skrivanek GD, Early JS, Wakefield C. The use of a continuous popliteal sciatic nerve block after surgery involving the foot and ankle: does it improve the quality of recovery? Anesth Analg 2003; 97: 1303–1309

# Index

Illustrations are comprehensively referred to from the text. Therefore, significant items in illustrations (figures and tables) have only been given a page reference in the absence of their concomitant mention in the text referring to that illustration.